COMBINING THE CREATIVE THERAPIES WITH TECHNOLOGY

COMBINING THE CREATIVE THERAPIES WITH TECHNOLOGY

Using Social Media and Online Counseling to Treat Clients

Edited by

STEPHANIE L. BROOKE, PH.D., NCC

(With 22 Other Contributors)

With a Foreword by Ellen G. Horovitz

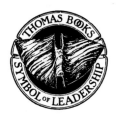

CHARLES C THOMAS • PUBLISHER, LTD.
Springfield • Illinois • U.S.A.

Published and Distributed Throughout the World by

CHARLES C THOMAS • PUBLISHER, LTD.
2600 South First Street
Springfield, Illinois 62704

© 2017 by CHARLES C THOMAS • PUBLISHER, LTD.

ISBN 978-0-398-09180-4 (paper)
ISBN 978-0-398-09181-1 (ebook)

Library of Congress Catalog Card Number: 2017018415

With THOMAS BOOKS *careful attention is given to all details of manufacturing
and design. It is the Publisher's desire to present books that are satisfactory as to their
physical qualities and artistic possibilities and appropriate for their particular use.*
THOMAS BOOKS *will be true to those laws of quality that assure a good name
and good will.*

Printed in the United States of America
MM-C-1

Library of Congress Cataloging-in-Publication Data

Names: Brooke, Stephanie L., editor.
Title: Combining the creative therapies with technology : using social
    media and online counseling to treat clients / edited by Stephanie
    L. Brooke ; (with 22 other contributors).
Description: Springfield, Illinois, U.S.A. : Charles C Thomas,
    Publisher, LTD., [2017] | Includes bibliographical references and
    index.
Identifiers: LCCN 2017018415 (print) | LCCN 2017018736 (ebook) |
    ISBN 9780398091811 (ebook) | ISBN 9780398091804 (paper)
Subjects: | MESH: Sensory Art Therapies--methods | Telemedicine--
    methods | Therapy, Computer-Assisted--methods | Internet
Classification: LCC R855.3 (ebook) | LCC R855.3 (print) | NLM WM
    450 | DDC 610.285--dc23
LC record available at https://lccn.loc.gov/2017018415

CONTRIBUTORS

Stephanie L. Brooke, PhD, NCC
Jennifer Byxbee, MPS, ATR-BC, LCAT
Joel Cahen
Lucía Casal de la Fuente
Rashmi Chidanand, PhD
Kate Collie, MA, MFA, PhD
Deborah Elkis-Abuhoff, PhD, LCAT, ATR-BC, ATCS, BCPC
John Farnsworth, PhD
Theresa Fraser
Morgan Gaydos, LCAT, ATR-BC
Hilda R. Glazer, EdD, RPT-S, PCC-S
Robert Goldblatt, PhD
Dalia Gottlieb-Tanaka, PhD
Peter Graf, PhD
Sara Prins Hankinson, RCAT
Ellen G. Horovitz, PhD, ATR-BC, LCAT, E-RYT, LFYP, C-IAYT
Kate Hudgins, Ph.D, TEP
Jeffrey Jamerson,M.S.
Brennan Jones, Bsc
Hilary Lee, MS
Dorothy A. Miraglia, PhD
Sheila Rubin, LMFT, RDT/BCT
Priyadarshini Senroy MA, CCC
Karette Stensæth, PhD
Amanda Zucker, MPS, ATR-BC, LCAT

FOREWORD

We keep moving forward, opening new doors, and doing new things, because
we're curious and curiosity keeps leading us down new paths.
                                                                —Walt Disney

It seems to be both paradoxical and fitting that Dr. Stephanie L. Brooke
asked me to write this Foreword to her latest book, *The Use of the Creative
Therapies and Technology.* I came to know her as a wide-thinking student,
whose first book, *Tools of the Trade: A Therapist's Guide to Art Therapy Assess-*
ments, was her master's thesis, later to be published by Charles C Thomas,
Publisher, Ltd. Doctor Brooke is currently working on a third edition of *Tools*
of the Trade (forthcoming). As her advisor, I encouraged Doctor Brooke to
present her opus to Charles C Thomas and to get her work published. Even
before her first book was printed, she had been an accomplished writer,
arriving to her art therapy training with a master's degree as a seasoned
counselor. Given her innate creativity and talent, art therapy seemed to be a
natural fit and the fields of creative arts therapy have been distinguished by
her profuse contributions.

This latest book arrives in good company (Garner, 2017; Grady, Myers,
& Nelson, 2009; Hines, 2016; Horovitz, 2011, 2014a, 2014b, 2015a, 2015b,
2015c, 2016a, 2016b, 2017a, 2017b; Krupinksi & Bernard, 2014). Fortunately,
such "forward" thinking on the subject of integrating technology into the creative art therapies is arriving at a time when the constituents of those fields
have finally cracked open. It wasn't so long ago (the 1990s) when conversations about my use of technology sent shudders down the spines of my more
conservative counterparts. They couldn't imagine themselves using digital
applications (e.g., the Adobe Photoshop, which is practically fodder for most
middle school aged children), let alone using digital applications in their sessions. I, on the other hand, ever curious (like Brooke), couldn't imagine not
moving forward and embracing these new palettes, the digital crayons of my
patients.

While my mentors, Dr. Laurie Wilson and the late (mother of Art Therapy), Edith Kramer, may have once balked at moving away from a fine arts platform, they instilled great principles in me as my supervisors: I recall Kramer saying to me that if a patient mentioned a book, movie, or other format with which I was unfamiliar, it was my duty as an art therapist to familiarize myself with what he or she was talking about. I have carried that message in my work and espoused that same ideology to the students who I mentored. It has served me well; but more importantly, it has aided my patients.

Considering that adolescents spend an estimated 7.5 hours per day using social media (almost as long as the workday of most adults), it behooves art therapists to not only embrace digital platforms, but to also be familiar with IAD (Internet Addiction Disorder). While one need not throw out the proverbial baby (fine arts media) with the bathwater (digital applications), it is pinnacle that health professionals embrace this new way of communication (Horovitz, 2016a, 2017b). In Brooke's opening chapter on Steampunk Art, she sets the stage showing how this vehicle can connect both the past and the future, thus laying out the idea of mixing riches from the past with the present and future. Indeed, in this book, Byxbee and Zucker aptly point out blogging as a vehicle to meet their patients where they maintain their safety and create a holding environment for them. While Miraglia, Cahen, and Fraser's respective chapters highlight the myriad ways of incorporating ethical principles into online therapy and into supervision, the chapters incorporating, music, drama, and mixed expressive therapies abound with rich ideas worth considering and implementing.

This book should serve as a springboard, propelling curiosity, seeding the minds of its readers, and offering not only suggestions for kneading digital applications into their toolbox, but also driving home the notion that flexibility is the hallmark of all great clinicians. Adaptation, after all, is the marching forward of our species, continually motivating us toward wellness.

ELLEN G. HOROVITZ, PhD, ATR-BC, LCAT, E-RYT, LFYP, C-IAYT

REFERENCES

Brooke, S. L. (in print). *Tools of the trade: A therapist's guide to art therapy assessments* (3rd ed.). Springfield, IL: Charles C Thomas, Publisher, Ltd.

Garner, R. (Ed.). (2017). *Digital art therapy* (2nd ed.). Philadelphia: Jessica Kingsley Publishers.

Grady, B., Myers, K., & Nelson, E. (2009). Evidence-based practice for telemental health. American Telemedicine Association, July. Retrieved September 1, 2015 from http://www.americantelemed.org/docs/default-source /standards /evidence -based-practice-for-telemental-health.pdf?sfvrsn=4

Hines, L. (2016). Media considerations in art therapy: Directions for future research. In D. E. Gussak & M. L. Rosal (Eds.), *The Wiley handbook of art therapy*. Malden, MA: John Wiley & Sons, Ltd.

Horovitz, E. G. (2011). *Digital image transfer: Creating art with your photography*. New York: Pixiq-Sterling Publishers.

Horovitz, E. G. (2014a). (Ed.). *The art therapists' primer: A clinical guide to writing assessments, diagnosis and treatment* (2nd ed.). Springfield, IL: Charles C Thomas Publisher.

Horovitz, E. G. (2014b). Expressive therapies summit: Family yoga therapy/art therapy with an ADD child and her family. November 9, 2014; New York.

Horovitz, E. G. (2015a). *Master lecture: Inside/outside with trauma survivors*. University of San Juan, Puerto Rico. April 30, 2015.

Horovitz, E. G. (2015b). *A guided practice: Combining art therapy and yoga therapy for mood management*. University of San Juan. May 2, 2015

Horovitz, E. G. (2015c). Common interest community presentation: Family yoga therapy treatment with a bipolar 11-year-old boy. *SYTAR 2015,* Newport Beach, CA. June 4, 2015.

Horovitz, E. G. (2016a). *Efficacy, apps, and telehealth: Treatment for a digital age*. American Art Therapy Association 47th Annual Meeting. Baltimore; July 9, 2016.

Horovitz, E. G. (2016b). Photography as therapy: Through academic and clinical explorations. In D. E. Gussak & M. L. Rosal (Eds.), *The Wiley handbook of art therapy*. Malden, MA: John Wiley & Sons, Ltd.

Horovitz, E. G. (2017a.) Efficacy, apps and telehealth: Treatment and ethical issues for a digital age. In A. Di Maria (Ed.), *Exploring ethical dilemmas in art therapy*. New York: Routledge.

Horovitz, E. G. (2017b.) *Art therapy materials and methods: A practical, step-by-step approach*. New York: Routledge

Krupinski, E. A., & Bernard, J. (2014). Review: Standards and guidelines in telemedicine and telehealth. *Healthcare, 2,* 74–93.

PREFACE

Combining the Creative Therapies with Technology is a comprehensive work that examines the use of art, play, music, dance/movement, and drama with technology, such as social media and online counseling in order to treat clients. The editor's primary purpose is to examine how the creative therapists use technology as part of their everyday practice with clients. Work with individuals, couples, and groups is considered. The collection of chapters is written by renowned, well-credentialed, and professional creative art therapists in the areas of art, play, music, dance/movement, and drama. In addition, some of the chapters are illustrated with photographs of client artworks, tables, and graphs. The reader is provided with a snapshot of how these various creative art therapies effectively use and incorporate technology to promote growth and healing for their clients. This informative book is of special interest to educators, students, and therapists as well as to people working with families and with children in need of counseling and clinical support.

CONTENTS

PART 3: MIXED EXPRESSIVE THERAPIES

PART 4: E-COUNSELING AND SUPERVISION

FIGURES AND TABLES

CHAPTER 1

CHAPTER 3

CHAPTER 4

CHAPTER 5

CHAPTER 6

CHAPTER 7

CHAPTER 8

CHAPTER 10

CHAPTER 13

COMBINING THE CREATIVE THERAPIES WITH TECHNOLOGY

Part 1

ART AND PLAY THERAPIES

Chapter 1

STEAMPUNK ART ADVENTURES

STEPHANIE L. BROOKE

Steampunk is . . . a joyous fantasy of the past, allowing us to revel in a nostalgia for what never was. It is a literary playground for adventure, spectacle, drama, escapism and exploration. But most of all it is fun!
−George Mann http://georgemann.wordpress.com/

This chapter will take a look at an evolving art form called Steampunk. It is a relatively new form in art, gaining media attention over the last decade. Oxford Dictionary (2016) defines Steampunk as "A genre of science fiction that has a historical setting and typically features steam-powered machinery rather than advanced technology." Starting as a fiction genre in the 1950s and 1960s, Steampunk has taken a variety of forms and shapes not only in art, but in fashion, in jewelry, and even as a cultural way of life. In the field of art, Steampunk can be as minute as pocket watches and redesigned laptops, to more grand forms such as redesigned vehicles and houses (VanderMeer & Boskovich, 2014). The media varies from glass, copper, leather, wood, and more. Images coincide with steam power technology so it is very likely that you will see gears, rivets, cogs, chains, and other industrial items (VanderMeer & Boskovich, 2014).

What Is Steampunk?

Steampunk is an eclectic world of cogs and rivets. It is airships, goggles and steam. It is romance. It is traveling on clouds and driving beneath rugged waves. It's an adventure.

−Aether Emporium

Steampunk is known as the art of Victorian futurism (Steampunk District, 2012). Originally, Steampunk was a literary genre. "Spurned on by so much fantastical and inventive imagery born from authors such as H. G. Wells, Jules Verne, Tim Powers, and K. W. Jeter, fans were inspired to bring life to the beauty and technology of the Steampunk genre by way of art and fashion" (Steampunk District, 2012, ¶ 1). Often, Steampunk has Victorian influences as "Steampunk art could often resemble what Victorian era dreamers would visualize when imagining what future technology might look like" (¶ 3).

History and Evolution of Steampunk

Reality provides us with facts so romantic that imagination itself could add nothing to them.
      –Jules Verne from the cover of his book, *The Fur Country*

According to Gross (2010), Steampunk began in the early years of scientific romances such as Verne's *Voyages Extraordinaires & Victorian Penny Dreadfuls*. Inspired by the works of Charles Cabbage, Thomas Edison, and Nikola Tesla, Gross writes that this form originally emerged in the literary works of Verne, Wells, H. Rider Haggard, George Griffin, Sir Arthur Conan Doyle, Garrett P. Serviss, Edgar Alan Poe, Mark Twain, and Edgar Rice Burroughs, so that their work focused on colonialism, the growing age of technology, heavy industry, and scientific exploration. "Yet the romance of the Victorian Era could not be escaped in its entirety, and several threads were fermenting that would, by the late 70's, mark the rebirth and eventual solidification of what would come to be known as Steampunk" (Gross, 2010, ¶ 17).

Steampunk emerged out of the Cyberpunk genre and the term was coined by the author K. W. Jeter in 1987 (as cited in Gross, 2010). In Jeter's words: "Personally, I think Victorian fantasies are going to be the next big thing, as long as we can come up with a fitting collective term for Powers, Blaylock and myself. Something based on the appropriate technology of the era; like 'steampunks,' perhaps. . . " (¶ 18).

According to Gross (2010), *The Different Engine* legitimized Steampunk. The co-authors Gibson and Sterling created a Victorian world where Cabbage, the mathematician-engineer, realized his plans for creating a programmable, analogue computer. "The Information Age met the Steam Age as the computer revolution happened a century earlier than it did in our world, with the consequent deleterious effects on society, politics and individuals" (Gross, ¶ 21). Many Steampunk authors set their stage in London. According to the science fiction writer Peter Nicholls, London signified the following for Steampunk authors:

In essence Steampunk is a US phenomenon, often set in London, England, which is envisaged as at once deeply alien and intimately familiar, a kind of foreign body encysted in the US subconscious. . . . It is as if, for a handful of writers, Victorian London has come to stand for one of those turning points in history where things can go one way or the other, a turning point peculiarly relevant to itself. It was a city of industry, science and technology where the modern world was being born, and a claustrophobic city of nightmare where the cost of this growth was registered in filth and squalor. (as cited in Gross, 2010, ¶ 22)

Starting with novels, Steampunk began to take other literature forms. *Steampunk Magazine* was first published in March 2008 (http://www.steampunkmagazine.com). As Gross notes, the first magazine issue described Steampunk as follows:

Steampunk is a re-envisioning of the past with the hypertechnological perceptions of the present. . . . Too much of what passes as steampunk denies the punk, in all of its guises. Punk—the fuse used for lighting cannons. Punk—the downtrodden and dirty. Punk—the aggressive, do-it-yourself ethic. We stand on the shaky shoulders of opium-addicts, aesthete dandies, inventors of perpetual motion machines, mutineers, hucksters, gamblers, explorers, madmen and bluestockings. We laugh at experts and consult moth-eaten tomes of forgotten possibilities. We sneer at utopias while awaiting the new ruins to reveal themselves. We are a community of mechanical magicians enchanted by the real world and beholden to the mystery of possibility. We do not have the luxury of niceties or the possession of politeness; we are rebuilding yesterday to ensure our tomorrow. Our corsets are stitched with safety pins and our top hats hide vicious mohawks. We are fashion's jackals running wild in the tailor shop. (as cited in Gross, 2010, ¶ 36)

Gross provides a detailed account of the literary and film movements in Steampunk that gave emergence to the art form. See his website for more information: http://steampunkscholar.blogspot.com/2010/08/history-of-steampunk-by-cory-gross.html

Steampunk Culture

She has halls and she has castles, and the resonant Steam-Eagles, Follow far on the directing of her floating dove-like hand, With a thunderous vapour trailing, underneath the starry vigils, So to mark upon the blasted heaven, the measure of her land.

—Edgar Allan Poe

Wren (2013) states that the culture of Steampunk, stylized corsets, aeronaut googles, clockwork gears, and industrialized pipes, typically displayed in art, has weaved its way through fashion, theater, novels, and contemporary ballet. "With its emphasis on craftsmanship, salvaged materials and do-it-yourself philosophies, the steampunk lifestyle rebukes our own era's mass-produced design and throwaway consumerist ethos—a point lucidly made in VanderMeer and Chambers's authoritative and handsomely illustrated nonfiction book, *The Steampunk Bible*" (Wier, 2013, p. 31). According to Wren, the Steampunk culture implies visible technology or seeing how objects work. In this culture, anyone can be an inventor. As Wren notes, the Steampunk culture is spiritually affirming and scientifically user-friendly; yet, it has darker sides. She states that "punk" suggests a rebellious, vaunting attitude. Also, Steampunk reflects the darker sides of the Industrial Revolution such as street urchins, smokestacks, and mills (Wren, 2013). "If steampunk provides a handy way to address weighty matters such as uncertainty, faith, science and aggression, it also can just be fun" (p. 32). She further notes that Steampunk culture is not just about lessons from the past, it indicates the instability and desuetude of our own times.

Steampunk collaborations have been taking off as a way to interest children and teens in school ventures. "When I saw how steampunk pulled students I'd never seen into the library, I was glad I ventured into this extraordinary world" (Hoppe & Wilson, 2012, p. 25). These teachers collaborated with librarians to create a Steampunk Ball that was promoted on Facebook. Departments of fine art, science, and media contributed to this unique project promoting the Steampunk culture.

With respect to the visual arts, Christians (2011) notes that the Steampunk culture "expresses itself as a low-tech survivalist attitude aspiring to artistic grace" (p. 18). This culture promotes the concepts of time, motion, assembly, and disassembly. Overall, it is a collaborative, imaginative, and participatory culture with rich allegory and metaphor. In many ways, Christians notes that the steampunk culture is the antithesis of the digital age. "Steampunk is steaming along, bridging old and new, and the ways in which it is transforming art with historical technology, quality fabrication, and attention to detail is progressing at lightning speed" (p. 19).

Steampunk in Higher Education Research

Tut, tut. We can't let mere sentiment intrude. This is Science.
                                                    —K. W. Jeter, *Infernal Devices*

The cutting edge of the research is in master's theses and in doctoral dissertations, often addressing the current gaps in the literature with the intention of promoting social change. This is where we can find the most recent focus on Steampunk in the literature. Briefly presented in this section is an evolutionary approach to the discussion of Steampunk in higher education.

Master's Research

Smith (2015) talks about the science fiction of Steampunk in her master's thesis. She views Steampunk as a countercultural movement rooted in science fiction. Additionally, she writes that Steampunk "looks to both the past that was–and the past that never was–for inspiration and guidance as to where the future is going and what it might hold" (p. 1). Additionally, Smith stated that the literary beginnings of Steampunk emerged with the works of Tim Powers, James P. Blaylock, and Jeter who challenged one another to write stories with alternate histories set in the Victorian era. The three authors were inspired by the science fiction author Phillip K. Dick who mentored and encouraged their efforts. Smith argues that Steampunk views motion as a humanizing force while rejecting the sterile, dull computer quoting Jake von Slatt, who stated that "current technology and engineering [are] 'jellybeans'–everything is different coloured, creating the illusion of difference, but it is actually executed in the same shape" (p. 7). Smith states that Steampunk embraces the beauty of machines while computers attempt to remove machinery from the material world. She makes the interesting argument that computers/modern technology break the connection with humanity in a way that makes its users less human. Steampunk creators, on the other hand, "are driven to find ways to fuse the objects and themes of the past with those of the present, so as to satisfy their need to connect and to reconnect with the people and the world around them, while simultaneously rejecting most of the "popular" fads and fashions–in both lifestyle and literary genre" (p. 8).

Doctoral Research

Perschon (2012) conducted his doctoral dissertation on the Steampunk aesthetic focusing on techno-fantasies in a neo-Victorian retrofuture. He writes: "Steampunk works share a fantastic aesthetic that separates steampunk from neo-Victorian writing or just alternate history" (p. 1). Instead of viewing Steampunk as a culture, he states that it should be considered an expression of features that constitutes a style or aesthetic surface. The focus of Perschon's dissertation was primarily focused on literature related to Steampunk. He tries to provide a surface aesthetic for Steampunk: "Steampunk does not seek to reconstruct the past in literature, art, or fashion, but rather constructs something new by choosing elements from the Victorian and Edwardian past to create a style which evokes those periods" (p. 4). He views Steampunk, not as a genre, but rather as a visual interface between retro-Victorian style and contemporary technology. According to Perschon, Steampunk is comprised of three components: neo-Victorianism, retrofuturism, and technofantasy. He states that the first wave of Steampunk in the 1970s and 1980s was expressed in writing and in cinema. The current wave of Steampunk has expanded into the visual arts, performing arts, fashion, and décor.

Young (2014) completed a dissertation allohistorical reconstruction of Victorian restrictions in young adult Steampunk. Young argued that Steampunk is more than technology's effect on humanity. Rather, Steampunk focuses on using technology to understand the nature of interpersonal relationships within humanity. He writes:

> Steampunk suggests we accomplish self-understanding by recognizing the contemporary self through connections with not only alternate pasts, but also the multitude of possible futures. In other words, it focuses on the idea that contemporary society is the future self of a past that was once contemporary and speculative of the future, just as it will soon become that speculative future's past. This trifecta of time is perpetually in flux with itself, but ultimately, as steampunk illustrates that man and woman–past, present, and future self–are relatively unchanging; what changes are the perceptions they cast upon who they are in relationship to the known past and the imagined future. (p. 1)

His work covers some of the historical Steampunk art images. First, he presents the work of John Coulthart featuring his graphic post, Steampunk Redux (see Fig. 1).

Coulhart's work combines the written word, according to Young, with visualization and mathematical concepts. In addition, Young states that Coulhart's work is the epitome of Steampunk. Each artist will represent an element of Steampunk more prominent than the others. Young discussed the work of Molly Fredrick's "Mechanical Womb with Clockwork Fetus" as combining two-dimensional Steampunk art using materials that were available during the 19th century while drawing on the feel of futuristic steam technology and Victorian images–see the image at https://www.flickr.com /photos/porkshanks/2779897894. Further, Young argues that Steampunk goes beyond science fiction. The heart of Steampunk, according to Young, is in the critical evaluation of contemporary society in light of the stark contrast of the romanticized images of the nineteenth century:

> Unlike traditional science fiction that questions the present through futuristic projections, steampunk questions what changed from the comparatively simple lifestyle and technologies of the nineteenth century to create the

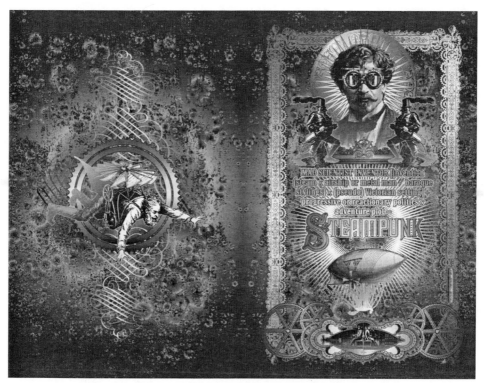

Figure 1. Steampunk Redux from www.JohnCoulthart.com.

complicated lifestyle and technologies of today. The simplified nature of the technology that assuredly the average person could not only create, but also operate and fix with minimal training, which is often found in steampunk, acts as a metaphor for the seemingly uncomplicated social relations of supposed days gone by. In other words, the more easily understood technologies of the nineteenth century represent a time when societal expectations were clearly defined, instead of the mixture of social structures that have become increasingly more indefinable. (p. 8)

Young views Steampunk as a vehicle to connect ourselves with our past and with our future that lends itself well to use in the creative therapies. Building on Young's idea, Steampunk can connect important social issues to one's personal development through art and through the creative therapies. For example, abused children were often marginalized so that Steampunk art can create a vehicle to represent their heart, and to empower that child to move from being a victim to a survivor. Steampunk can help create a dialogue between the client's present self, with that child of the past, to the survivor of the future.

Steampunk and the Creative Therapies

Many great things have been accomplished by the careful combination of keen minds and ardent spirits.

–G. D. Falksen, *Blood in the Skies*

There is a current gap in the literature with respect to the use of Steampunk in the creative therapies, but the potential uses of Steampunk lends itself well to the creative therapies–art, play, dance/movement, drama, poetry, and music. In May of 2013, the *Globe* correspondent Taryn Plumb, talked about the use of Steampunk in art therapy for autistic teens (see Fig. 2). The article talks about the use of Steampunk in art therapy with fifteen young adults on the autism spectrum. It was a one of a kind art therapy program called: Steampunkinetics: Building Art into Science, and was held at the University of Massachusetts, Lowell. One nineteen-year-old young man commented: "I like the process of going from sketch to reality" (¶ 4).

Plumb said this project combines antique mechanical and industrial objects, and "incorporates Janusian thinking, a paradoxical perspective based on Janus, the Roman god associated with doorways, beginnings, and transitions" (¶ 6). Given that those on the autism spectrum often excel in tasks centered around technology, mechanics, and kinesthetics, this project emerged

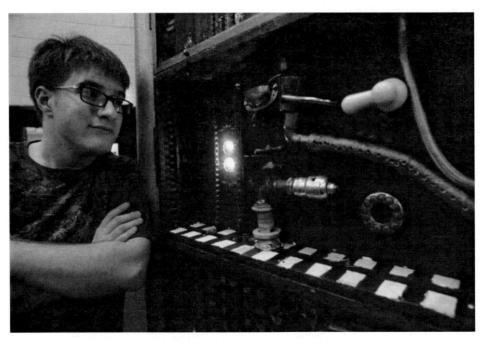

Figure 2. Steampunk Redux from www.JohnCoulthart.com.

from the work of the Steampunk artist and designer Bruce Rosenbaum, and the assistant professor of psychology Ashleigh Hillier. Over the years, Hillier has worked with young adults on the autism spectrum and notes their high creativity and attention to detail: "[they] have piecemeal cognitive processing style that supports divergent thinking—the very essence of the steampunk design process" (¶ 10). The participants were broken down into small groups and were working on separate boxes which would then be structured in one cohesive tower or "steampunked" house. Hillier explained, "the goal was to help the participants increase self-esteem, improve attitudes toward peers, reduce feelings of stress and anxiety, and foster collaboration, communication, and the sharing of ideas—things that don't always come easy to those on the autism spectrum" (¶ 16). The entire project took nine weeks and resulted in a grandfather clock like tower based on group efforts (see Fig. 3).

In another article by Pho (2014), she interviewed Bruce Rosenbaum about the Steampunkinetic's collaboration. With respect to the project, Rosembaum said: "When I saw how Steampunk art and design could help to

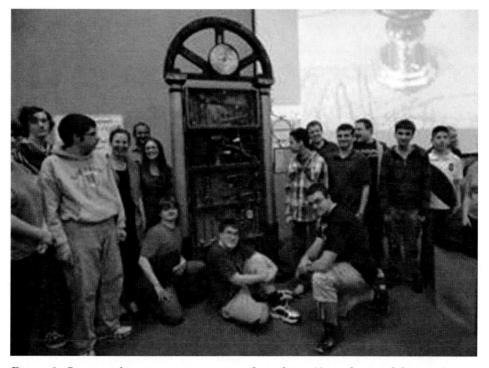

Figure 3. Steampunkinetics group creation from https://www.bostonglobe.com/metro/regionals/north/2013/05/25/steampunk-art-therapy-for-autistic/3TSOCFHa0K65f8wduW52IK/story.html.

improve the lives of kids with Autism–I thought that Steampunk has the power to be a game changer in how people can view themselves, others and the world around them" (¶4).

Pho noted that Bruce and Melanie Rosebaum have been involved in several collaborative projects to help different people with disabilities. Their organization, ModVic, is currently working on Steampunk to help people with assisted living devices to help empower them. For instance, they partnered with Make-A-Wish Foundation to help develop a Steampunk themed bedroom for a 14-year-old with muscular dystrophy. The Rosebaums also designed a Steampunked wheel chair for the 14-year-old boy. ModVic sponsored a contest for designers who wanted to contribute their ideas of a steampunk wheelchair (see Fig. 4). Out of eighteen possible designs, Greg Hurley, a designer from Michigan, was the

Recently, Turner (2016) covered a story on a teen who fractured a vertebra in her spine. As a result, she had to wear a body brace for two months. Maddie Cable was in a car crash that resulted in her injury. In Figure 5, she took the body brace and made steampunk art.

It took Maddie five hours to make this transformation into "a Victorian era warrior princess." It represented her battle to heal from her injuries as well as to give people a reason to smile instead of staring.

My Personal Experience Using Steampunk

> *To survive, to avert what we have termed future shock, the individual must become infinitely more adaptable and capable than ever before. We must search out totally new ways to anchor ourselves, for all the old roots–religion, nation, community, family, or profession–are now shaking under the hurricane impact of the accelerative thrust. It is no longer resources that limit decisions, it is the decision that makes the resources.*
> —Alvin Toffler, *Future Shock*

When I was in junior high and high school, I was an avid reader. I would save any money I earned from babysitting and from summer jobs and buy books. One day, I bought this neon green used book called *Future Shock,* by Toffler (1970). When I picked it up in the early 1980s, I could not put it down. When I was in high school, I remember the time that our family got our first Apple computer with the black and green screen. Technology was taking hold and it would become an integral part of my education and later career. With respect to the Toffler text, my interest grew in the field of sociology and I went on to teach courses on the introduction to sociology and the social problems at the undergraduate level. I would often discuss this text with my

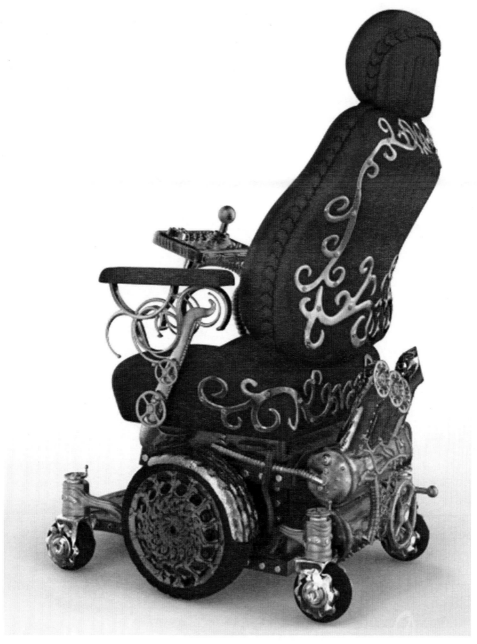

Figure 4. Steampunked wheelchair from https://www.keyshot.com/steampunk-wheel chair-design winner. "Steampunk design celebrates the past, present and future–at the same time–creating functional art and a pathway to re-imagination and new purpose. Steampunk does not hide from the technology–but brings it forward for everyone to see" (¶5).

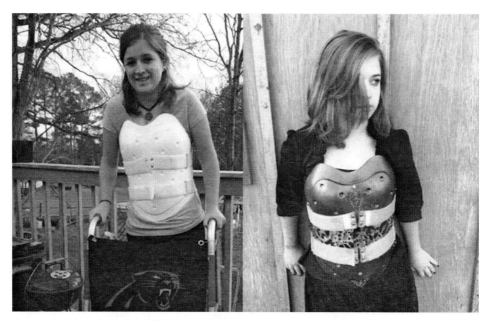

Figure 5. Steampunked backbrace from http://www.epbot.com/2016/01/this-steampunked-back-brace-looks-like.html

students in light of the rapidly changing technology that was impacting all of our lives.

I met a Centenarian when I lived in Lakeville, New York. He was 100 years old in 2013. The amount of change that he had seen in his lifetime seem beyond me but then thinking about our generation, we will see even more technological change at an ever increasing rate. Toffler talked about Future Shock as the anxiety and sometimes, inability, to keep up with the fast pace of technological change in our culture. I remember feeling this stress and anxiety when I had to learn how to use a computer. So, I forced myself into it and set up small businesses on their computers when I was an under-graduate student–setting up databases, spreadsheets, and so on. It was a learn by doing, Bau Haus, sort of method, but I did it. I could find glitches in computer programs, it seemed, like no one else, but I got over my fear of "the computer'."

Later in my education, I began to take online classes as a PhD student and then went on to become a certified online instructor and built a suc-cessful career at Capella University teaching PhD counseling students, men-toring PhD learners (with 25 graduates to date), and conducting scientific merit reviews. When I first started teaching online in 2000, only IBM com-puters were compatible with that type of work. Later, Apple computers adapted, so I was once back with that familiar family computer that we had in our home in the early 1980s. Over the course of the last 16 years, I have seen rapid change in the platforms used for the online delivery of educational courses and had to adapt quickly or perish.

I had the honor of mentoring master's art therapy students at Nazareth College in 2015 and I incorporated technology into my work with them. For instance, I was not able to be present with them for one class due to an upcoming geographical move, so I used Zoom.us to remotely connect with them. I was pretty comfortable with Zoom but it was their first time and it was fun. With each giggle and slight sound, the focus of the image would move to that person. We connected as a group and I was able to answer any questions they may have had about their research, even though each person was in a different location. Each of us was in our home which made it comfortable. A few of my cats video bombed the session and they thought that was fun–they showed me their dogs and cats, as well so it was a means of connecting that would not have been possible in the classroom. I am sure technology will continue to change throughout my career, but as a certified art and play therapist, I wondered how technology impacts our field and our work with clients. This is what lead to the inception of this book.

VanderMeer and Boskovich (2014) wrote a wonderful user's manual on Steampunk. They wrote: "On the technology side, Lev Rosen, author of the well-received debut *All Men of Genius,* believes that Steampunk allows us to work out our own anxieties, using the lens of the past" (p. 142). This linked in directly to my reading of Toffler's work because technology is advancing at such a rapid speed that ethics and legal issues cannot even catch up and for many, this it is intimidating and creates fear of the future. Rosen wrote:

> But if you take that tech and you put it in a fantastical, mad-science past . . . it becomes a way to interact with the ideas of advancing technology without being afraid of them. And I think that with us moving forward so quickly, a lot of people want to hold on to the past, too–there's a fear we could lose the past altogether, that e-books will somehow cause all paper books in the world to burst into flame. Steampunk lets us hold on to that past while still moving forward." (as cited in VanderMeer & Boskovich, 2014, p. 142)

I can see a venue for creative art therapists to address this fear and anxiety of the future in their work using the arts and combining that with technology. This is especially true for those working with young people who use technology as their main means of communication. For them, technology is second nature.

VanderMeer and Boskovich (2014) had this section in their work called "Finding the Path to Steampunk." I suppose that is what I have done not only in my own life and art, but with this book. I truly identified with Pho (2014), the founder of the popular Steampunk block—Beyond Victoriana. She talked about being an avid reader as a teen, just like myself. "My obsession with nineteenth-century literature started in high school with my passion for Jane Austen and the Bronte sisters, and my love for sci-fi has gone on much longer than that. . . " (p. 143). Much like Pho, I have loved sci-fi since I was a child—it inspired my imagination. Pho felt Steampunk is best expressed through storytelling (VanderMeer & Boskovich). For my Steampunk path, it combined art and storytelling as the two were inseparable.

Figure 6 is depicted on the cover of this book. It was my first two-dimensional Steampunk piece.

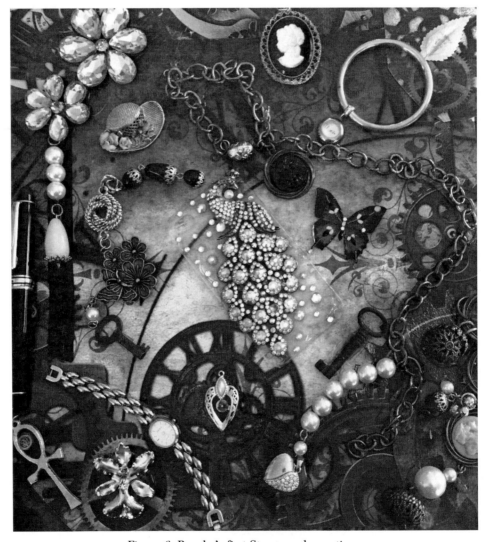

Figure 6. Brooke's first Steampunk creation.

I suppose this one tells a story. I have a cameo on here that was given to me by my maternal grandmother and also a gold flower pendant given to me by my paternal grandmother after they both passed away. It was a way that I could stay connected to them each day as I pass this art piece in my hallway. I have the fountain pen representative of my identity as a writer. The centerpiece, the peacock cell phone cover, is the tech part, but also represents my identification with this bird. The peacock symbol is represented in a tech/abstract form. The Ahnk was a necklace that I wore that represents my spirituality and my belief that we are all connected to one another. The butterfly is also something that appears quite a bit in my art as I view it as a symbol of beauty, fragility, transformation, and freedom. The other items represent my long attachment to the Victorian era and my love for pursuing antique stores. This is what led to my three-dimensional steampunk creation in Figures 7 and 8–Steampunked Antique Wheel.

My love for the Victorian era has led me to collect antiques like cameos, boxes, antique lanterns, steamer trunks, and spinning wheels. This spinning wheel was in very poor condition so it was hiding in a closet for years. In following my Steampunk path, I transformed this into a work of beauty. I am

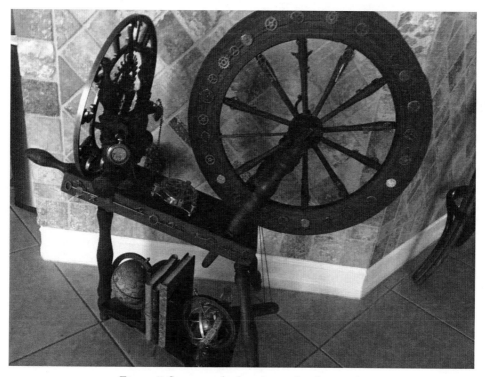

Figure 7. Steampunked antique wheel–view 1.

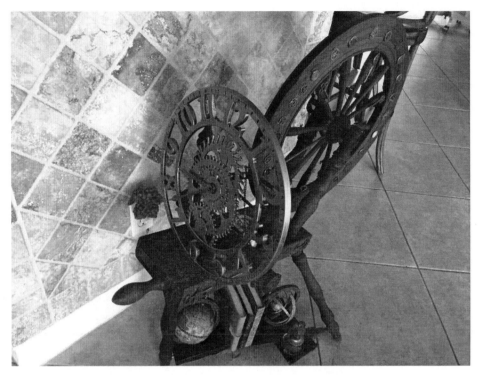

Figure 8. Steampunked antique wheel–view 2.

an avid journal writer, so I included those as a means of expressing my voice, which I can do so often in writing rather than speaking. I have my antique lanterns, globe bookends, nautical compass, and Steampunk gear clock with functions, gears, and skeleton keys. I was missing a wooden spoke on this wheel, but fortunately, when I bought this wheel years ago, it actually had the original spinning needle, so I made this into a spoke to replace the missing wooden piece. I think this Steampunked spinning wheel reflects my focus on reading, expressing myself in writing, and my love for the Victorian era. It reflects my love for world travel with the globes, and my focus on time as that seems to be critical to my career. I continued with my Steampunk creations making masks out of a surgical gaze on my own face and then decorating them in Figures 9 and 10. This was a very empowering process, not only trying to make them beautiful, but powerful. This can also be a process of trust building between the counselor and therapist or using it in group work so that they can make masks on one another.

With the spinning wheel, I think I took something that most would have discarded because it was not in perfect condition and made it into something beautiful and personally meaningful. We are not all perfect, but just like the

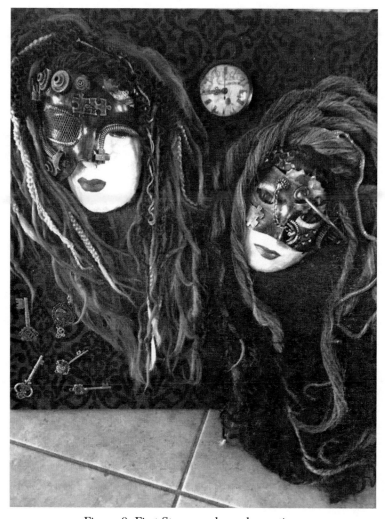

Figure 9. First Steampunk mask creation.

girl with the back brace, we can take that imperfection and transform it through Steampunk to create something that empowers us. Not only did this piece link me to the past and to my love for the Victorian era, but it linked to my writing, to my desire to travel, and to my desire to transform something that someone would have discounted into something beautiful. So, I will end this chapter with a quote from Suna Dasi, the founder of Steampunk India: "I am one of those people who, after a lifetime passion for all things Victorian; a lifetime love of the macabre; of alternative ways of living and thinking outside the box, not to mention a taste for vintage sci-fi, were searching for community. Well, we suddenly looked up to find the world had

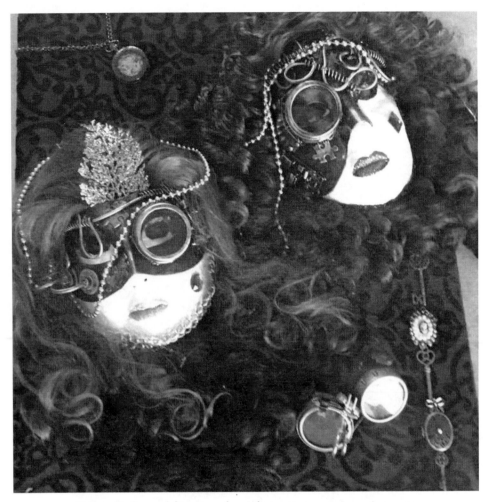

Figure 10. Second Steampunk mask creation—warrior princesses.

conveniently lumped the whole shebang into one genre that encompassed all of the above!" (VanderMeer & Boskovich, 2014, pp. 146–147). And now on to the creative art therapists who gratefully contributed to this book on using the creative therapies and technologies to help their clients. Onward and upward!

REFERENCES

Christians, K. (2011). Steampunk future past. *Metalsmith, 31*(3), 18–19.
Gross, C. (2010). History of Steampunk. Retrieved on March 13, 2015 from http://steampunkscholar.blogspot.com/2010/08/history-of-steampunk-by-cory-gross.html

Hoppe, K. M., & Wilson, J. (2012). Steampunk collaboration. *Library Media Connection, 31*(1), 24–26.

Oxford Dictionary. (2016). Steampunk defined. Retrieved on September 28, 2016 from https://en.oxforddictionaries.com/definition/steampunk

Perschon, M. D. (2012). *The steampunk aesthetic: Technofantasies in a neo-victorian retro-future* (Order No. NR89296). Available from ProQuest Dissertations & Theses Global. (1151509327). Retrieved from http://search.proquest.com.library. capella.edu/docview/1151509327?accountid=27965

Pho, Diane M. (2014, February 3). Steampunk hands around the world: Good gears good works. Retrieved from http://beyondvictoriana.com/2014/02/03/steampunk-hands-around-the-world-good-gears-and-good-works/

Plumb, T. (2013, May 26). Steampunk as art therapy for the autistic. *Boston Globe.* Retrieved from https://www.bostonglobe.com/metro/regionals/north/2013/05/25/steampunk-art-therapy-for-autistic/3TSOCFHa0K65f8wduW52IK/story.html

Smith, K. K. (2015). *Everything old is new again: The Victorian roots of the Steampunk movement* (Order No. 1526762). Available from ProQuest Dissertations & Theses Global. (1720330213). Retrieved from http://search.proquest.com.library.capella .edu/docview/1720330213?accountid=27965

Steampunk District. (2012). What is Steampunk art? Retrieved on March 13, 2015 from http://steampunkdistrict.com/what-is-steampunk-art/

Toffler, A. (1970). *Future shock.* New York: Random House.

Turner, T. (2016, February 1). Teen turns body brace into steampunk fashion statement. GoodNewsNetwork. Retrieved from http://www.goodnewsnetwork.org/teen-turns-her-body-brace-into-steampunk-fashion-statement/

VanderMeer, J., & Boskovich, D. (2014). *The Steampunk user's manual: An illustrated practical and whimsical guide to creating retro-futurist dreams.* New York: Abrams Image.

Wren, C. (2013). You've been steampunked. (Cover story). *American Theatre, 30*(2), 30–33.

Young, B. C. (2014). *Contemplating "what if?": Allohistoric reconstructions of Victorian restrictions in young adult Steampunk* (Order No. 3711411). Available from ProQuest Dissertations & Theses Global. (1703025259). Retrieved from http://search.proquest.com.library.capella.edu/docview/1703025259?accountid=27965

Biography

Stephanie L. Brooke has her MS degree in Community Agency Counseling, a PhD in Organizational Psychology, and Certifications in Art Therapy, Play Therapy, and Leadership in Higher Education. Additionally, she is a nationally certified counselor–NCC 31267. She is a dissertation mentor in the Counseling Department at Capella University, with twenty-five graduates to date. Dr. Brooke received five Steven Shank Awards at Capella University for her teaching and mentoring excellence. She has served as the comprehensive exam lead and is currently a scientific merit reviewer. In April of 2016, she became the course lead for Quantitative Methods for Counselor Education Research as well as for Tests and Measurements. Dr. Brooke has written three books on art therapy, edited several works on the creative therapies, written chapters in texts in her field, and has published several professional, peer-reviewed journal articles. For more information on Dr. Brooke, visit her website at: http://stephanielbrooke.com/

Chapter 2

PLAY THERAPY IN THE DIGITAL AGE: PRACTICE AND TRAINING

HILDA R. GLAZER

Ashley sits across from me not saying a word and says she can sit here for the entire session. She had just come into the room. The presenting problem was anger and not getting along with her family. Her mom said she spends every minute she can on the computer and gets angry when they limit her time.

My computer is on my desk but turned away from her. I turn the computer to Ashley and ask her to find a website that showed how she was feeling right now. She immediately engaged and after a few minutes of searching and talking, shared a video of a lonely girl sitting alone in a room. After a few more searches, we were talking. Each session after that, began with searching for a website or an image that represented how she felt that day. Homework was usually computer related. This is a positive example of how the computer can be used to connect with a teen. The next example illustrates a different outcome.

While sitting in the waiting room, Terry asked his mom for her phone and she obliged. Terry immediately began playing a game, but when it was time to go to the playroom, he refused to stop his game and proceeded to scream at his mother. His mom was powerless to handle this public display of anger.

These two examples illustrate both ends of the continuum for the impact and for the use of technology in therapy. In the first case, the computer allowed the teen to engage and to move onto other games and activities in the playroom. In the second one, the child's engaging with the game on the phone became the primary focus of his activity and because more important than anything else.

Technology enhanced toys (augmented toys) are part of the child's play experiences (Bergen, 2012). The variety and types of toys expand for children of all ages, even toddlers and many have design elements that are in common with traditional age appropriate toys (Bergen, 2012). However, there is little research on the augmented toys (Bergen, 2012).

Photography has been part of play therapy practice for many years. My clients often ask for pictures of their sand trays or want to be in a picture doing something in the playroom that they want sent to their parent or guardian immediately or want me to keep as a reminder of them. I have also had requests for videos of puppet plays.

For the generation in which computers are integral to play and found in all parts of the environment, using computers as a playful intervention seems to be a natural addition to the toolkit of the play therapist. In an early review of the uses of computer in play therapy, Aymard (2002) found that computers were not contraindicated in therapy for children and adolescents. The can be a "hook" to engage them in counseling or in play therapy. Second, there was evidence that the presenting problems remitted. Aymard described the use of a computer game with children and with adolescents. He has successfully used the computer for drawing, storytelling, craft-making, puppetry, creating animated therapeutic metaphors, and gaming. He concluded that the value of a computer game is the same as that of any toy as the child can use it as an integral part of the play therapy journey. Other have documented the use of computers in psychotherapy with specific aspects of an intervention including an interactive website or photos in systematic desensitization of a phobias. Research has also been done on computerized cognitive behavior therapy (Bouchard, 2011; Richardson, Stallard, & Velleman, 2010) and the use of virtual reality for treating specific phobias (Bouchard, 2011). Virtual reality (VR) is an application that lets users navigate and interact in real time with a 3D computer-generated environment. Bouchard suggested that the use of virtual reality in therapy with children will increase and that it will become an empirically validated intervention.

A guideline for using any technology is whether it helps meet a therapeutic goal with the client. For example, with a teen with abandonment issues, who had trouble verbalizing the components of her issue, developing a collage using the computer might prove to be more effective and be more portable than trying to do this with cutouts from magazines. Here, there is a direct line between the use of the computer and the therapy. Allowing children to bring a handheld game or phone into the playroom may disrupt the therapeutic process.

WebCam

Using the WebCam in the playroom was suggested by Chlebowski and Fremont (2011). The WebCam is seen as nonjudgmental by the child and may encourage expression. They developed the following technique using the WebCam for preschool-to-early school-age children who appear to be hesitant or shy. The intervention begins with the child being asked to assume another role. Once the child appeared comfortable with the computer screen and with the microphone, the therapist invited the child to watch himself or herself. The WebCam may function as part of play and engagement in the preschooler and give the child a sense of control and mastery. The therapist later introduces himself or herself as a friendly interviewer or reporter and asks identifying questions to engage the child. Depending on the reaction of the child and the responses to the questions, the therapist can continue the questioning. Alternately, the WebCam has the potential to be used in a more nondirective way in the playroom with the therapist engaging the child therapeutically without asking questions. The saved video can be used in parent or family sessions or just with the child.

In another intervention developed by Chlebowski and Fremont (2011), the WebCam was used as a mirror, letting the child see how he or she looked. Their example was a child with temper tantrums. The child has no way of seeing how frightening or scary he or she seems to others. The WebCam can show the child that image. They gave the example of a child who was surprised to see how angry he looked during a tantrum and decided he did not want to look like that again.

Video Games

The use of the various technologies to play games is often a source of contention in families. While children may become engrossed in the games and not engage with others, they can also improve visual and spatial attention skills (Meszaros, 2004). How children and their caretakers regard the use of video games is one consideration in treatment planning. Other considerations include the presenting problem, the intended uses of the game, and the ability of the child to use the technology.

While we often use therapeutic games in the playroom that are age and problem specific, we may find that computer versions will be developed that will be more engaging for today's children. The format for the games can vary from simulated game shows, computerized therapy games, and therapeutic video games.

Violence is part of many of the published video games. Children "can be encouraged to use this safer alternative to expressing anger as a way to test limits and rebel that may have fewer social consequences, and counselors can ask questions to help clients distinguish between the real world and the virtual experience" (Perkins, Brumfield, Collins, & Morris, 2010, p. 7).

The Virtual Play Therapist

The use of robotics has application in the playroom. An example of a robotic companion is Paro, which looks like a baby seal and is programmed to respond to sound and touch, to show different emotions, and is able to learn information about its environment, such as the name of its person (https://www.ai-therapy.com/articles/computers-and-therapy). When Animal-Assisted Therapy is not an option, a robot may be an option.

Virtual counseling for play therapists may take on some interesting possibilities. One is a virtual playroom in a virtual world such as Second Life (http://secondlife.com/) where the therapist and child interact in the virtual world in a virtual playroom. I spent a month overseas and a few of the parents and I talked about ways to keep in touch. While email for questions was not an issue, none of the children or parents thought the use of synchronous sessions was a viable option. Rather, referral to another play therapist was seen as the optimal solution. The therapeutic value of the therapist and child in the playroom was recognized. That is not to say that if online therapy were the only option, that it would be rejected outright, but when therapy began in the playroom, online was not an option.

Guidelines for the ethical and legal practice of virtual therapy are a concern of the major professional organizations. Being aware of these issues and professional and legal requirements and guides is important. A National Institute of Health Study published in 2012, concluded that "Ethical and legal issues in virtual environments are similar to those that occur in the in-person world. Individuals represented by an avatar have the rights equivalent to the individual and should be treated as such." (http://www.ncbi.nlm.nih.gov/pubmed/22823138)

A related issue is using social media. Who is your friend on Facebook (https://www.facebook.com)? What limits do you set on your privacy? What boundary issues are there? With asynchronous communication, there is the potential for entering the life of the other in ways typically reserved for friends and for family. How does this impact the relationship between client and therapist (Drum & Littleton, 2014)? Social networking may create ethical dilemmas in the areas of privacy, confidentiality, and informed consent (Harris, Robinson-Kurpius, 2014). When clients and former clients have found me, I always ignore the friend requests, but use it as an opportunity to talk about safety and boundary issues for both of us.

I often use texts to set and to verify dates and times of the session. One preteen noticed a text from me on his mother's phone and initiated a conversation with me; the first time it was fine. Then every time he could, he texted me as he would a friend. This became a topic of the next session, and we worked to figure out the rules for communicating so that he did not feel rejected but understood the boundaries.

When making the decision about using the Internet to interact with clients, it is important to consider the ethical, HIPPA, and other legal implications. Boundary crossings and unintentional disclosures should be considered. With email and sending texts, security and privacy issues should also be taken into consideration.

Many professional associations have ethical guidelines on the use of technology in therapy and in therapeutic relationships, including The American Psychological Association, the National Association of Social Workers, the American Counseling Association, and The American Association for Marriage and Family Therapy (Hudspeth & Davis, 2015).

Technology and Play Therapy Training

Watching and listening to lectures and to demonstrations online for continuing education credits, is quite common, as is the use of technology to enhance teaching and learning. The Association for Play Therapy (APT) has an extensive video collection showing the classic play therapists in action as well as interviews of many of the prominent people in play therapy. Bringing in a speaker via the Internet is also quite common.

Taking a course or enrolling in an educational program at an accredited university is relatively new. There are a number of models that exist to do this, including adding an online lab or discussion to a face-to-face class, combining online and face-to-face sessions (blended classroom), and the totally online class.

Extending didactic training in play therapy to those who are not near a university with a play therapy center or courses was the goal of Capella University in creating the Certificate in Play Therapy. Capella University is a regionally accredited online university. The challenge was to create a program which would meet the rigors and depth of coursework required by the Association for Play Therapy and to accomplish this in the online environment. The space in which learning occurs encourages learning from each other, each constructing his or her own meaning within the scope of the practice of play therapy (Stein, Wanstreet, & Calvin, 2009).

One of the challenges is to provide the interaction necessary for learning and skill building. Interaction is a key variable in learning and in satisfaction with distance education courses (Fulford & Zhang, 1993; Gunawardena & Duphorne, 2001). Engaging the adult learner so that he or she takes an active part in learning, remains motivated, and takes responsibility for learning, is part of the strategy for course development and for teaching in the online environment. An extensive body of literature in online and distance learning addresses concerns with interaction from three perspectives: interaction as an instructional exchange, interaction as computer-mediated communication, and interaction as a social/psychological connection (Wanstreet, 2009). Interaction as an instructional exchange between entities includes learner-content, learner-instructor, and learner-learner (Moore, 1989). It is how we include these elements that becomes critical to learning in the instructional space that we provide. Applying social constructivist theory, people learn best when they actively construct their own understanding through interaction with their peers (Sthapornnanon, Sakulbumrungsil, Theeraroungchaisri, & Watcharadamrongkun, 2009).

Within the learning platform, the student is encouraged to engage with the content, with the faculty, and with the other students. The requirements for engagement do not let the student hide in the back of the classroom. Writing skills and critical thinking skills are essential to having your voice heard in the online classroom. Students interact in the learning platform with the faculty, and with other students through the discussion boards and in weekly synchronous sessions. Lack of participation results in outreach to the student to encourage engagement or to help in problem solving as needed.

Using the technology in the courses can be a challenge for some students who do not have the technology experience. Assessing the online library, writing center, and other resources can initially be challenging. Learning to navigate in the learning platform becomes the first task faced by many learners. Providing access to the university orientation has provided additional support for those less comfortable with the learning platform and with online support services.

Including weekly synchronous face-to-face sessions using technology was an essential part of the program. It was hoped that adding this element to the learning space would reduce some anxiety about the learning tasks and make the learning less distant therapy (Stein, Wanstreet, & Calvin, 2009). It was also seen as meeting the requirement of the Association for Play Therapy for interaction between student and faculty. While the requirements for students as well as for faculty to respond to each other in the discussion boards is seen as been critical to learning and encouraging critical thinking, there was a concern voiced by APT that discussion boards were not sufficient, but that live interaction between faculty and learners and learners and learners was required. To meet this need, in four of the five classes, learners and faculty meet synchronously for two hours per week in the virtual classroom. This space is used for answering questions, for sharing techniques, for presenting papers, and for having discussions.

Students have the opportunity to make comments as part of the end of course evaluations. While some of the learners had problems with the technology and did not like the synchronous nature of the sessions, there were more positive than negative comments. Here are some of the recent comments:

- I really liked the ability to interact with other students for the assignments. This is the first course I have taken in the Play Therapy Certificate program where we did this. After speaking to other students, this interface has been a requirement with other instructors. It should be required for every course.
- The live sessions. It made me feel like more a part of the class.
- The adobe connect does not work half the time, live or recorded. I gave up trying to watch a recorded session.
- Once I was on the live sessions, the experience was very helpful.
- I think there should be one weekly live session rather than two.
- I was disappointed when my life got in the way. Additionally, this is supposed to be an online course and I think two sessions is one too much.
- I liked the visual aids and the dialogue during the live chats and on the discussion board.

Learners did find that the blended model using synchronous and asynchronous interaction was beneficial for the most part. For some, there were issues with the timing of the classes because they lived in time zones or had work schedules that made attendance impossible. To meet the needs of those learners, the faculty have developed an alternative plan which includes viewing the recordings of the sessions. When papers are to be presented in class, the learners are able to prerecord their presentations. The faculty show that the videos and the learners are able to comment, knowing that the presenter will listen to this later.

Enhancing the online classroom through the use of technology and media can improve the learning experience for the student. Engaging increases the opportunities for learning and for the enjoyment of the experience. For example, interactive activities can be included in which the students drag an icon to match it with a definition or description. Interactive media pieces can be developed in which there are pull-down menus providing details. One example is the use of an interactive timeline. Short interviews can be included allowing the learners to hear from experts. Videos demonstrating skills can be included. Case studies can be presented in an animated format or with actors giving the student a better feel for the case. All of these can be done in ways that allow for alternative formats making the content available to people with disabilities. Internet sites such as https://community.articulate.com/ offer a variety of interactive games and activities that can be used in the online environment to enhance learning.

Students can submit videos of skill practice allowing for feedback from faculty members or from other students. This is similar to what is being done in traditional classes where sessions are taped and reviewed. As in the traditional setting, the same ethical concerns apply.

Conclusion

Technology is a part of the world of the child. Play therapists have opportunities to enter the world of the child by using technology as part of their toolkit. The therapist should be mindful of the impact on the therapeutic process and how it relates to therapeutic goals as well as ethic and legal considerations. Play Therapy training is being enhanced in the online environment. Re-conceptualizing what it means to interact online and how that relates to skill learning and developing a professional identity, is part of this.

REFERENCES

Aymard, L. L. (2002). Funny Face: Shareware for counseling and play therapy. *Journal of Technology in Human Services, 20*(1/2), 11–29.

Bergen, D. (2012). Play, technology toy affordances, and brain development: Research needs and policy issues. In L. E. Cohen, & S. Waite-Stupiansky (Eds.), *Play: A polyphony of research, theories and issues* (pp. 163–173). Lanham, MD: University Press of America.

Bouchard, S. (2011). Could virtual reality be effective in treating children with phobias? *Expert Review of Neurotherapeutics, 11*(2), 207–213. doi:http://dx.doi.org/10.1586/ern.10.196

Chlebowski, S., MD, & Fremont, W., MD (2011). Therapeutic uses of the WebCam in child psychiatry. *Academic Psychiatry, 35*(4), 263–267. Retrieved from http://search.proquest.com.library.capella.edu/docview/888685451?accountid=27965

Drum, K. B., & Littleton, H. L. (2014). Therapeutic boundaries in telepsychology: Unique issues and best practice recommendations. *Professional Psychology: Research and Practice, 45*(5), 309–315. doi:10.1037/a0036127

Fulford, C. P., & Zhang, S. (1993). Perceptions of interaction: The critical predictor in distance education. *The American Journal of Distance Education, 7*(3), 8–21.

Gunawardena, C., N., & Duphorne, P. L. (2001, April). *Which learner readiness factors, online features, and CMC related learning approaches are associated with learner satisfaction in computer conferences?* Paper presented at the Annual Meeting of the American Educational Research Association, Seattle, WA.

Harris, S. E., & Robinson-Kurpius, S. E. (2014). Social networking and professional ethics: Client searches, informed consent, and disclosure. *Professional Psychology: Research and Practice, 45*(1), 11–19. doi:10.1037/a0033478

Hudspeth, E. F., & Davis, P. (2015). Ethical web-based play therapy supervision. *Play Therapy, 10*(2), 16–20.

Meszaros, P. S. (2004). The wired family: Living digitally in the postinformation age. The American Behavioral Scientist, 48(4), 377-390. Retrieved from http://search.proquest.com.library.capella.edu/docview/214760390?accountid=27965

Moore, M. G. (1989). Three types of interaction. *The American Journal of Distance Education, 3*(2), 1–6.

Perkins, G. W., Brumfield, K. A., Collins, E. N., & Morris, N. T. (2010). Working with gamers: Implications for counselors. Retrieved from http://counselingoutfitters.com/vistas/vistas10/Article_65.pdf

Richardson, T., Stallard, P., & Velleman, S. (2010). Computerised cognitive behavioural therapy for the prevention and treatment of depression and anxiety in children and adolescents: A systematic review. *Clinical Child and Family Psychology Review, 13*(3), 275–90. doi:http://dx.doi.org/10.1007/s10567-010-0069-9

Stein, D. S., Wanstreet, C. E., & Calvin, J. (2009). How a novice adult online learner experiences transactional distance. *Quarterly Review of Distance Education, 10*(3), 305–311, 319–320. Retrieved from http://search.proquest.com.library.capella.edu/docview/89167435?accountid=27965

Sthapornnanon, N., Sakulbumrungsil, R., Theeraroungchaisri, A., & Watcharadamrongkun, S. (2009). Social constructivist learning environment in an online professional practice course. *American Journal of Pharmaceutical Education, 73*(1), 10.

Wanstreet, C. E. (2009). Interaction in online learning environments: A review of the literature. In A. Orellana, T. L. Hudgins, & M. Simonson (Eds.), *The perfect online course: Best practices for designing and teaching* (pp. 425–442). Charlotte, NC: Information Age Publishing.

Biography

Hilda R. Glazer, EdD, RPT-S, PCC-S is director of the Center for the Study of Play Therapy and Coordinator of the Teaching Assistant Program in Psychology at Capella University, Minneapolis. Dr. Glazer has a small private practice and works as a bereavement counselor for Mount Carmel Hospice in Columbus. Her primary clinical and research area is grieving children. She has over fifty referred articles and book chapters. Dr. Glazer has over sixty workshops and presentations including invited workshops in Ireland, Germany, Indonesia, and most recently in China.

Chapter 3

ADAPTING ART THERAPY
FOR ONLINE GROUPS

Sara Prins Hankinson, Brennan Jones, and Kate Collie

Adapting Art Therapy for Online Groups

In a culture that is increasingly reliant on computers and at a time when technology is advancing quickly, therapists have wonderful opportunities to use technology to improve the services we offer as well as to expand access to them. As an international team of art therapists, computer scientists, and others with a shared goal of using the Internet to expand access to art therapy, we developed online art therapy groups for young adults with cancer. In this chapter, we discuss our development process, the online art therapy techniques we created, preliminary findings, and plans for further development. Hankinson, an art therapist working in cancer care, wrote the first part of the chapter. She worked with Collie and others to explore digital art therapy techniques up to the present time, and with the help of Jones, Collie, and others, devised a method of hosting art therapy groups online, using the platform of www.cancerchatcanada.ca as a base. Jones, a computer science student who studied our process and has been exploring and designing possibilities for the future of online art therapy, wrote the second part of the chapter.

Cancer Care

At the time of this article, Hankinson and Collie were working as art therapists within cancer care centers in Canada. (Hankinson at the BC Cancer Agency in Vancouver, Canada, and Collie at the Cross Cancer Institute in Edmonton, Alberta.) There is a great need for art therapists to work within cancer care, as cancer is an intense illness that brings up many emotions, reactions, fears, and fantasies. It produces more metaphorical thinking than any other illness, and a diagnosis often brings up fears of death and existential questions (Driefuss-Kattan, 1990). Cancer treatments are sometimes considered worse than the disease itself, causing patients to suffer through body and weight changes, hair loss, fatigue, nausea, headaches, scars, and other physical symptoms, along with host of emotional side effects. The field of psycho-oncology was created, recognizing the unique psychological needs of cancer patients.

Young adults with cancer have high levels of unmet psychosocial needs (Giese-Davis et al., 2012) but much less access to age-appropriate psychosocial support than children or older adults (Zebrack & Isaacson, 2012). They are significantly more likely to report distress than other age groups and to report problems such as delayed social maturation, mood disturbances, academic difficulties, career and insurance discrimination, and relationship problems (Kelly & Gibson, 2008). Psychological difficulty may stem from the fact that young adults can feel caught between the worlds of children and adults. They are on the cusp on autonomy–gaining success at making decisions independently, honing interpersonal and social skills, mastering new roles, and discovering their vocation and sexuality (Bleyer & Barr, 2007; Bleyer, Viny, & Barr, 2006). Being diagnosed with cancer can make them lose control and impose dependence back on them, threatening their personal development, peer relationships, and development of realistic goals in the life. It can lead to uncertainty, a search for meaning, social stigma, and isolation. Particularly if a young adult's cancer continues to advance, there is a heightened awareness of death, feelings of helplessness, loss of control, and an intensified search for meaning.

The increasing incidence of cancer in this age group, unique psychological needs, and lack of improvement in survival (Bleyer & Barr, 2007; Bleyer, Viny & Barr, 2006) has created interest in developing age-specific group support for people diagnosed with cancer in their twenties and thirties. Topics brought up in support groups for young adults may include body image, health-related anxiety, concerns about fertility and child-rearing, relationship problems, returning to work, and financial concerns.

Art Therapy in Cancer Care

Art therapy uses fine art materials and activities within the context of a therapeutic relationship to encourage expression and well-being and foster relationships. Goals can include the expression and release of feelings (discharge), creating an alternative place for these feelings to be (in the art rather than in the person), stress reduction, and discovering inner strengths. It is a creative approach that can be more inviting than other forms of psychosocial support.

Art therapy has been found to support cancer patients both emotionally and physically (e.g., Nainis et al., 2006; Wood, Molassiotis, & Payne, 2011). Making art is a way to reveal unspoken truths and the creative work may become a container for all of the shifting emotions that a person with cancer may experience, holding the fear, grief, and aggression, which may be projected instead of kept inside. People with cancer often think that they need to be positive or "strong" for themselves and for everyone around them. Because of its ability to foster expression, art therapy might be the only place where some cancer patients express their negative emotions.

Art making can be empowering as it gives patients something that they can control, even in the last stages of their life (Malchiodi, 1999, 2000). Self-efficacy, self-mastery, and self-awareness can be fostered by the arts, allowing patients to move toward an empowered state and away from feeling dependent or like a victim. Art making can be a powerful method for dealing with physical changes, emotional trauma, interpersonal problems, and spiritual dilemmas for persons in advanced stages of cancer.

For young adults with cancer, an art therapy group can be a place to connect with others who understand the experience of cancer. The group can be a place to share and to normalize experiences and to provide mutual support. Through their art, members of an art therapy group can express grief and difficult feelings in a safe place, while improving self-esteem, communication and socialization, and promoting whole-person healing.

Art Therapy Online

Art therapists began experimenting with using computers in the 1980s. Weinberg (1985) was an early explorer of the potential for computers to be used for patients with physical limitations. Subsequent work has shown that computers are powerful instruments for rehabilitative art therapy for physically and mentally disabled patients (Kuleba, 2008). They can be helpful for making art, especially for for people with certain disabilities and people experiencing fatigue, weakness, or compromised dexterity. Digital art tools can be user-friendlier than traditional art materials, particularly for people who frequently use computers. Parker-Bell (1999) advocated for the use of computers in art therapy, stating several advantages including the ability to track the progress of an image by being able to save multiple copiest; to make art therapy accessible to people with disabilities; to supply an endless source of collage material; and to provide a natural container for imagery and image making.

In the late 1990s, Collie and Davor Čubranic began researching ways of providing group art therapy via the Internet using voice communication and shareable images (e.g., Collie & Čubranic, 1999). Through their research, they identified issues to consider for developing Internet art therapy services and found that potential problems, such as confidentiality, are best addressed by establishing practice guidelines and group protocols. They note that art therapy lends itself to online delivery because visual images can be transmitted so easily from place to place and because art images made during online art therapy provide rich nonverbal information that can enhance communication between people who cannot see one another. One of their findings was that online art therapy might be particularly appropriate for younger people. We have added to the early work done in distance and computer art therapy to create methods and clinical guidelines for online art groups customized for the needs and preferences for young adults with cancer.

CancerChatCanada

We developed the groups to be offered through CancerChatCanada, a pan-Canadian program of online psychosocial support (see Fig. 1). CancerChatCanada was established as a way to extend the known health benefits of professionally led cancer support groups to more people in Canada. It began at the British Columbia Cancer Agency in Vancouver, in partnership with The Wellness Community in the United States. A fully Canadian CancerChatCanada service was launched in 2010. Since 2015, it has been hosted by the De Souza Institute (https://cancerchat.desouza institute.com/). CancerChatCanada includes an online registration and enrollment system with an integrated Canadian-based chat platform. The site incorporates the most up-to-date security for the protection of identifying information (Secure Socket Layer or SSL) and is password protected. Participants register online and information is stored and downloaded by a site administrator through a content management system.

The groups that CancerChatCanada offers are 90 minutes in length, occur on a weekly basis, and generally include 6–10 participants and one or two professional counselors who may be anywhere in Canada. At the time we were developing our different methods of working on this platform (2012–2013), CancerChatCanada also offered a discussion board and a private messaging for group members to connect outside of the chat room. Confidentiality is maintained, and members are known to each other only through their first name or through a chosen screen name.

Evaluations of CancerChatCanada have shown that these online groups do indeed improve access to psychosocial support for people with cancer. The evaluations indicate that the online groups, which use live chat and are professionally led, are as effective as in-person groups. In some ways they can even be more effective, such as for facilitating the expression of difficult emotions and of addressing difficult topics (Stephen et al., 2013).

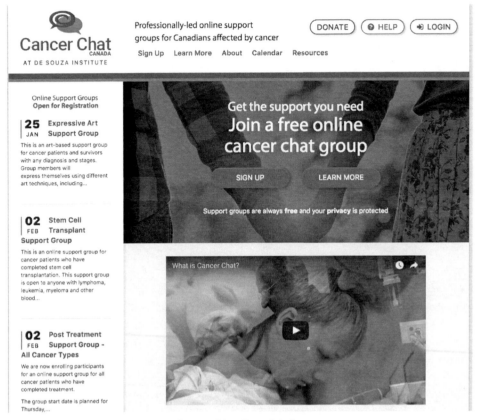

Figure 1. CancerChatCanada's home page.

CancerChatCanada participants have reported feeling psychologically safe because they are able to access the group from their home. They have also reported being more honest and emotionally expressive with people they get to know but do not see. Some have noted that they preferred writing to talking because they could articulate themselves more, reflect while they were typing, and cry and write at the same time. They have described how deep emotional connections can form in professionally led online cancer support groups (Stephen et al., 2014).

Developing Online Art Therapy Methods for CancerChatCanada

Seeing the need for distance art therapy services for young adults with cancer and the success of the online support groups already being offered on CancerChatCanada, we decided to use this site as a platform for hosting online art therapy groups. In 2012, Collie and Hankinson began collaborating with Jones and with other art therapists and health professionals on this project. Our goals were (1) to create art groups for young adults with cancer on CancerChatCanada, (2) to formulate clinical procedures and guidelines for online art-based therapeutic groups in general, and (3) assess digital technology already in place and begin designing new digital art therapy tools.

Our project began with much experimentation with different online digital art tools and techniques. Hankinson found and trialed various online art-making programs. For websites to be functional for us, they needed to be free for use, easy to learn, and the images created needed to be saved and not distributed publicly. The websites we used at first were http://pencilmadness .com, http://graffiter.com, and http://www.polyvore.com/cgi/app (see Fig. 2). We also developed exercises that used digital photography or traditional art materials for images that could then be photographed. The images in this chapter are examples of artwork that was created within our trial groups. The artists have consented to showing their work within this chapter.

We looked briefly into apps and programs that would create art on a tablet (e.g., iPad or smart phone), but decided that for the purpose of our group on CancerChatCanada, we needed to keep the technology we used, free and simple to use. CancerChatCanada is a low-tech website (with high security) that uses text (no video or voice) so that it can operate at a low bandwidth and be accessible to users even in remote locations. We decided that the websites we used, needed to be equally accessible.

Collie and Hankinson, along with the art therapists Mady Mooney and Gretchen Miller, began running our own mock art therapy groups where we took turns facilitating and experimenting with different formats for online art therapy. We tried Skype and Google Hangouts, but favored the security of CancerChatCanada as a site for online art therapy.

Throughout our development process, we were aware of tension between group members wanting to "see" each other figuratively without being seen physically. Because people with cancer often experience bodily changes and fatigue, many enjoy being able to be a part of a support group from the comfort of their own home where they do not have to go out, and it does not matter what they look like. Many also enjoy the semianonymity of a group where people just know them by their first names. Yet, participants in our trial groups said they were very curious about what other people looked like, and therapists said they would have liked to be able to see more nonverbal cues, like how the participants create their art. As we developed different modes of working online we strove to create an environment where people could "see" each other through their artwork, yet retain their privacy. One example of how we did this was by asking participants to introduce them-

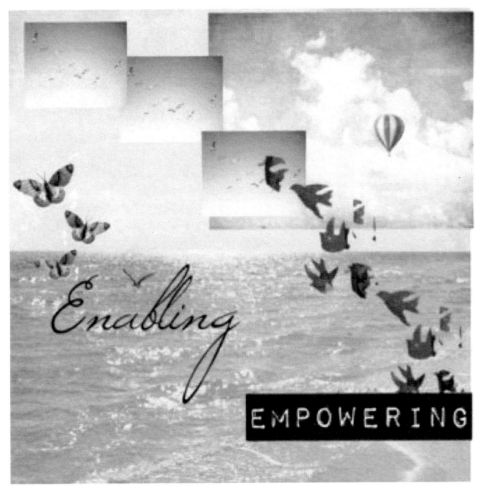

Figure 2. A collage made using Polyvore.com.

selves to each other by posting a photograph that represents something about who they are—without including themselves or any other person.

Through our experimentation, we discovered three basic formats for hosting online art therapy sessions on CancerChatCanada: synchronous, asynchronous, and mixed. In the synchronous sessions that we led, we posted an introduction to an art therapy exercise on the discussion board well in advance of each weekly session, telling participants what they could expect. For example, one session included an introduction to mandalas and instructions on how to use the drawing website, PencilMadness.com. We encouraged participants to prepare for the session by making themselves comfort-

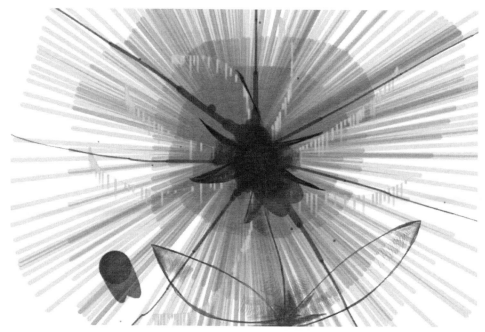

Figure 3. A mandala created using Pencilmadness.com.

able with the medium (PencilMadness). While together in the chat room, the art therapist (Hankinson in this case) typed instructions for the participants to follow in the Pencil Madness program (e.g., "Draw a circle. . . . Now, fill it in. . . ") (see Fig. 3). Once the exercise was completed, participants saved and posted their images onto the discussion board. Hankinson then led the group through looking at each person's images and discussing the process using text communication.

Using the asynchronous method, the art therapist would post an activity on the discussion board weeks in advance of when it needed to be completed. The activity would include thorough instructions for what the participants needed to do to complete their artwork, which they would do on their own time and then post their image on the discussion board when they had finished. Group members would then respond to each other's art on the discussion board, all on their own time. The asynchronous format worked well for activities involving physical art materials. For example, one session we led included a link to a YouTube video about how to create wish dolls. Hankinson mailed each participant a package containing a piece of fabric and yarn for their use and they followed the video, creating a doll out of the supplied materials along with items in their own home. They posted photographs of their dolls on the discussion board, and then responded to each

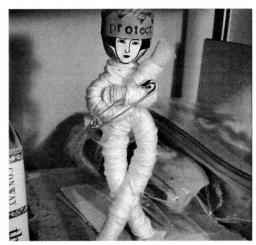

Wrapped in light to guide my journey,
Guarding my safety . . . protecting it with my
shield
I protect the integrity of my intentions:
Stillness, simplicity, service, trust, light, and
honor.

Standing tall and strong, I watch over to protect
What's in my heart
And to trust my heart and crown to guide me
to safety.

I feel & carry pure protection of love & radi-
ance among me
As I strongly, yet softly gaze ahead
In my journey.

Figure 4. One participant's wish doll and poem.

other's dolls with a phrase. These phrases were then compiled by each artist into a poem to accompany their wish doll (see Fig. 4).

Using the mixed method that we devised, the art therapist would post an art exercise on the discussion board, again well in advance of the session. Participants would complete their art on their own time, and meet in the chat room to discuss their art in real time. For example, for one session we focused on graffiti art and posted an introduction to this on the discussion board along with instructions on how to create graffiti using the program, www.graffiter.com (see Fig. 5). Participants painted their "tag" or some type of social commentary, and discussed this in the text within the chat room.

After our initial group of art therapists (Collie, Hankinson, Mooney, & Miller) became comfortable with the three different modes we devised of working on CancerChatCanada, we invited many other professionals to participate in three mock online art therapy groups. Participants in these mock groups included other art therapists, clinical counselors, and social workers with an interest in working online; health professionals working within cancer care; computer scientists; and a young adult in remission from cancer. Participants were mostly located across Canada, but also in the United States and the United Kingdom. Overall, the feedback we received from these groups was positive. One participant said, "There was a quality of relating online that was incredibly human and potentially very profound that would allow a group to benefit very much, despite physical isolation." The positive feedback and helpful suggestions encouraged us to continue developing the methods we had begun using.

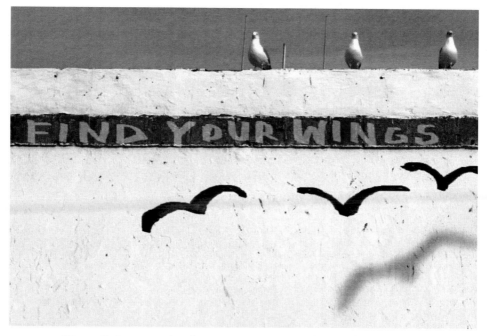

Figure 5. An example of a commentary created using Graffiter.com.

In the fall of 2013, we led our first online group for young adults with cancer on CancerChatCanada. There were seven participants in this group, which lasted for eight sessions. Our sessions included all of the art therapy exercises mentioned in this chapter, plus a self-portrait as a tree exercise, body image, and self-care collages, as well as an assignment to create a treasure box. The group was very lively and supportive of each other, relating instantly to each other's interests and experiences. They were inquisitive about each other's art and illnesses, and connected so deeply that they exchanged contact information (on their own) and one member decided to host a gathering for them all to meet in person.

Since 2013, our practice has evolved due to changes in CancerChat-Canada's website. The discussion board that we relied heavily on for our art therapy groups had to be removed from the website for security purposes. We have had to adapt our process so that the participants receive their instructions to their art exercise in a Word document emailed to them the week before they meet in the chat room. They email their art back when it is completed, and the CancerChatCanada site administrator compiles the art into a password-protected document. This is emailed back to the group members and everyone opens up this file while they are dialoguing via text in the chat room. We have also opened our art groups up to all cancer patients–not just young adults.

With these changes, we have not yet used the asynchronous and synchronous techniques that we previously developed–for now the groups are just using our mixed method. The site has retained its high security but remains low-tech for now. Regardless, we are running art therapy groups online, and they are full. The groups are lively and very emotional. Group members have expressed how grateful they are to meet other cancer patients who understand them, and how much they look forward to receiving their art assignment for the week, as it takes their mind away from their tests and treatments.

CancerChatCanada has plans to update their platform soon. It may include video or voice or other technologies. It may also remain low-tech, just including the chat function. While we hope at some point to try digital tools that feel more like paint brushes and markers, we have discovered that as long as the proper security measures are in place, simple technology can be powerful for giving group members a feeling of togetherness and for allowing freedom of emotional expression. Participants have reported being grateful for the opportunity to be creative and to engage in a form of support that might not otherwise be available to them.

Computers were useful for art therapy in the 1980s, and will continue to be useful regardless of the specifics of the technology in place. However, well-designed art-making tools and online platforms can enhance the experience of distance art therapy. Moving forward, there is much potential for technology to adapt to the needs of cancer patients and of others using distance art therapy services.

Part II: Explorations into the Future of Online Art Therapy Groups

Technology evolves rapidly. The technology that many of us have in our homes today is not the same as what we had ten to twenty years ago. Technological innovations and infrastructure upgrades are making a greater number of activities possible through technology-mediated communication.

Of course, this trend will likely continue over the next ten to twenty years. With these advancements, it makes sense to explore what online group art therapy could be like then. In this section, we explore the future of online group art therapy. We outline the benefits and limitations of current technologies, discuss how future technologies could address those limitations while still retaining the benefits of current technologies, and discuss the implications of future technologies on art therapy groups.

In general, the participants from our mock art therapy groups were aware of being apart from their fellow group members. For some, this provided comfort. Group members could express themselves in whatever way they desire, through their artwork rather than through photos or through video streams of themselves.

In addition to the benefits provided, the reduced awareness in the chat room and in the discussion board also brought a level of discomfort to some. For example, some mentioned there being "more moments of distraction" and "often wondering who [their] group members really were." Some mentioned discomfort with "waiting for long periods of time" and having "uncertainty of who was there and what was going on." One group member thought that being able to pair off into smaller groups during the sessions might make the connections feel more interpersonal.

The purpose of art therapy groups in general is to bring people in similar circumstances together to engage in art activities that provide a therapeutic benefit to the individuals in the group. Being able to actively connect with the people in the group is beneficial, because it allows one to share their experiences with, and to take in experiences from others who are in a similar circumstance. In the mock art therapy groups we conducted, most of the art exercises were individual exercises. The creation of art was an individual activity, whereas the sharing of the art was a group activity. On the one hand, this can be beneficial because it allows individuals to separate themselves from others while focusing on their artwork and exploring and expressing themselves as individuals. On the other hand, combining the art-making realm and the chat realm in some cases might add some benefit by making communication richer and more interpersonal, and it might increase feelings of connectedness and group presence, thereby potentially creating more opportunities for shared experiences and for increasing the benefits of social support within the group.

When asked what they imagined (and wanted) the technology to be like in twenty years, a general trend was that people wanted communication among the group to be more interpersonal. Participants mentioned "virtual reality," "video chatting," and "simulation of physical-based presence."

Research and Exploration through Design

We took a research-through-design (Frayling, 1993; Zimmerman, Forlizzi, & Evenson, 2007) approach to explore the future of online group art therapy by designing a set of art therapy prototypes. These were very simple, yet novel prototypes of art-creation tools, each designed and built in a short amount of time. The purpose of designing these prototypes was not to eventually deploy them for real-world use in online group art therapy, but to spark ideas on (1) how art therapy can be delivered online in the relatively near future with the technology that might be commonplace, (2) what kinds of art therapy activities such future technologies could support, and (3) what implications these technologies could have on art therapy group members and on facilitators.

Our initial ideas were inspired by our experiences with the mock art therapy groups; interview comments from other participants in the mock groups; and previous research in art therapy, psychotherapy, distance delivery of therapy, and Human Computer Interaction. Our ideas progressed through our group discussions involving all three authors, the second author's thesis supervisor (Dr. Anthony Tang), and occasionally another expert.

At the beginning of the design stage, we derived a set of four design goals to address in building our prototypes: (1) promote shared creative experiences; (2) promote a sense of connectedness between individuals; (3) allow for meaningful interaction through nonverbal communication; and (4) allow group members to be aware of each other without actually seeing each other. Several design iterations were built. We will briefly go through the iterations here—they are discussed in greater detail in another paper (Jones, Prins Hankinson, Collie, & Tang, 2014).

Shared Drawing Space with Improved Nonverbal Awareness

One of the participants in our mock groups, as a therapist herself, mentioned that she values some of the subtle nonverbal cues that she gets in face-to-face art therapy sessions, such as pen and brush pressure. In an attempt to satisfy this need in an online setting, we built a shared painting tool, utilizing tablets with pressure sensitivity that reveals basic nonverbal information such as pen pressure and finger contact area (see Fig. 6).

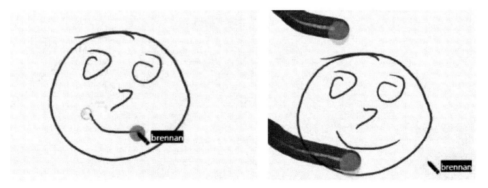

Figure 6. A prototype of a shared drawing tool that improves awareness of other users by showing their cursors, pen pressures, finger contact areas, and paths.

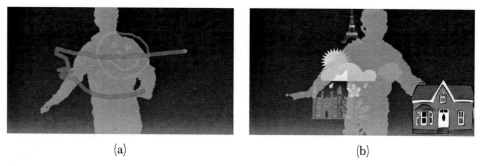

(a)   (b)

Figure 7. A series of tools, utilizing a commodity depth camera, that represent the user as a silhouette in a shared virtual art-making space.

Providing Awareness of the Body

Many of our participants mentioned that they wanted to be able to "see" others or at least to be more aware of their presence, but participants also said that they found value in remaining hidden. With this as inspiration, we created a series of tools (see Fig. 7), utilizing Microsoft Kinect commodity depth cameras, that represent users as silhouettes (to hide their faces) and place them in a virtual environment where they could interact with each other by moving their bodies.

Using the Body as a Canvas

To give users more freedom in controlling their identities, we also explored the idea of allowing users to paint on their own silhouettes and to use their painted silhouettes as digital avatars (see Fig. 8). This idea was inspired by the body outline art therapy activity described by Luzzatto, Sereno, and Capps (2003) and by Luzzatto and Gabriel (2008).

Stick Figures as Simple Representations

During our brainstorming sessions, it was brought up that some people can express deep emotions more easily when doing so as someone (or something) else, and that this is why puppetry is common in some therapy exercises (Ginott, 1961). Based on this, we came up with the idea of representing users as stick figures rather than as silhouettes (see Fig. 9).

Discussion

Each of the design ideas discussed share the same goals. While currently deployed technologies bring groups together during the discussion and

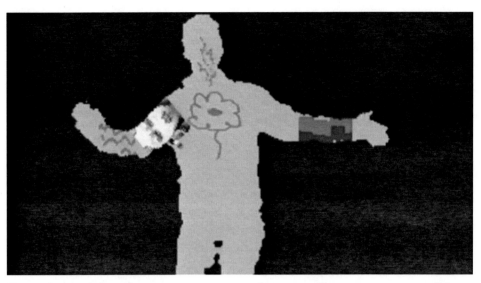

Figure 8. A tool that allows a user to paint on their own silhouette as a means of decorating their avatar and controlling the expression of their identity.

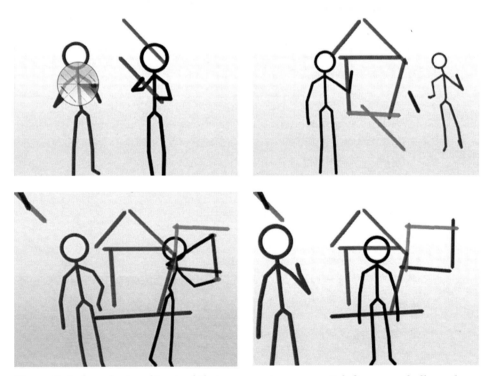

Figure 9. A shared art-making tool that represents users as stick figures and allows them to create "stick art" in a shared virtual space.

reflection phase of an art therapy session, these tools aim to bring the group (or a subset of the group) together during the art-making phase. They also aim to support richer communication and experience sharing between group members.

We are not necessarily promoting the idea that these specific design concepts are the "right" designs. We do, however, believe that the four goals that we listed earlier–the goals that these designs aim to satisfy–are worth pursuing in the development of online group art therapy technologies. Our prototypes serve as examples of how researchers and developers *could* (but not necessarily *should*) achieve these goals. Perhaps those who work on building the future of online group art therapy could iterate on these design ideas in the same ways that we did to create even better designs–perhaps ones that could eventually be deployed in real online art therapy groups.

If such technologies become commonplace in online group art therapy in the future, we could see exercises that focus on group communication and team work become more common in online art therapy programs. Fostering this type of interaction could potentially help break barriers between group members and make seeking and giving support within the group much easier and richer.

Conclusion

Art therapy is a relatively young profession that has been changing and adapting ever since its inception. Additionally, art therapists have been continuously pushing the boundaries of their profession, discovering new populations to work with and new ways to use artistic expression to promote healing. Art therapy has proven to be of great value in helping cancer patients relax, mobilize their personal resources, identify and express difficult emotions, and gain new strength. Furthermore, art therapy groups may be especially beneficial for young adult cancer patients–a small population with great needs and few resources available to them. Many young adult cancer patients struggle to find others who are their age, and are looking for alternatives to traditional therapy models. Online art therapy groups, led by art therapists who have been trained to work online, provide a unique opportunity for young adult cancer patients to feel connected with one another and to receive age-appropriate psychosocial support.

Art therapy is also proving to work well when used with digital technology. The use of computers for art therapy is still a relatively new idea, and one that has developed and will continue to develop over time. In order to provide distance art therapy services to young adults with cancer, we (with the help of many people) devised a method of working online, using www.cancerchatcanada.ca as a platform. We created a method for hosting arts-based activities on a discussion board, and dialoguing about the art within a chat room. We began offering art therapy groups in three different methods, using many different digital tools for creating artwork to be used within our online art therapy groups. Also, we found several websites that worked well for this, as well as digital photography and traditional art exercises that were then photographed. Through our trials we were also developing clinical guidelines for practicing art therapy within an online support group.

Our trial art therapy groups and art groups for young adults with cancer have received much positive feedback. However, we realize that there is great potential for growth in this field, and that the technology we currently use, can be greatly improved. We hope that those with an interest in using technology to provide art therapy services will be inspired to see that it can be done successfully with limited technology. As shown in the prototypes offered, the future could include creating more user-friendly tools, which allow group members to "see" each other more while retaining their privacy. Regardless of the specifics, continued development in this field will allow young adult cancer patients and potentially many others to access art therapy services, all from the comfort of their own homes.

REFERENCES

Bleyer, A., Viny, A., & Barr, R. (2006). Cancer in 15-to 29-year-olds by primary site. *The Oncologist, 11*(6), 590–601.

Bleyer, W. A. & Barr, R. A. (2007). Cancer in adolescents and young adults. Heilderberg, Germany: Springer.

Collie, K., & Čubranic, D. (1999). An art therapy solution to a telehealth problem. *Art Therapy, 16*(4), 186–193.

Driefuss-Kattan, E. (1990). *Cancer stories: Creativity and self-repair.* Hillsdale, NJ: The Analytic Press.

Frayling, C. (1993). *Research in art and design.* London: Royal College of Art.

Giese-Davis, J., Waller, A., Carlson, L. E., Groff, S., Zhong, L., Neri, E., Bachor, S. M., Adamyk-Simpson, J., Rancourt, K. M. S., Dunlop, B., & Bultz, B. D. (2012). Screening for distress, the 6th vital sign: Common problems in cancer outpatients over one year in usual care: Associations with marital status, sex, and age. *BMC Cancer, 12*(1), 441.

Ginott, H. G. (1961). *Group psychotherapy with children: The theory and practice of playtherapy.* McGraw-Hill Book Company.

Jones, B., Prins Hankinson, S., Collie, K., & Tang, A. (2014). Supporting non-verbal visual communication in online group art therapy. In *CHI'14 Extended Abstracts on Human Factors in Computing Systems* (pp. 1759–1764). ACM.

Kelly, D., & Gibson, F. (2008). *Cancer care for adolescents and young adults.* Oxford, UK: Blackwell Publishing.

Kuleba, B. A., (2008). *The integration of computerized art making as a medium in art therapy theory and practice.* (unpublished master's thesis). Drexel University, Philadelphia.

Luzzatto, P. (2005). Musing with death in group art therapy with cancer patients. In D. Waller, & C. Sibbett (Eds.), *Art therapy and cancer care* (pp. 163–171). New York: Open University Press.

Luzzatto, P., & Gabriel, B. (2000). The creative journey: A model for short-term group art therapy with post-treatment cancer patients. *Art Therapy: Journal of the American Art Therapy Association, 17*(4), 265–269.

Luzzatto, P., Sereno, V., & Capps, R. (2003). A communication tool for cancer patients with pain: The art therapy technique of the body outline. *Palliative & Supportive Care, 1*(02), 135–142.

Malchiodi, C. (1999). Art therapy, arts medicine, and arts in healthcare: A vision for collaboration in the next millennium. *International Journal of Arts Medicine, 6*(2), 13–16.

Malchiodi, C. (2000). Medical art therapy: Contributions to the field of arts medicine. *International Journal of Arts Medicine, 2*(2), 28–31.

Nainis, N., Paice, J. A., Ratner, J., Wirth, J. H., Lai, J., & Shott, S. (2006). Relieving symptoms in cancer: Innovative use of art therapy. *Journal of Pain and Symptom Management, 31*(2), 162–169.

Parker-Bell, B. (1999). Embracing a future with computers and art therapy. *Art Therapy: Journal of the American Art Therapy Association, 16*(4), 180–185.

Stephen, J., Collie, K., McLeod, D., Rojubally, A., Fergus, K., Speca, M., Turner, J., Taylor-Brown, J., Sellick, S., Burrus, K., & Elramly, M. (2014). Talking with text: Communication in therapist-led, live chat cancer support groups. *Social Science & Medicine, 104,* 178–186.

Stephen, J., Rojubally, A., MacGregor, K., McLeod, D., Speca, M., Taylor–Brown, J., Fergus, K., Collie, K., Turner, J., Sellick, S., & Mackenzie, G. (2013). Evaluation of CancerChatCanada: A program of online support for Canadians affected by cancer. *Current Oncology, 20*(1), 39.

Waller, D. & Sibbett, C. (Eds.). (2008). *Art therapy and cancer care.* New York: Open University Press.

Weinberg, D. (1985). The potential of rehabilitative computer art therapy for the quadriplegic, cerebral vascular accident and brain trauma patient. *Art Therapy: Journal of the American Art Therapy Association, 2*(2), 66–73.

Wood, M. J., Molassiotis, A., & Payne, S. (2011). What research evidence is there for the use of art therapy in the management of symptoms in adults with cancer? A systematic review. *Psycho-Oncology, 20*(2), 135–145.

Zebrack, B., & Isaacson, S. (2012). Psychosocial care of adolescent and young adult patients with cancer and survivors. *Journal of Clinical Oncology, 30*(11), 1221–1226.

Zimmerman, J., Forlizzi, J., & Evenson, S. (2007, April). Research through design as a method for interaction design research in HCI. In *Proceedings of the SIGCHI conference on human factors in computing systems* (pp. 493–502). ACM.

Biographies

Sara Prins Hankinson, RCAT, graduated from Vancouver Art Therapy Institute in 2007, completing her thesis on art therapy within cancer care. In 2010, she began working for the BC Cancer Agency, primarily leading art therapy groups for families and for young adults with cancer, and researching online art therapy.

Brennan Jones, BSc, at the time of this writing, was an MSc student studying Computer Science and Human-Computer Interaction at the University of Calgary. Jones worked with Sara and Kate Collie to help develop procedures for online art therapy groups on CancerChatCanada. As part of his undergraduate thesis work, Jones worked with the Collies to design and to evaluate tools that could be used by online art therapy groups in the future (see Jones, Hankinson, Collie, & Tang, 2014).

Kate Collie, MA, MFA, PhD, is a registered psychologist and art therapist. At the time of this writing, this she was working in the Department of Psychosocial & Spiritual Resources at the Cross Cancer Institute and was also an assistant professor in the Department of Oncology at the University of Alberta in Edmonton. She began developing online art therapy in the late 1990s, at the University of British Columbia, in collaboration with members of their computer science department.

Chapter 4

USING TABLET TECHNOLOGY
AS A MEDIUM FOR ART THERAPY

Deborah Elkis-Abuhoff, Morgan Gaydos, and Robert Goldblatt

Introduction

Collaborative efforts in the field of medicine have strived to incorporate alternative treatment methods for practitioners in order to better address an individual's need for treatment as a whole. Complementary therapies, such as art therapy, have been shown to produce positive outcomes on quality of life, enhanced mind-body connections, and can provide a noninvasive approach to coping with a medical diagnosis and treatment interventions (Elkis-Abuhoff, Goldblatt, Gaydos, & Convery, 2013; Malchiodi & Goldring, 2013a; Warson, 2013). The application of art therapy has been found to assist in the decrease of not only somatic dysfunction, but also emotional distress in individuals with a medical diagnosis, specifically neurodegenerative disorders (Elkis-Abuhoff, Goldblatt, Gaydos, & Corrato, 2008). Bridging a patient's treatment experience with a non-invasive treatment approach, such as art therapy, can be adjunctive to standard medical procedures and can help physicians assess the psychological needs of an individual undergoing cancer treatment (Elkis-Abuhoff, Gaydos, Goldblatt, Chen, & Rose, 2009). As advancements in the field of art therapy continue to grow, adaptations through tablet technology can engage an individual undergoing treatment without compromising the restrictive, clean environment or the art therapy process.

Art Therapy and Technology

Art therapy within the medical population has been found to help patients cope with their length of treatment stay, physical symptoms, and psychological factors associated with their diagnosis (Malchiodi & Goldring, 2013). Therapeutic art making within medical settings has been found to promote insight relating to the overall experience of critical illness and its treatment (Elkis-Abuhoff, Goldblatt, Gaydos, & Corrato, 2008). Arnett and Malchiodi (2013) believe that art expression can help patients convey any symptoms or treatment experiences that they may not be able to verbalize directly. However, not all art materials are appropriate for specific medical settings where infection control policies and protocols are practiced. Due to the rise of art therapy in medical settings, researchers have explored a wider range of creative materials, most recently, including computer technology.

Within the past decade, researchers in the field of art therapy have begun to truly explore the application and benefits of technology with the creative process. Peterson, Stovall, Elkins, and Parker-Bell (2005) suggest that technology can enhance the art making process by offering a solution to the inability of utilizing art mediums in specific medical settings. Despite past approaches to art therapy, current trends suggest that technology can enhance the art therapy process by offering adaptations to a restricted environment (Peterson, Stovall, Elkins, & Parker-Bell, 2005). Pratt (2004) found that computer-based art therapy programs offered an appropriate means of self-expression to individuals who suffered traumatic brain injuries. Individuals were able to utilize the computer-based art therapy program to compensate for neurological and physical impairments resulting in an accident (Pratt, 2004).

More recently, the use of technology within art therapy has become slightly more mainstream due to the rise and the scope of technology as a whole. Art therapists have taken pride in exploring adaptive and cutting-edge techniques to not only engage an individual on multiple levels, but to do so with appropriate alternatives and safer materials, which are associated with technology (Peterson et al., 2005). Individuals with physical disabilities or with a limited range of motion/flexibility can have the opportunity to participate in an art therapy session through the use of an iPad by using slight movements with a finger on a touchpad that translate to magnified brush strokes or scribbles on the computer screen (Waller, 2014). Although some may argue that the elimination of art materials takes away from the art therapy process, creating art through the use of technology that can accommodate those with a limited range of motion or for those who are unable to contaminate their environment. For those undergoing chemotherapy, where all of these examples apply to their treatment process, individuals can not only directly engage in art therapy during their chemotherapy sessions, but can do so while maintaining a clean environment through the use of tablet technology.

The treatment environment can significantly influence multiple factors of infection; therefore, it is important that treatment centers require that sanitary conditions in patient care areas are maintained (Abreu, Tavares, Borges, Mergulhau, & Simoe, 2013). By incorporating art therapy and tablet technology, individuals can have their creative needs met while maintaining the clean environment necessary to carry out their treatment. Furthermore, technology-based adaptations can be seen and greatly utilized within a chemotherapy session where an individual has limited movement due to being connected to the chemotherapy machine and to the monitoring system.

Exploring Tablet Technology with Adults Diagnosed with Colon Cancer

Colon cancer ranks as the top third cause of cancer deaths in both males and females worldwide (Ferlay et al., 2015). Colon cancer, along with that of rectal cancer, is currently the number two cause of cancer deaths in males, following that of prostate cancer, and is the number third cause of cancer death in females, following that of breast and uterine cancer, within the United States. As of 2014, these statistics suggest that an estimated 1.2 million people, both men and women, will be living with a diagnosis of colon cancer (DeSantis et al., 2014). Colon cancer is typically diagnosed to those over the age of 50, but as seen in other forms of cancer, the onset can occur at a younger age. Although survival rates for colon cancer vary depending on the stage of diagnosis and on the severity of the affected area, colon cancer continues to be a leading cause of death among other cancers (Ferlay et al., 2015).

It is believed that the most common development of colon cancer is caused by the adenoma-carcinoma sequence (Matsumoto et al., 2011). This process occurs when carcinoma develops from an adenomatous polyp. Due to their ability to mutate, these polyps are more likely to become cancerous and form a tumor (Matsumoto et al., 2011). Although researchers have been striving to investigate molecular markers and gene expression profiles present in colon cancer, it is still difficult to determine if this type of cancer can be predicted (Marisa et al., 2013). Risk factors for the development of colon cancer include genetic history, obesity, having a sedentary nature, and diabetes (American Cancer Society, 2015).

As colon cancer progresses into an advanced stage, physical symptoms can include rectal bleeding, bloody stool, cramping in the lower abdomen, and symptoms associated with anemia, such as weakness and fatigue due to blood loss (American Cancer Society, 2015). Physical symptomology can greatly vary patient to patient, with the most common symptom being rectal and gestational tract bleeding (Hreinsson, Jonasson, & Bjornsson, 2014). As seen within other forms of cancer, psychological symptoms can also be present within a diagnosis of colon cancer; Anxiety, depression, and feelings of distress are commonly reported by patients undergoing treatment for colon cancer (Shun et al., 2014). Alongside coping with the initial diagnosis, undergoing invasive and time-consuming treatment protocols, even with a prospectively positive prognosis, can be emotionally overwhelming and physically exhausting.

The most common treatments for colon cancer are surgery, chemotherapy, and radiation. It has been suggested that individuals who receive chemotherapy post-surgery are more likely to survive colon cancer (American Cancer Society, 2014). Chemotherapy and surgical procedures for those diagnosed with stage III of colon cancer have an increased survival rate and can lead to curative results before the cancer reaches a stage IV diagnosis (ACS, 2014). Chemotherapy treatment for colon cancer, although recommended, has been found to impact an individual's quality of life and can lead to overall physical and mental deterioration (Graca, Figueiredo, & Fincham, 2012). Due to the invasive nature of chemotherapy, patients undergoing colon cancer treatment are likely to experience feelings of depression and anxiety due to the unknown outcomes of treatment (Graca, Figueiredo, & Fincham, 2012). Treatment methods including surgery and chemotherapy have been found to affect the physical well-being of an individual through invasive measures that are likely to cause physical discomfort (Elkis-Abuhoff et al., 2009). The application of art therapy, through the use of tablet technology, can be applied while also maintaining the clean environment that is essential during the chemotherapy process. Through the use of tablet technology, art therapy can be brought into a space that has previously been restricted to any and all outside materials, and can assist in the overall medical and emotional evaluation of the individual. The therapeutic application of tablet technology, as a catalyst for therapeutic art expression for those diagnosed with colon cancer, can allow an art therapist to work alongside medical clinicians to assess a patient, in real-time, without disrupting their chemotherapy treatment session.

Therapeutic Applications of Tablet Technology within a Chemotherapy Setting

As just illustrated, the use of tablet technology as a therapeutic art intervention has great potential with an ill patient who requires the maintenance of a clean environment to create. One area for adults, where tablet technology could help to support patients during their treatment, is with those receiving chemotherapy. The work currently being completed by Elkis-Abuhoff, Goldblatt, Gaydos, & Convery (2013a) brought tablet technology directly into the chemotherapy room. This ongoing study focuses on adults receiving chemotherapy for a diagnosis of colon cancer. The protocol consists of 8–12 treatment cycles, one cycle every 2 weeks, which theoretically becomes a 16-24 week study. However, consideration is taken for any possible delays due to toxicities requiring drug delivery delays and illnesses such as colds or flu that would then extend the study period beyond the 24 weeks. Participants for this research study are being recruited through the cancer center at a major metropolitan health care system in the Northeast.

This study utilizes a specific method of recruitment, referred to as a Modified Zelen Design, to recruit patients and to select the experimental and control groups. A Modified Zelen Design is applied when patients undergoing the study wish to receive their preferred method of treatment as opposed to the alternative treatment asked by the research team (Torgerson & Roland, 1998). This design has been proposed to "encourage physicians to participate in random trials because it would help to overcome the difficulties that health professionals can experience in explaining equipoise, and reduce the discomfort for both clinician and patient in acknowledging uncertainty" (Campbell, Peters, Grant, Quilty, & Dieppe, 2005, p. 2). A Modified Zelen Design was suggested because clinicians can often feel reluctant to participate in randomized clinical trials due to the notion that the physician-patient relationship can be compromised if the patient realizes his or her inability to select a preferred method of treatment (Zelen, 1990). By incorporating a Modified Zelen Design in this study, the research team is able to offer an alternative treatment to the experimental group while also providing patients in the comparison group with their preferred method of treatment with including only the addition of the assessments. This eliminates the placebo effect within the control group, which has been notoriously found to be a concern in research regarding medical treatment (Zelen, 1990). This research study has received IRB approval from the health care system where the protocol is being administered, as well as from two universities.

The materials in this study include a tablet, stylus brush, demographic sheet, the Perceived Stress Scale (PSS-4), the Functional Assessment of Cancer Therapy (FACT-C), and a self-report questionnaire to assess the quality of life for patients diagnosed with colon cancer. Three art applications are downloaded onto the tablet for easy access, along with a video tutorial for each to help the participant engage in their app of choice with ease and with understanding. The self-report questionnaire will be based off of the PSS-4 and off the FACT-C assessments, which has been standardized for use with adult cancer patients.

To ensure the application of the Modified Zelen Design, two phases are being used for this research study. For Phase 1, participants are recruited, informed of the assessments, and are asked to fill out the initial consent form which grants permission to be a part of the Phase I of the 8–12 cycle research study. After the initial informed consent, all of the patients are equally randomized (25/25) into two groups: the control group and the experimental group. For those randomized into the control group, participants will follow the PSS-4 and FACT-C assessment schedule while undergoing their chemotherapy treatment. Those randomized into the experimental group will have the opportunity to enter into the Phase II component of the study. Those who agree to enter the Phase II component will receive additional information on the art therapy component of this research, the opportunity to engage in tablet technology while undergoing their prescribed chemotherapy treatment, and a second informed consent granting permission to enroll in this protocol is secured. If the patient declines the second informed consent and does not wish to participate in the experimental group, he or she becomes a participant in the comparison group where they will receive only the assessments and their standard chemotherapy treatment.

Participants in the experimental group are supplied with tablets that contained three graphic/design application. The first application is similar to a Japanese ink brush, creating a very relaxing and Zen-like engagement. This app is nonthreatening and inviting for anyone, especially those who who become anxious when asked to create art. The second application is similar to an art studio, with the ability to create in different types of media, from pencil to watercolor, to airbrush, to oil pastels, and to oil paints. The app allows for color blending and smudging among other fine art techniques. Finally, the third application mimics the 3D medium of clay; this medium was based on the work of Elkis-Abuhoff, Goldblatt, Gaydos, and Convery (2013) which focused on patients diagnosed with Parkinson's Disease. Although it is a 2D electronic format, this app allows for pushing and pulling a clay shape and results in a 3D image that can be rotated to see all sides and surfaces of the clay creation.

The following is the layout for the 12-cycle research protocol (see Table 1):

Table 1
12-CYCLE CHEMOTHERAPY PROTOCOL

Cycle 1	Demographic information, pre-assessments (PSS-4 and FACT-C), and orientation to the tablet technology
Cycle 2	Tablet engagement and post-assessments (PSS-4 and FACT-C)
Cycle 3	Tablet engagement
Cycle 4	Pre-assessments (PSS-4 and FACT-C), tablet engagement, and post-assessments (PSS-4 and FACT-C)
Cycle 5, 6, 7	Tablet engagement
Cycle 8	Pre-assessments (PSS-4 and FACT-C), tablet engagement, and post-assessments (PSS-4 and FACT-C)
Cycle 9, 10, 11	Tablet engagement
Cycle 12	Pre-assessments (PSS-4 and FACT-C), tablet engagement, post-assessand ments (PSS-4 and FACT-C) with exit information

Throughout the data collection period, participants are asked to save at least one piece of artwork per session and to give it a title for collection by the researchers. If there is a specific piece of artwork that the participant would like to keep, the researcher will directly email it to them. All collected artwork will be evaluated within 24 hours of submission by one of the licensed research team members for any significant distress (i.e., suicidal ideation). Although this has not been an issue, if there is any indication of risk, the researchers would immediately contact the treatment team at the cancer center so that the patient can be further evaluated for emotional state and risk factors. The following is a case example of an adult patient's experience with the table technology.

Case Illustration 1: Adults Receiving Chemotherapy

Kaleena is a 46-year-old Native American female, diagnosed with Stage III colon cancer. She is married and is a mother of 19-year-old and 16-year-old daughters. Kaleena disclosed that although her marriage "wasn't always the most loving," her husband and daughters have been very supportive and encouraging of her treatments, taking on many responsibilities that were hers before her illness. She has two older brothers and both of her parents are healthy, living in Minnesota. There has been no family history of any type of cancer and she has been healthy until her recent diagnosis. Additionally, Kaleena has an MBA in accounting from a large midwestern university, and is currently on sick leave from her job as an accountant at a large medical supply company, for which she has worked for the past eleven years. She has lived in the Northeast since being recruited for the job at the medical supply company and says she and her family enjoy the Northeast and its proximity to the "big cities and the ocean." Kaleena describes her social life as "average" with friends, family, and coworkers. Her hobbies include baking, gardening, and "shopping."

Kaleena was diagnosed with colon cancer four months before starting her chemotherapy treatment. When discussing her decision to undergo chemotherapy, she appeared very anxious about her diagnosis and about the treatment methods that would follow. She understood her prognosis to be "guarded" and realized that the treatments were her best option at the present time. Kaleena stated that she has "good days," where she described herself as positive and strong, and "bad days," where she described herself as feeling negative and depressed.

When Kaleena arrived for her initial chemotherapy intake session, she was accompanied by her husband and by her two daughters. She appeared subdued and quiet, and allowed her husband to speak to the receptionists and to the intake nurses. As is standard in this cancer center, each patient is set up in a private cubicle that contains a recliner chair, a small table, and possibly one additional chair for the person who may accompany them. After initially being quiet, she began to appear more open to answering questions directly without the help of her husband. Upon filling out medical forms, which took about twenty minutes. The research team introduced themselves and asked if she would like to be a part of the study. After some thought and discussion with her family, Kaleena agreed to participate.

Kaleena was provided with the initial consent form and the research protocol, as described in the methods section, began. She was randomized into the experimental group and was invited to enter the tablet technology component of the study. Kaleena agreed and was consented into Phase II. Her husband and daughters left for lunch and informed Kaleena that they would be back in three hours when she finished her chemotherapy for the day. While she was being prepared for her chemotherapy by the nurses, the research team provided Kaleena with instructions about the tablet and about the art therapy programs available at her disposal. During this period, she stated that she was "pleased to be distracted from what was going on." Kaleena engaged in conversation with the researchers and with the nurses and was extremely cooperative throughout. She was then given the instructions and assessment forms, including the demographic, FACT-C, and PSS-4 to fill out before engaging in the tablet artwork.

When Kaleena was given the tablet to produce her first drawing, she immediately smiled and said that this experience was "fun." She started using the drawing and painting application, experimented with the stylus brush, and explored how the medium responded. After about ten minutes, Kaleena asked if she could erase her doodle and start over. After reassuring her that she could, she said, "I know what I am going to draw." It was at that point that she seemed to focus and was able to work steadily for about twenty-five minutes. Kaleena didn't speak much while engaging in her creation, but appeared to be enjoying the art experience. When she completed her artwork, Kaleena looked up at the researcher and looked for reassurance that she did it "right" by asking the researcher if her art (see Fig. 1) looked like "a sunrise or a sunset."

During Kaleena's final cycle of chemotherapy, she produced her final piece of artwork utilizing the Japanese brush-painting application (see Fig. 3). She was very pleased to be finished with her chemotherapy regimen and her oncologist indicated to her that her treatment seemed to be effective. Kaleena produced smooth and fluid brushstrokes, showing a growing and forward-leaning flower, which may indicate the forward direction where she feels she is heading. Additionally, the ground appears uneven at the start and moves toward a smoother surface.

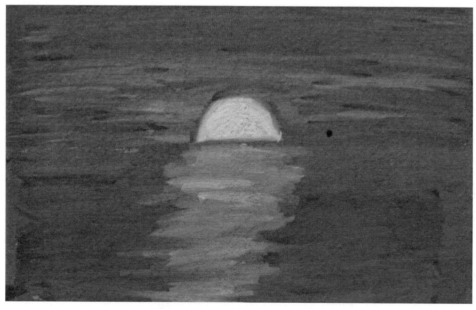

Figure 1. Kaleena's tablet drawing.

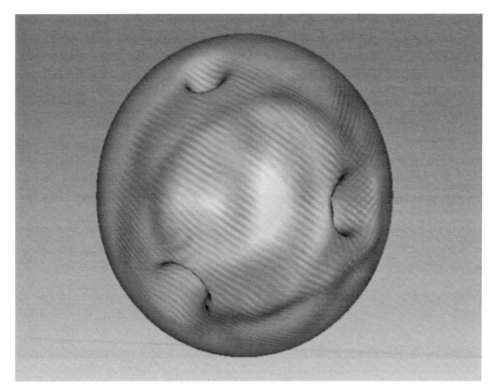

Figure 2. Kaleena's exploration with the clay manipulation app.

Kaleena completed her 12-week cycle of chemotherapy and her work on the tablet. She was asked to complete her final assessments (FACT-C and PSS-4). During the debriefing, she was eager to convey that she was aware of the serious nature of her illness and the promise of the potential of her medical treatment. She smiled and said that the drawing will be a "sunrise on her future" if the medicine and the treatment remain effective. Additionally, Kaleena then became teary, somber, and could not speak. After somewhat regaining her composure, she explained that "it will be a sunset if the treatment doesn't work." She talked about the chemotherapy experience as "scary" and talked about the tablet work as a "good distractor." At that point, she realized that her chemotherapy regimen for the day was almost done and she was looking forward to seeing her family and going home.

As illustrated in this case illustration, utilizing tablet technology as way to provide art therapy in medically restricted environments, holds great benefits to adults receiving chemotherapy treatment for cancer. Considering the advancements, applications, and potential for tablet technology, children receiving medical treatments within restricted environments could also greatly

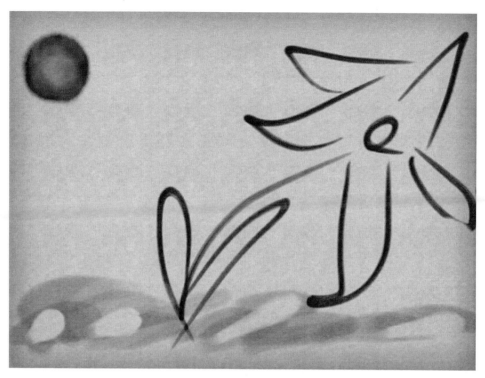

Figure 3. Kaleena's Japanese brush painting on the tablet.

benefit from an art therapy experience through tablet engagement. Children receiving blood transfusions, specifically through an outpatient clinic, can engage in the art therapy process utilizing a tablet during their treatment session.

Exploring Tablet Technology with Children Receiving Blood Transfusions

Blood transfusions have been described by physicians as one the greatest contributions to modern medicine (Istaphanous, Wheeler, Lisco, & Shander, 2011). Although blood transfusions have historically been associated with a number of risk factors and complications, advancements in procedures, techniques, and overall treatment have benefited the lives of many individuals and decreased chances of mortality (Shander, Gross, Hill, Javidroozi, & Sledge, 2013). Blood transfusions are a relatively simple procedure, which provides a patient with either a whole blood mixture or a specific type of blood cell, such as red, white, platelets, or plasma, intravenously (Shander et al., 2013).

Medical conditions that require blood transfusions include, but are not limited to, anemia, sickle cell disease, loss of blood from an accident or surgery, and an individual's ability to produce an adequate amount of blood cells (Hulbert et al., 2011; Ware et al., 2011). The most well-known type of transfusion is that of red blood cells; approximately half of all critically ill patients, including children, admitted into a medical setting for more than 48 hours, will be administered a red blood transfusion (Karam et al., 2010).

Although blood transfusions have been found to be favorable in treating children with medical diagnosis, infectious and noninfectious complications still exist and can lead to prolonged medical admissions (Istaphanous, Wheeler, Lisco, & Shander, 2011). Risks can include transmitted infections, further medical complications such as acute lung injury and a compromised immune system, and pain which can bring about psychological symptoms such as anxiety and emotional distress (Hassan, Winters, Wintenhalter, Reischman, & El-Borai, 2010; Landier & Tse, 2010). Anxiety disorders, including stress, are considered one of the most common psychiatric diagnoses in children and in adolescents experiencing chronic medical illness (Pao & Bosk, 2011). Recently, clinicians addressed the need for quality of life measures with medically ill children as a subjective means of reflecting present lifestyle, past experience with diagnosis and treatment, hopes for the future, and life ambitions (Klaassen et al., 2013). Multimodal approaches, such as outpatient treatment, offer a variety of medical resources, specialized therapies, and continued support for children with medical diagnoses (Hechler et al., 2011). Rao, Nainis, Williams, Langner, Eisen, & Paice (2009) states that individuals undergoing medical procedures often seek alternative treatment methods, besides pharmacology, to help relieve symptoms and to distract from treatment protocols.

Collaborative efforts in the field of medicine can help incorporate alternative treatment methods, such as therapeutic art, to help medically ill children cope with not only their length of treatment stay, but also with physical and psychological symptoms associated with their diagnosis (Malchiodi & Goldring, 2013). Therapeutic art making within medical settings has been found to promote insight relating to the overall experience of critical illness and of its treatment (Elkis-Abuhoff, Goldblatt, Gaydos, & Corratun, 2008). Arnett and Malchiodi (2013) believe that art expression can help medically ill children convey any symptoms or treatment experiences that they may not be able to verbalize directly. Children receiving lengthy treatment protocols within an outpatient setting can utilize therapeutic art as healthy stimuli to not only distract from the overall treatment, but also gain a sense of tolerance to the treatment experience (Madden, Mowry, Gao, Cullen, & Foreman, 2010).

Therapeutic art making includes a wide range of creative materials, including that of tablet technology. The treatment environment in medical settings can significantly influence multiple factors of infection, a known risk with blood transfusions, and requires sanitary conditions within patient care areas to be maintained (Easa, Abdou, Mahmoud, & El-Meseiry, 2008). Peterson, Stovall, Elkins, and Parker-Bell (2005) suggest that technology can enhance the art-making process by offering a solution to the inability of utilizing art mediums in specific medical settings. Young individuals are also more likely to welcome technology as a means to engage in art therapy because it has been present in the world around them (Waller, 2014). A child's mind also allows for easy exploration; a child is more likely to become excited, curious, and creative when navigating tablet technology compared to an older individual. Children also have a natural tendency to want to engage in an activity when sitting still; for those undergoing routine and scheduled medical procedures, where they have limited mobility and access to outside materials, incorporating tablet technology can therapeutically engage on multiple therapeutic levels. By incorporating art therapy and tablet technology, medically ill children receiving blood transfusions can have their creative needs met while maintaining the clean environment necessary to carry out the treatment protocol.

Ilkis-Abuhoff, Goldblatt, Gaydos, Corvery, Gleason, & C'Olmiploi (2014) has been involved in bringing art therapy through tablet technology to children receiving blood transfusions. Children in this study are receiving transfusions on an outpatient basis, most diagnosed with sickle cell, and receiving transfusions on a regular basis. All of the children in this study are being recruited through the children's hospital within a metropolitan health care system.

Therapeutic Applications of Tablet Technology within an Outpatient Medical Setting

This research study utilizes a pre-post design and participants are assigned to either the experimental or the control group based on their day of treatment. After consent and assent, participants in the experimental group receive information and the opportunity to be included in the therapeutic art component of the project. The art component includes the tablet experience, along with their standard transfusion treatment, and a pre- and post-assessment to evaluate their perceived stress, hope, and a pain scales (Elkis-Abuhoff et al., 2014). For this project, two applications have been chosen due to being child-geared and friendly and are available to participants. One application mimics finger paint and the participant can fully engage in the medium without the mess typically involved in painting. The second application allows for drawing and painting, slightly similar to the application used with adults with colon cancer, with a basic and vibrant presentation that is appropriate for children. A child-participant also has access to the stylus brush for painting with the tablet. The control group within this research study only completes the pre- and post-assessments along with their standard blood transfusion protocol.

At the end of each treatment session, participants in the experimental group are asked to save at least one piece of artwork created during that session and to give it a title for collection by the researchers. Once again, if there is a specific piece of artwork that the participant would like to keep, the researcher will email them the chosen image when they leave the treatment session.

All collected artwork and assessments will be evaluated within 24 hours of submission by one of the New York State- licensed research team members for any significant emotional distress (i.e., extreme depression or anxiety). If there is any indication of risk, the researchers will immediately contact the child's treatment team. In addition, the pain-rating scale will be evaluated at time of collection and outcomes that score high will be reported to the physician on record and on the registered nurse (RN).

Case Illustration 2: Blood Transfusions with Children

Harrison is a 10-year-old, African American male diagnosed with Sickle Cell anemia. He is in the 5th grade and comes from a low-income family, with a household income of less than $24,000 a year. Harrison receives blood transfusions on a regular basis and has had more than 10 blood transfusions before the commencement of the research protocol. As the treatment team prepared him for the transfusion, Harrison appeared anxious and very restless. Harrison was approached by the researcher and asked if he would be interested in participating in this one session research experience. After the protocol was explained to him and to his mother, they both eagerly agreed. Consent and assent were secured prior to issuing him the tablet. Once the tablet was available to him, the researcher reviewed the two apps and gave him full access to the tablet and stylus brush.

During Harrison's blood transfusion regimen, he produced two pieces of artwork. His first piece of artwork was completed immediately after his transfusion started (see Fig. 4). Harrison created the artwork with the finger paint application and as he finished it, he appeared to be immediately calmed down. It is interesting to notice that the artwork may represent Harrison's experience with the transfusion. For example, if the red area represents the blood vein, and the purple area the sickle cell, the green area could be interpreted as representing the transfusion addressing the illness.

After his blood transfusion was completed, Harrison appeared stronger and eager to leave the treatment area. He completed the second artwork from the drawing application showing an image of a boy with a smile on his face surrounded by a background of deep red (see Fig. 5). This could represent the healthy blood that Harrison just received. The strong stance of the boy in the image may indicate the renewed energy that the healthy blood provided. The object that appears to be a weapon in his left hand may further indicate power and strength.

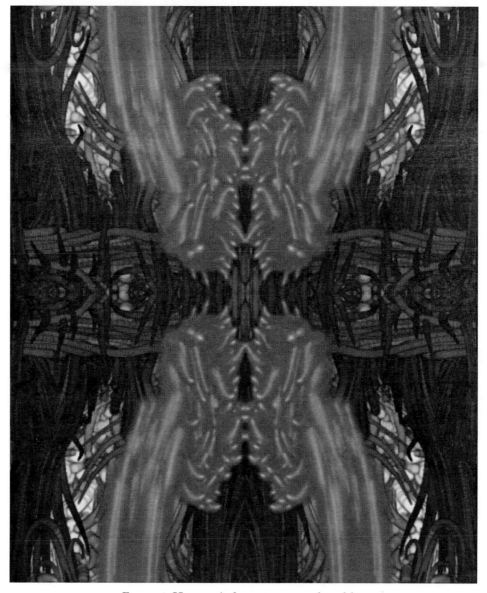

Figure 4. Harrison's finger paint on the tablet.

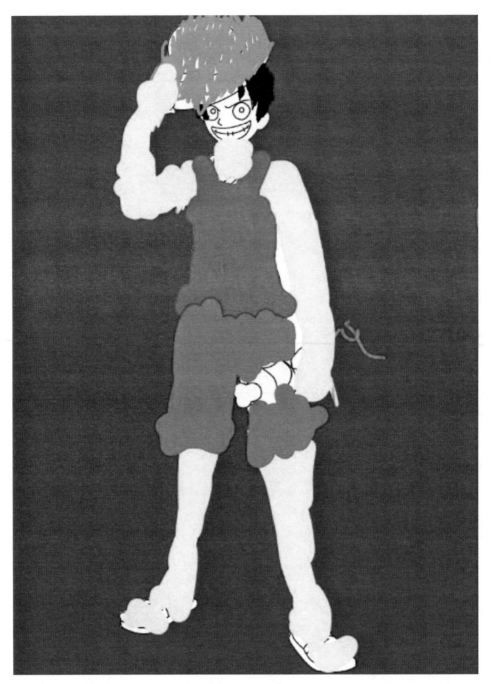

Figure 5. Harrison's artwork created on the drawing tablet.

Discussion and Conclusion

The application of tablet technology has supported the use of art therapy with medically ill adults and children. In many facilities, art therapy is extremely limited by an organization's requirements to limit art materials that can be brought into a treatment room. These case illustrations depict how art therapy can be incorporated into medical facilities and to designated treatment areas, even under the restrictions of a limited clean environment. This allows the patient to engage in a creative manner with the ability to express himself in a nonverbal manner, and even to serve as a distraction from the stressful treatment experience. The use of the tablet, along with the available art applications, could allow the patients to virtually experience an array of art media. As the patient becomes engaged, it is not uncommon to see him or her dip their brush in the virtual color, but dab it on the side as one would do in real life when painting. Another example is watching a patient create with virtual oil pastels and to see them smudge the colors on the tablet, then switch to another finger so that the two colors do not mix, as someone would do when engaging in oil pastels. However, no paint will drip and no oil residue will linger on their fingers, so that their hands are kept clean when using the tablet.

Moving forward, the use of tablet technology allows for the continued expansion of art therapy in various settings and with populations that have been difficult to directly engage in the past. The virtual engagement in different, more advanced media, although not the actual art medium, could still give the artist a close facsimile of the feel and properties of the material. In addition, it allows the patient to express himself or herself in a nonverbal manner in a place where words may not be easily available.

REFERENCES

Abreu, A. C., Tavares, R. R., Borges, A., Mergulhao, F., & Simoes, M. (2013). Current and emergent strategies for disinfection of hospital environments. *Journal of Antimicrobial Chemotherapy, 68*(12), 2718–2732.

American Cancer Society. (2014). *Colorectal Cancer Facts and Figures 2014–2016.* Atlanta: American Cancer Society, Inc.

American Cancer Society. (2015). *Cancer Facts & Figures 2015.* Atlanta: American Cancer Society, Inc.

Arnett, M. C., & Malchiodi, C. A. (2013). Understanding children's drawings in medical settings. In C. A. Malchiodi (Ed.), *Art therapy and health care* (pp. 33–47). New York: The Guilford Press.

Campbell, R., Peters, T., Grant, C., Quilty, B., & Pieppe, P. (2005). Adapting the randomized consent (Zelen) design for trials of behavioural interventions for chronic disease: A feasibility study. *Journal of Health Services Research & Policy,* *10*(4), 220–225.

DeSantis, C. E., Lin, C. C., Mariotto, A. B., Siegel, R. L., Stein, K. D., Kramer, J. L., Alteri, R., Robbins, A. S., & Jemal, A. (2014). Cancer treatment and survivorship statistics, 2014. *CA: A Cancer Journal for Clinicians, 64*(4), 252–271.

Easa, B. A. Y. A., Abdou, M. H. M., Mahmoud, A. H., & El-Meseiry, M. A. (2008). Environmental assessment of Alexandria Medical Research Institute. *Journal of King Abdulaziz University, Meteorology, Environment and Arid Land Agriculture Sciences, 20,*1, 83–103.

Elkis-Abuhoff, D., Gaydos, M., Goldblatt, R., Chen, M., & Rose, S. (2009). Mandala drawings as an assessment tool for women with breast cancer. *The Arts in Psychotherapy, 36*(4), 231–238.

Elkis-Abuhoff, D. L., Goldblatt, R. B., Gaydos, M., & Convery, C. (2013). A pilot study to determine the psychological effects of manipulation of therapeutic art forms among patients with Parkinson's disease. *International Journal of Art Therapy, 18*(3), 113–121.

Elkis-Abuhoff, D. L., Goldblatt, R. B., Gaydos, M., & Convery, C. (2013a). *A pilot study to examine the effects of art therapy during chemotherapy on stress and quality of life in patients with stage 3 colon cancer.* Research presented at the The Culture Health and Wellness International Conference, Bristol, UK.

Elkis-Abuhoff, D., Goldblatt, R., Gaydos, M., & Corrato, S. (2008). The effects of clay manipulation on somatic dysfunction and emotional distress in patients with Parkinson's disease. *Art Therapy: The Journal of the American Art Therapy Association, 25*(3), 122–128.

Elkis-Abuhoff, D. L., Goldblatt, R. B., Gaydos, M., Convery, C., Gleason, K., & D'Olmipio, J. (2014). *Pilot study to examine the effects of art therapy during chemotherapy on stress and quality of life in patients with colon cancer.* Research presented at the 45th American Art Therapy Association Annual Conference, San Antonio.

Ferlay, J., Soerjomataram, I., Dikshit, R., Eser, S., Mathers, C., Rebelo, M., Parkin, D. M., Forman, D., & Bray, F. (2015). Cancer incidence and mortality worldwide: Sources, methods and major patterns in GLOBOCAN 2012. *International Journal of Cancer, 136*(5), E359–E386.

Graca, M., Figueiredo, A. P., & Fincham, F. D. (2012). Anxiety, depression, traumatic stress and quality of life in colorectal cancer after different treatments: A study with Portuguese patients and their partners. *European Journal of Oncology Nursing,* 1–6.

Hassan, N. E., Winters, J., Winterhalter, K., Reischman, D., & El-Borai, Y. (2010). Effects of blood conservation on the incidence of anemia and transfusions in pediatric parapneumonic effusion: A hospital perspective. *Journal of Hospital Medicine, 5*(7), 410–413.

Hechler, T., Martin, A., Blankenburg, M., Schroeder, S., Kosfelder, Hoscher, L., Denecke, H., & Zernikow, B. (2011). Specialized multimodal outpatient treatment for children with chronic pain: Treatment pathways and long-term outcome. *European Journal of Pain, 15,* 976–984.

Hreinsson, J. P., Jonasson, J. G., & Bjornsson, E. S. (2014). Bleeding-related symptoms in colorectal cancer: A 4-year nationwide population-based study. *Alimentary Pharmacology and Therapeutics, 39*(1), 77–84.

Hulbert, M. L., McKinstry, R. C., Lacey, J. L., Moran, C. J., Panepinto, J. A., Thompson, A. A., Sanaik, S. S., Woods, G. M., Casella, J. F., Inusa, B., Howard, J., Kirkham, F. J., Anie, K. A., Mullin, J. E., Ichord, R., Noetzel, M., Yan, Y., Rodeghier, M., & DeBaun, M. R. (2011). Silent cerebral infarcts occur despite regular blood transfusion therapy after first strokes in children with Sickle Cell Disease. *Blood, 117*(3), 772–779.

Istaphanous, G. K., Wheeler, D. S., Lisco, S. J., & Shander, A. (2011). Red blood cell transfusion in critically ill children: A narrative review. *Pediatric Critical Care Medicine, 12*(2), 174–183.

Karam, O., Tucci, M., Bateman, S. T., Ducruet, T., Spinella, P. C., Randolph, A. G., & Lacroix, J. (2010). Research association between length of storage of red blood cell units and outcome of critically ill children: A prospective observational study. *Blood, 15,* 18.

Klaassen, R. J., Alibhai, S., Allen, M. K., Moreau, K., Pulcini, M. M., Forgie, M., Blanchette, V., Buckstein, R., Odame, I., Quirt, I., Yee, K., Rieger, D. W., & Young, N. L. (2013). Introducing the Tran Qol: A new disease-specific quality of life measure for children and adults with Thalassemia Major. *Journal of Blood Disorders & Transfusion, 4*(4), 1–5.

Landier, W., & Tse, A. M. (2010). Use of complimentary and alternative medical interventions for the management of procedure-related pain, anxiety, and distress in pediatric oncology: An integrative review. *Journal of Pediatric Nursing, 25,* 566–579.

Madden, J. R., Mowry, P., Gao, D., Cullen, P. M., & Foreman, N. K. (2010). Creative arts therapy improves quality of life for pediatric brain tumor patients receiving outpatient chemotherapy. *Journal of Pediatric Oncology Nursing, 27*(3), 133–145.

Malchiodi, C. A., & Goldring, E. (2013). Art therapy and child life: An integrated approach to psychosocial care with pediatric oncology patients. In C. A. Malchiodi (Ed.), *Art therapy and health care* (pp. 33–47). New York: The Guilford Press.

Marisa, L., de Reyniès, A., Duval, A., Selves, J., Gaub, M. P., Vescovo, L., Etienne-Grimaldi, M.C., Schiappa, R., Guenot, D., Ayadi, M., Kirzin, S., Chazal, M., Fle?jou, J-F., Benchimol, D., Berger1, A., Lagarde, A., Pencreach, E., Piard, F., Elias, D., Parc, Y., Olschwang, S., Milano, G., Laurent-Puig, P., & Boige, V. (2013). Gene expression classification of colon cancer into molecular subtypes: Characterization, validation, and prognostic value. *PLoS Medicine, 10*(5), e1001453.

Matsumoto, M., Nakajimi, T., Kato, K., Kouno, T., Sakamoto, T., Matsuda, T., Kushima, R., & Saito, Y. (2011). Small invasive colon cancer with systemic metastasis: A case report. *BMC Gastroenterology, 11*(59), 1–8.

Parker-Bell, B. (2005). Art therapists and computer technology. *Art Therapy: Journal of the American Art Therapy Association, 22*(3), 139–149.

Peterson, B. C., Stovall, K., Elkins, D. E., & Parker-Bell, B. (2005). Art therapists and computer technology. *Art Therapy: Journal of the American Art Therapy Association, 22*(3), 139–149.

Peterson, B. C., Stovall K., Elkins, D. E, & Pao, M., & Bosk, A. (2011). Anxiety in medically ill children/adolescents. *Depression and Anxiety, 28*(1), 40–49.

Pratt, R. R. (2004). Art, dance, and music therapy. *Physical Medicine and Rehabilitation Clinics of North America, 15,* 827–841.

Rao, D., Nainis, N., Williams, L., Langner, D., Eisin, A., & Paice, J. (2009). Art therapy for relief of symptoms associated with HIV/AIDS. *AIDS Care, 21*(1), 64–69.

Sanoff, H. K., Carpenter, W. R., Sturmer, T., Goldberg, R. M., Martin, C. F., Fine, J. P., McCleary, N. J., Meyerhardt, J. A., Niland, J., Kahn, K. L., Schymura, M. J., & Schrag, D. (2012). Effect of adjuvant chemotherapy on survival of patients with stage III colon cancer diagnosed after age 75 years. *Journal of Clinical Oncology,* 1–15.

Shander, A., Gross, I., Hill, S., Javidroozi, M., & Sledge, S. (2013). A new perspective on best transfusion practices. *Blood Transfusion, 2,* 193–202.

Shun, S. C., Yeh, K. H., Liang, J. T., Huang, J., Chen, S. C., Lin, B. R., Lee, P-S., & Lai, Y. H. (2014). Unmet supportive care needs of patients with colorectal cancer: Significant differences by Type D personality. *Oncology Nursing Forum, 41*(1), E3–E11.

Torgerson, D. J., & Roland, M. (1998). What is Zelen's design? *British Medical Journal, 316*(7131), 606–608.

Ware, R. E., Schultz, W. H., Yovetich, N., Mortier, N. A., Alvarez, O., Hilliard, L., Iyer, R. V., Miller, S. T., Rogers, Z. R., Scott, J. P., Waclawiw, M., & Helms, R. W. (2011). Stroke with transfusions changing to hydroxyurea (SWiTCH): A phase III randomized clinical trial for treatment of children with sickle cell anemia, stroke, and iron overload. *Pediatric Blood & Cancer, 57*(6), 1011–1017.

Waller, D. (2014). *Group interactive art therapy: Its use in training and treatment.* New York: Routledge.

Warson, E. (2013). Healing across cultures: Arts in healthcare with Native American Indians and Alaska native cancer survivors. In C. A. Malchiodi (Ed.), *Art therapy and health care* (pp. 162–183). New York: Guilford Press.

Zelen, M. (1990). Randomized consent designs for clinical trials: An update. *Statistics in Medicine, 9,* 645–656.

Biographies

Deborah Elkis-Abuhoff, PhD, LCAT, ATR-BC, ATCS, BCPC is an associate professor teaching in the Creative Arts Therapy program at Hofstra University. She holds both Creative Arts Therapy and Psychology licenses in New York State, is a registered and board certified art therapist, is an art therapist certified supervisor, and a board certified professional counselor. She also holds her teacher certification in Art Education (K-12). Her research interests bring together behavioral medicine and creative/medical art therapy and neuroscience. Her recent research projects connect art therapy with those diagnosed with Parkinson's disease, those with cancer, and connecting the creative process to neurological response. She and her research team have published in peer-reviewed journals, and have presented to national and international audiences. Dr. Elkis-Abuhoff's diverse experiences include medical geriatric, psychiatric, child, adolescent, and family populations. She holds an appointment to the North Shore/Long Island Jewish Health System's, Feinstein Institute for Medical Research as an assistant investigator in the Center for Neuroscience. She holds memberships in the American Art Therapy Association (AATA), the New York Art Therapy Association (NYATA), the American Psychological Association, the American Psychotherapy Association, and Arts in Health South West, UK. She is active in the community and serves as a member of Hofstra University's Faculty Affairs Committee, is the School of Health Professions and Human Services Institutional Review Board (IRB) representative for Hofstra University and a member of the Interdisciplinary Research Committee for her school. She also sits on the Research Committee for the American Art Therapy Association, and as an editorial board reviewer for *Art Therapy: Journal of the American Art Therapy Association.*

Morgan Gaydos, LCAT, ATR-BC, is a registered and board certified art therapist in New York State. She currently practices art therapy within a forensic psychiatry unit in a hospital setting. Her work experience also includes art therapy with clinical psychology, inpatient/detoxification chemical dependency programs and children diagnosed within the autism spectrum. Gaydos's past and current research efforts, as a member of an interdisciplinary research team, focus on art therapy with Parkinson's Disease, neuroscience and cancer. She has been an active contributor to both international and national journal publications, book chapters within the field of art therapy in collaboration with neuroscience and education, as well as national conference presentations pertaining to mental health, medicine, and art therapy.

Robert Goldblatt, PhD has taught in the medical school and in the school of health professions at the New York Institute of Technology. He received his doctorate at the University of Connecticut and is a licensed psychologist in the State of New York. He has served as the chair of the behavioral sciences department and at the medical school, was affiliated with the Department of Psychiatry, and taught the course entitled, Behavioral Medicine. As a clinical psychologist he has worked and continues to work in the Academic Health Care Center in Old Westbury and in the Family Health Care Center in Central Islip. His clinical focus is on the issues of young adults dealing with medical and psychological challenges and he works with those individuals diagnosed with Parkinson's Disease and their psychological adjustments. His research expertise with Art Therapy and Parkinson's Disease has resulted in many publications and presentations at national conferences.

Chapter 5

EXPRESSIVE REMIX THERAPY: USING DIGITAL MEDIA ART AS A THERAPEUTIC INTERVENTION WITH TRANSITION-AGE YOUTH (TAY)

JEFFREY JAMERSON

There is no greater agony than bearing an untold story inside you.
                                                    −Maya Angelou

Introduction

This chapter explores how to use digital media art as an intervention in therapeutic sessions with Transition-Age Youth (TAY); the process or engagement is called expressive remix therapy. This chapter also draws on my background in behavioral modification work with children, as well as my work as a videographer and my experience in the realm of hip-hop culture as a disc jockey (DJ). An emphasis is placed on the idea of the remix; DJs use remixing as a standard technique of expression, taking existing records and mixing them up (blending, cutting, fading, and scratching) to create something new and powerful (changing the groove, if you will). This chapter uses the word remix as a metaphor for therapeutic techniques that play with the idea of transformation. It will explore and discuss the use of digital art and digital play as therapeutic interventions, in particular, iPad app exploration and digital storytelling using audio and video formats and laptop computers as techniques used to evoke a client's personal story construction and story transformation. Two underlying themes will comprise the framework of this chapter: (1) the construction of narratives and (2) the remix (or creative transformation) of narratives using various forms of digital media. I frame the construction and remix of narratives as a client's "expressive life performance."

Topic Background and Inspiration

Part of my inspiration for expressive remix therapy comes from my experience as a disc jockey (DJ). When I first began to DJ, the whole idea of mixing or remixing was fascinating to me because it embodies a sense of creativity and imagination. The first person credited with inventing our current form of club mixing is DJ Kool Herc from the South Bronx.

In the early 1970s, DJ Kool Herc had a vision to change the apparently unchangeable: he had a vision to change the groove on a record. When he peered down at his spinning turntable, he asked, "How can I change this song? How can I make it sound different?" DJ Kool Herc dared to inquire, or perhaps more adequately put, he dared to "creatively inquire," and through his inquiry, he concluded that by adding another turntable and a "mixing" device, he could blend the two immutable songs together and create a new rendition of the song in the process. Thus was born the art of modern-day DJing.

My personal journey with DJing and remixing began one summer day in 1979, when a friend, invited me to his house to show off his new stereo setup. I was in awe sitting in his room watching him play vinyl records on two turntables with a small mixing board between them. He demonstrated how to mix two different songs together, playing them at the same time, by manipulating the mixing board. I still remember the feeling when he said, "Do you want to try?" He stepped back and motioned for me to take control. I put on headphones, cued a record, and began mixing songs. The first two songs I mixed were from a group called Kraftwerk and another from the Rolling Stones. The experience was pure magic! From that day forward, I would never be the same. I got two turntables and a mixer for Christmas and eventually began a young career as a DJ.

You might ask what DJing and remixing have to do with therapy and with mental health. I would respond that they have everything to do with therapy and mental health–especially *my* mental health. The most joyful moments of my life have occurred during this creative and expressive time, and these experiences still impact the approach and process I use in mental health treatment today.

Remixing is a powerful metaphor that I draw upon and use for a new form of therapy that places the client in the position of a DJ. Instead of mixing records, the client mixes narratives. The essential idea of remix therapy is to remix narratives that appear in the form of writings, speeches, pictures, video clips, and images, regardless of where the narrative comes from. In remix therapy, remixing is conducted through the use of digital technology. Participants use digital technology to manipulate narrative assets (collected narratives in the form of poetry, interview questions, song lyrics, stories, etc.). The final product of expressive remix therapy is an artistic creation.

I often wonder whether therapy is in need of a technological upgrade, or a remix, particularly therapy with children, as most children today are born and reared in a digital world. They are familiar and comfortable with digital media as an extension of the self. This is important because it potentially opens up another avenue for reaching and for treating children who have experienced trauma and life crises. Many forms of therapy utilize techniques with children that were developed decades ago. I am hoping that the use of a novel approach in therapy, such as digital media art, will create a healing space for children to express their stories. I contend that the field of psychotherapy is ready for a shift and an upgrade in its therapeutic approach with children and adolescents. My contention is based on the digital shift that is occurring throughout the world today.

Transition-Age Youth

With over 20 years of working with children and with adolescents in the foster care system, I have developed a soft spot in my heart for youths who fall between the ages of 16 and 25. Foster youth within this age range are called *transition-age youth* because at 16 they are on the brink of emancipating from the foster care system (this usually occurs at 18 years of age). I have developed this soft spot due to seeing how unprepared TAY are for an independent life of emancipation. Over the years, research studies have been conducted that affirm this apparent reality of TAY. Because these studies have revealed a major gap in TAY preparedness for independent living, administrators of child welfare agencies and mental health programs and policy makers have attempted to meet the challenge by developing and offering a service called *independent living program* (ILP). In ILP, the TAY learn basic life skills, like how to grocery shop, open a bank account, fill out an employment application, and maneuver through the financial aid process of a collegiate system. In a research study titled, "Transitional Youth Services: Practice Implications from a Systemic Review," by Naccarto and DeLorenzo (2008), the authors stated:

> In 2005, according to the Adoption and Foster Care Analysis Reporting System (AFCARS), there were 24,407 adolescents who "aged out" of the foster care system into independent living (U.S. Department of Health and Human Services 2006). These foster youth often lack support from family and social systems and may often experience a more difficult transition to independent living than non-foster youth. (Courtney et al., 2004, p. 287)

DeLorenzo and Naccarato (2008) also said, "Because youth who are transitioning to independent living are extremely vulnerable and experience many negative outcomes, it is imperative that researchers make it a priority to provide practitioners with guidelines for providing effective independent living services" (p. 288).

More purposeful guidelines are important as well as figuring out a way to include TAY in having a voice and a choice on what the ILP guidelines and curriculum looks and feels like. Without a voice and choice by TAY on these important shifts, the question remains about how effective ILP will be with TAY. After all, during the time of ILP many of the TAY are dealing with life problems related to whatever landed them in foster care in the first place. Needless to say, focusing and concentrating on ILP then becomes a challenging task, and hence, many never complete the program. If TAY are not getting the independent living skills offered by the program, what happens at the age of 18 when they emancipate? My direct experience has revealed that they slowly deteriorate into a life of homelessness, crime, and abuse (as both perpetrator and victim).

I believe that a creative form of ILP curriculum would engage TAY in a positive way that helps them acquire and use life skills more purposefully. This creative form of ILP curriculum could come from a shift in how it is taught to TAY. In other words, imagine ILP curriculum being taught through the avenue of the expressive remix therapy groups (using digital media art). TAY could utilize expressive remix as a tool to help reframe their foster care experience. I also believe ILP could utilize these digital art tools to reframe how youths enhance life skills.

Generation D and the Birth of the Expressive Remix Group

Baby Boomers, Generation X, and Generation Y (or "Millennials") are names for generational cohorts. I call the kids of today, Generation D, where the D stands for *digital.* It is not a stretch to say that youth are more comfortable texting than chatting on the phone or in person. Kids today are natural experts when it comes to social media; it is second nature for them to navigate Twitter, Facebook, Instagram, Tumblr, YouTube, Flickr, and so forth. I began to see this shift while working with clients in school settings about five years ago and asked myself, "Why not use the technology that youths are connected to, to deliver service?" My imagination began to explode with ways of engaging youth therapeutically with digital media.

After all, traditional art therapy asked similar questions decades earlier and discovered ways to integrate common artistic practices (painting, drawing, and collage) in a therapeutic manner. I began to envision different ways in which art could be explored and created in therapy using digital media technology. The fun part of this journey was discovering a metaphor (remixing), a mechanism (use of digital technology), and a theory (constructivism, social constructionism, narrative therapy, and expressive art therapy) to guide the process.

Narratives as a Theoretical Framework

Discovering and researching the philosophies of constructivism, social constructionism, language, and storytelling, were critical to the theoretical framing of this treatment approach, and also helped explicate why narrative remixing was a progressive step in narrative work. Humans connect to the world through language and through conversation, and the idea pattern of language is story. As stated earlier, the premise for expressive remix therapy has been influenced by narrative therapy (NT) and expressive arts therapy (EAT). NT is a psychotherapeutic orientation that relies strongly on altering a participant's narrative in a therapy session. In their seminal book, *Narrative Means to Therapeutic Ends,* White and Epston state that a person's identity and beliefs are held within the stories that person thinks and speaks (Epston & White, 1990). A major aim of NT is to externalize the problem (usually as a story) and then to find ways to express the problem differently. "As alternative stories become available to be performed, other "sympathetic" and previously neglected aspects of the person's experience can be expressed and circulated. Inviting persons to be an audience to their own performance of these alternative stories enhances the survival of the stories and the sense of personal agency" (p. 17).

NT is based on a constructivist paradigm which states that reality is not something outside of us, but that the perception of the outside world is constructed within. This construction is accomplished through language and narrative—through the internal and external conversations that people have with themselves and others. In their book, *Narrative Therapy,* Combs and Freedman show how "realities are organized and maintained through stories" (Combs & Freedman, 1996, pp. 28–29), giving rise to therapies focusing on shifting the internal narrative of clients.

The narrative-therapist is not as concerned with setting goals to solve problems as are proponents of other schools of therapy. Rather, he or she is more engaged in listening to clients' stories and then helping those clients re-author their stories and connect with their intentions, values, hopes, and commitments. When clients achieve this connection, they experience their lives in a different manner and, consequently, experience their problems in a different light. In many instances, the problems go away altogether, as the client begins to live out a new self-image and future (Combs & Freedman, 1996).

Narrative therapists encourage their clients to give names to themes that occur within the clients' narratives or stories. These themes can take the form of problems or projects. Giving names to problems and projects creates a space in which they can be objectified and viewed as existing outside of the self, leading to the notion that problems are separate from people (Freedman & Combs, 1996). Remix therapy is a progressive step in therapeutic narrative work: the client has the opportunity to progress from the realm of narrative creation, to the realm of narrative performance through the use of digital media art.

The Performance of Narrative Remixing

For the past few years, I have facilitated a workshop called the Expressive Remix Group (ERG), a weekly group that explores different ways of storytelling and story meaning. ERG uses the metaphor of the "remix" as an example of how to transform stories. Participants are youths from Los Angeles County who have been identified as being at-risk for joining gangs in their neighborhoods. The two overarching goals of the group are to increase participants' skills in digital media technology and to practice the skill of narrative making and narrating expression (or performance). While the capacity to create narrative is vital to mental health, the ability to change pre-existing narratives may be even more important. This ability to change narratives is a vital coping skill.

Within the group, facilitators raise a number of questions to participants, such as, "What is your story?" "Who controls the story (in the individual, in culture, and in society)?" "Are you and your story one and the same?" These questions are generally posed in two ways: in an informal manner through dialogue between facilitators and participants, and more formally via therapeutic worksheets. Stories and narratives are formulated from the client's responses to both the formal and informal questions. The narrative can be as concise as a word or a symbol, or as extensive as a poem or an essay. Stories do not have to come from the client's life; they can come from culture, communities, and society, and they can reflect a current or a past event. Once the narratives are gathered, the clients are encouraged to remix the narratives using digital media tools (iPads, laptops, smart phones, etc.) in the same way that a DJ remixes a song.

ERGs meet for a 13-week cycle, divided into 4 mini-cycles of three weeks each, called creative excursions. At the end of the fourth creative excursion, there is a final session called creative showcase theater, in which participants exhibit their digital works of art for family and for friends.

Expressive Remix Group Curriculum

*Creative Excursion 1 (CE 1): Digital Storytelling**

Week 1: Discuss group dynamics, make rules, explain and demonstrate digital stories.

Week 2: Begin digital storytelling projects.

Week 3: Complete digital storytelling projects.

*Creative Excursion 2 (CE 2): Animated Mask***

Week 4: Complete CE1, begin creating masks after group facilitator demonstrates process..

Week 5: Paint masks.

Week 6: Complete therapeutic worksheets, use answers as a script to animate the masks.

Creative Excursion 3 (CE 3): Comic Voice, Magazine Cover, and Movie Poster

Week 7: Complete CE2. Facilitator demonstrates creation of a comic strip utilizing an informative theme (e.g., bullying, gang violence, and teen pregnancy). Participants create their comic strip storylines with the theme as a backdrop.

Week 8: Create mock magazine cover based on their theme from the previous week or on storyline of digital story from CE1.

Week 9: Create mock advertising poster for digital story.

Creative Excursion 4 (CE 4): Virtual World Creation

Week 10: Complete CE3. Facilitator shows examples of virtual world creation. Participants work with software to create a positively themed virtual world.

Week 11: Participants begin to create their own virtual worlds.

Week 12: Continue virtual world creation; complete project.

---

*An example may be found at http://youtu.be/TD02w83CSWo.

**Examples may be seen at http://youtu.be/aSp2DJ6Hl84 and http://youtu.be/31qaicf9eoU

Creative Showcase Theater

Week 13: Complete CE4. Family and friends invited to session to observe and to admire the creative art participants have designed.

Alternative Creative Excursions

- Graffiti Creator
- Magazine Cover
- Movie Poster
- E-book Publishing
- Logo Design
- Poetry in Motion
- Digital Collage
- Video Asset Remixing
- Digital Music Remixing

Participant Goals and Objectives

- Become familiar with digital media art as a mode of creative expression.
- Learn new skills using iPads, smart phones, and digital software.
- Discuss and practice the art of remixing (reframing) stories and ideas.
- Become engaged in strategic and empowering dialogue with peers and with group facilitators.
- Complete a digital story from beginning to end.

Resources

- Hardware: iPads, laptop computers, smart phones, and digital cameras
- Various forms of creative software
- Links to digital art websites

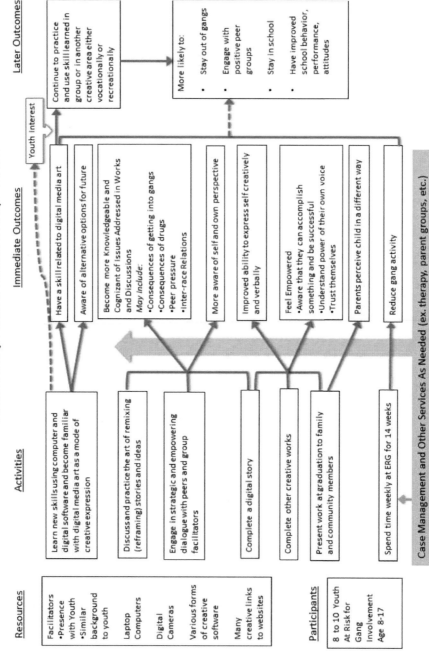

Figure 1. Expressive remix group pilot study logic model (Jamerson, 2013).

Implications and Applications

The personal, social, and professional implications of using digital media as a tool are life altering. One can pitch a persuasive argument that modern-day technology in the form of computers has directly influenced the evolutionary trajectory of humanity like no other tool in our history. If technology in the form of of digital computers or digital media has wielded this much influence, why not utilize it more, albeit in a positive and advantageous manner in the therapeutic context? Digital art through computers is an approach to therapy that is overdue. In the coming years, as more people become acclimated with the digital world, we will see various disciplines and domains following suit to be a part of this revolution or digital movement. Children and adolescents in particular, in some respects, are wired cognitively and neurologically to the digital world. This makes a natural fit with therapeutic approaches that use digital media and digital media art as a tool of engagement. My focus and approach to applying digital media art in the therapeutic context is predicated on using narrative as a foundation or as a starting point. As there are many ways to therapeutically approach treatment, so too are there many different ways to therapeutically use digital media with clients and with participants. I can envision psychodynamic, family systems, and cognitive behavioral therapists using digital media in unique ways to augment their already familiar modes of practice. I look forward to the future when therapeutic professionals will utilize digital media technology as a standard tool in their therapeutic practice.

Conclusion

Expressive remix can be used across many therapeutic models. Whether in cognitive behavioral, or in psychodynamic, humanistic, or family systems therapy, expressive remix can augment the existing techniques relied on by the therapist or modality as therapists become familiar with using digital expressive technologies in their sessions. A psychodynamic therapist who is doing work with dreams might encourage a client to keep a dream journal and assist him or her in remixing portions of that journal into a "digital dream"–a voice-over narration of the dream accompanied by pictures and by music. A family systems therapist might consider helping a client remix a genogram into a digital collage, helping the client process any underlying issues that might arise from the task. A cognitive behavioral therapist might consider using digital media expressive technology to expand specific skill-building exercises that address various cognitive deficiencies and behavioral challenges. For example, video game play or online digital game play could help a client practice actions that help overcome phobias or compulsions.

The future of expressive remix is still unfolding, and will become brighter as mental health professionals and their clients experiment with using digital media as a tool in therapy. I see a future in which digital therapeutic art expands to include video work, digital music production, and possibly video game design. The sky is truly the limit for digital art in therapy.

REFERENCES

Combs, G. F., & Feedman, J. (1996). *Narrative therapy: The social construction of preferred realities.* New York: Haddon Craftsman.

Epston, D., & White, M. (1990). *Narrative means to therapeutic ends.* New York: Norton Professional Books.

Jamerson, J. L. (2013). Expressive remix therapy: Using digital media art in therapeutic group sessions with children and adolescents. *Creative Nursing, 19*(4).

Naccarato, T., & DeLorenzo, E. (2008). Transitional youth services: Practice implications from a systematic review. *Springer Science-Business Media,* 21.

Biography

Jeffrey Jamerson, MS has over twenty years of experience in the public sector. He has served at-risk youths in various capacities, most recently as the vice president of programs and services at Aviva Family and Children's Services in Hollywood. Jamerson holds a master's degree in Counseling Psychology from National University and is a PhD candidate in Transformative Studies at the California Institute of Integral Studies. Jamerson's early work as a filmmaker, disc jockey, and break dancer showed him the power of story and creative self-expression to heal the psyche. His exploration of spirituality and consciousness led him to believe that the images and stories we hold in our imaginations have a powerful effect on how we live our lives. Hoping to create a shift in how therapy is conducted with foster children, he has integrated Narrative and Expressive Arts modalities with Digital Media Art, which he calls, Expressive Remix Therapy. The objective of Expressive Remix Therapy is to facilitate a child or youth's ability to revision a life story into a transformational narrative of strength and survival, utilizing digital media assets (I-Pads, laptops, digital pictures, music, and voice-over). Blending solid theoretical approaches with cutting edge audiovisual technologies, Jamerson hopes to engage these young people who are often resistant to traditional talk therapy.

Chapter 6

ART THERAPY BLOGGING
WITH ADOLESCENTS

Jennifer Byxbee and Amanda Zucker

Introduction

In this chapter, we will discuss the use of the Internet and how it can serve as a therapeutic holding environment for middle school-aged adolescents as they explore issues of identity, relationships, and communication. We will talk about how adolescents are using social media as a form of expression and will offer ideas for leveraging this phenomenon as a means for helping adolescents therapeutically. Examples of work created by student clients form a blogging project the authors initiated. Additionally, we will discuss ethical concerns and precautions one must take when setting up a therapeutic project with young people and with the Internet through a monitored blog with multiple contributors. By the end of this chapter, we hope to supply readers with thought provoking ideas and actionable information for integrating technology into their therapy practice.

For the purpose of this chapter, we must first define social media. According to Wikipedia, "Social media are media for social interaction, using highly accessible and scalable communication techniques. Social media is the use of web-based and mobile technologies to turn communication into interactive dialogue."

Adolescents spend an estimated 7.5 hours per day using social media, almost as long as the workday of most adults. In 2012, 95% of adolescents ages 12 to 17, used the Internet (Office of Adolescent Health, 2013). This shift is not only changing their maturation process, but also our future. During adolescence, the brain becomes wired to seek novelty (Siegel, 2014). This makes teens particularly attracted to a changing technological world. Teens are also more likely to take risks, reacting to their world without fully taking time to understand the consequences (Siegel, 2014). The center of their social worlds has shifted from their neighborhoods, schools, and group affiliations, to the Internet. Facebook, Instagram, and Twitter have become platforms for teens to express ideas; to create, to maintain, and to end relationships; and to develop online identities. Lonely teens are more likely to use online media (Grohol, 2010).

In this rapidly changing society, therapy continues to follow the same old model. We have not kept up with the times and in many cases ignore the new Internet norms. Furthermore, we are not using technology as a vehicle for connecting, understanding, or helping our youths. Even worse, we do not educate adolescents on the threats and issues they face online. Instead, we ignore the fact that adolescents spend so much time online, pretending everything is as it was a decade ago. As art therapists, we have the unique opportunity to utilize these tools to encourage community, connection, expression, and identity formation. We can give adolescents freedom of expression in a medium that comes naturally to them. Additionally, we can collaborate with them to discuss and to analyze what this expression means and how it affects their lives. In doing so, we not only help them develop skills that are valuable to today's ever-changing workforce. We also help them understand what it means to be a positive contributor to the web and society.

Furman (2013) states in her book, Ethics in *Art Therapy: Challenging Topics for a Complex Modality,* ethical guidelines do not always address the gray areas of important issues in art therapy practice. Art therapists have unique ethical considerations to their field considering the complexity of using art and materials alone (Furman 2013). As our world changes so rapidly in this digital era, the complexities are only compounded. It is necessary that we constantly evaluate the ethics of using technology within our field as we can no longer practice in a world untouched but digital innovation.

Blogging and Adolescent Use of Social Media

Adolescents are drawn to social media because it validates their presence. Postings on Facebook, Tumblr, and Instagram allow teens to assert themselves through posts and to receive feedback from their peers via posted comments, "likes," "favorites," and other signals. Social media is accessible and it provides instant gratification. In addition, social media is an integral space for building meaning and for forming relationships. As therapists, we believe it is our job to connect with our clients where they are, and today that is online.

The population we will discuss range in age from 12 to 15 years old. This generation, born after the Millennials, is called Generation Z (Benhamou,

2015). Generation Z is the first generation of people to have only known the world post-Internet. They are considered the first true digital natives (Benhamou, 2015). Working with this generation of children requires that we understand the challenges and the possibilities of technology in therapeutic care (Malchiodi, 2013). It is our responsibility to find a way to work in their space using their language.

Status Update Group

Status Update is a mixed-media program designed to help students explore and to understand what it means to use social media and the web as a means for identity formation, expression, and connection. In the Status Update pilot program, middle school students and art therapists collaborated in a school environment to create a multiuser interactive blog. Group members from two different schools used the blog as a vehicle for interacting and for responding to art therapy directives. We chose to host this program via a blog (instead of a Facebook group or other social networking site) because blogs are flexible, involve a long form if necessary, and a more thoughtful form of interactive social media. Blogs require students to press publish, and every time a student sent their work out into the world, we wanted them to consider the weight and meaning behind their actions. Throughout the Status Update program, students posted updates and responded to one another in a moderated environment that safely mimics their regular online use. Two client groups comprised of 10–12 adolescents, ages 13–15, participated in the Status Update group. Each group met for 8 weeks in conjunction with their typical art therapy and counseling sessions. The student clients were known to the art therapists at each site. Additionally, the student clients volunteered for the group and their guardians signed consent forms for their participation and for their permission for content to be posted online.

In addition to engaging with regular creative arts therapies groups, participants used visual art, photography, and writing to express feelings and reactions regarding identity, safety, and relationships. Before posting, teens discussed the content and purpose of their posts with the art therapist and with their peers. Working in this way allowed for teens to have space to think critically about not just their sessions, but also about the meaning and implications of what they were sharing online. Using the blog in this manner mirrors the adolescent process of posting to social media, but with more intentionality.

In the planning stages, the art therapist surveyed the students to find out what topics they wanted to discuss in the Status Update group. In this case, the topics included identity, digital footprint/internet safety, bullying/cyber-bullying, violence in the community, social status/material status, and relationships. Participants explored how these topics are experienced both in real life and across social media channels. Once the topic or focus was determined for the project, we set up a blog to display the students' thoughts throughout the program. Since the messages published online live forever (either live on the site or as an archive via portals like TheWayBackMachine [http://archive.org/web/], this blog still serves as a platform for reflection. This addition of the interactive blog breathed life into these students' work in a way that was unexpected. In what follows, you will find anecdotes around identity, bullying, and internet safety. Above all, we hope to supply thoughts, learning, and implications for integrating technology into therapeutic practice.

Thoughts and Implications of Integrating Technology into Therapeutic Practice

The following steps were taken in order to initiate and to survey the groups as well as to start the blog project:

- Consent was given from the site directors, in this case the school principals.
- The students were identified and releases fully explaining the project were sent home and collected.
- The students met in small groups or individually to discuss relevant topics.
- The space was secured that had internet access.
- The students were given surveys to measure their baseline mental status, their attitudes toward school, toward their community, and toward their level of resiliency.
- The students were consulted in picking the blog's theme.
- The students were made aware of the process of purchasing a domain name and setting up the site.
- The students created blog accounts as contributors in order to post work and for comments for review by the site monitors. In doing this, they learned basic Wordpress skills (Choe, 2015). W3Techs, a website which provides information about the usage of technologies on the web, reports that 24% of websites today are built using the Wordpress content management system (W3Techs, 2015). Based on the growing statistics, it can be concluded that learning these skills will be helpful for these students in the future.

Identity

When the art therapist leading group A gave the first directive to the students, they were shown a small piece of paper that looked like an Instagram picture. "You're going to create a "selfie using art–There will be no photos for this directive so try to think of how you want to represent yourself on the blog." The students appeared to pick up on this directive and to connect with it in a meaningful way, a contrast to the directive used under a different context. The students quickly moved into sketching their ideas to show themselves to the world in a symbolic way.

Kay, an 8th grader who recently lost a family member to gang related violence asked, "How would you show that you're upset inside but you're really good outside, like you don't want people to see the inside part" (see Fig. 1).

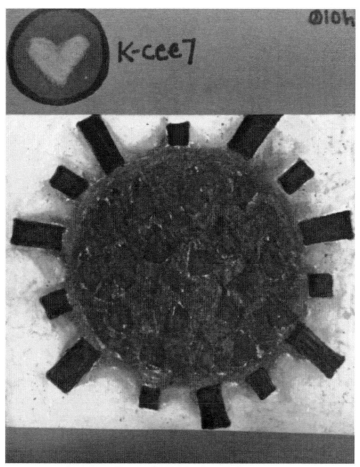

Figure 1. Kay's painting.

Another 8th grader, Sam, who describes herself as a former bully as well as an ongoing victim of being bullied due to her religious beliefs asks, "What colors would make you think of happiness and hope? A bright one, like this blue maybe?" and later, "I want to show the brightness pushing away the darkness" (see Fig. 2). These students have been working with the art therapist for two years, but it was only then that they understood what was meant by "self-portrait." They seemed to understand the context of sharing themselves with people as a post far more quickly than they could understand sharing themselves visually in therapy.

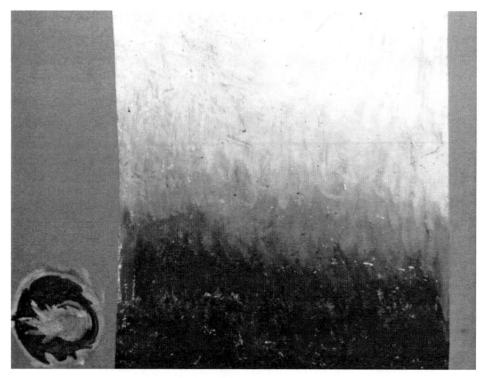

Figure 2. Sam's painting.

Bullying

After discussing bullying and cyberbullying experiences in group B, the art therapist encouraged the group to think about the feelings that come up when bullying occurs and to let their colors and lines tell the story. The clients understood that their work would be posted to the blog. Initially, the clients questioned how they would portray feeling without using words. The art therapist reminded students about filters that they used on Instagram and how a filter might alter a photo. Some participants worked together creating individual and collaborative pieces. Participants shared their work and discussed how the images that they created represent the bully's feelings, and how they looked similar to the sadness that the person being bullied might experience. "Hurt people often hurt people," one participant stated. She held up an abstract water color painting that had mostly dark browns and black with lines of red that bled into the black (see Fig. 3).

Figure 3. Hurt people–bullying.

The art therapist asked the participants how they felt when they looked at the painting, and they responded with words like, "sad, overwhelmed, angry, and ashamed." Another participant, created a figure without a mouth (see Fig. 4), explaining that when she was bullied she felt like she did not have a voice. Creating this piece and sharing it with others allowed for this student to be heard and be seen. Participants were eager for their work to be photographed and displayed on the blog.

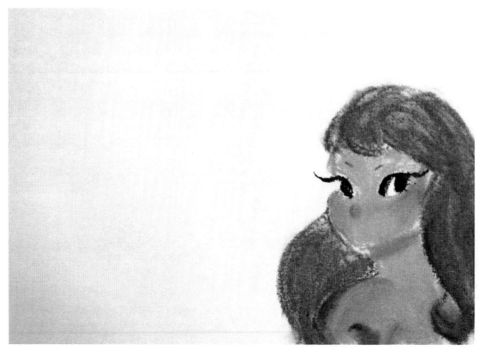

Figure 4. No voice.

Internet Safety

We are constantly talking with our young clients about their "digital footprint," but the argument is changing. Teens are no longer in a position to choose whether or not to leave a digital footprint but rather what type of footprint they want to leave. Scaring kids into social media abstinence is no longer an option as more than 9 out of 10 teenagers use social media today (Blaszczak-Boxe, 2014). Blogging enables students to experiment with the dangers of online safety and to build better-informed decisions on how to protect themselves while using the Internet (Educational Technology and Mobile Learning, 2013). Instead of asking adolescents to stop using social media, it is important to help them understand how to use social media in a way that fosters real connection, safety, and awareness of their audience.

During week 3, the group discussed their use of social media and their digital footprints. Participants were asked to consider their own social media posts and to think about how they present themselves. When asked about the content and the nature of their typical social media posts, most of the participants admitted that their posts or comments did not always reflect on them or on their peers in a positive way. The group discussed why it was important to consider who was looking at their posts and how to manage privacy settings. Participants shared their family guidelines around social media use which varied from guardians' monitoring their profiles, to complete freedom to post the content of their choice. Group members shared how they were conscious of how their peers would respond to a particular post. One client claimed that if she did not get at least twenty "likes" on a post within five minutes of posting, she would take it down. Others in the group quickly agreed. This led to the discussion about validation, and about how social media allows for people to quickly validate one's content. Participants claimed that the validation or lack of validation would alter the content that they would post. Sometimes this meant posting provocative comments, photo, and/or videos. When using the blog, the clients were allowed to validate one another's post through comments. The art therapists encouraged participants to think of positive comments for their group and the other participating group, thus modeling healthy online communication.

Moderating a Therapeutic Blog and Ethical Considerations

The most crucial considerations of integrating technology in therapeutic practice are safety and liability. When the project creators extended the Status Update group to online channels, they opened up a new means for interacting. As a result, it is crucial that the therapist finds a way to moderate online communication. When moderating a therapeutic site, one must consider risks such as posts containing suicidal or homicidal ideation. One must also consider how to respond or to moderate posts that are potentially offensive. The Status Update blog was, and continues to be, moderated by the art therapist facilitators. Participants are not allowed to post directly to the site. Their comments and entries must be approved by the art therapists. This allows participants to consider their intentions when posting. Wordpress in particular, lends itself to this kind of moderation. By designing this project on Wordpress (Choe, 2015), the project creators were able to maintain administrator access and to give students contributor access to the blog. This created a dynamic where students had to submit their drafts to the administrators for final approval. The project creators also turned on comment moderation, meaning that every comment required approval before actually going live to the site.

When thinking about integrating the web into a program, program moderators must consider participants' access to the Internet itself. As of 2013, 74% of households reported access to the Internet (Census). We chose not to extend the technological side of this program beyond school hours because not all participants had access to the web in their home, but we are sure that the project would have taken on new life if students could post at any time throughout the day or night.

When therapists integrate an online component to their practice, everyone should consider what it means to publish something to the Internet. Should the participant use their actual name or a pseudonym? Do pseudonyms actually equate to true anonymity? In this case, we opted to have participants use pseudonyms. This helped protect their identity, but also forced the students to understand how everything posted online has implications and that people can still deduce someone's online actions and identity even if they do not actually use their name when acting online. Using pseudonyms modeled safe use of social media, and generated a dialogue about privacy and one's digital footprint.

Conclusion

The Internet is changing how people spend their time, socialize, and develop. As therapists, it is our duty to address and to understand our clients' lives as they live them and to support them as they develop their most authentic selves. We are responsible to meet our clients where they are and to maintain their safety. Extending our work into the online space allows us to leverage new therapeutic methods for engaging with a medium familiar to our adolescent clients. Extending programs to the digital space successfully, means that we have a responsibility for moderating and for modeling safe use and awareness. Art therapy has been used a vehicle for self-expression, helping to increase the client's feelings of accomplishment and self-worth (Malchiodi, 1998). By blogging, the images created in groups, we are increasing their audience and thus the positive reinforcement that comes with seeing your creation exhibited. Blogging enhances the building of social identity and provides clients with a venue to practice their social skills before using them in the real world.

REFERENCES

Blaszczak-Boxe, A. (2014, October 8). Teens ditch Facebook for new social media favorite. Retrieved May 5, 2017 from www.cbsnews.com/news/kids-social-media-survey-instagram-twitter-facebook/

Benhamou, L. (2015). Everything you need to know about Generation Z. Business Insider. Retrieved from http://www.businessinsider.com/afp-generation-z-born-in-the-digital-age-2015-2

Choe, N. (2015, January 25). Why cultural competence is important for art therapists in this digital age. Retrieved from https://arttherapytech.wordpress.com/2015/01/25/cultural-competence-digital-age/

Educational Technology and Mobile Learning. (2013, March 8). Retrieved from http://www.educatorstechnology.com/2013/03/8-reasons-why-you-should-create-blog.html

Furman, L. (2013). Electronic transmission of confidential information and artwork. In *Ethics in art therapy challenging topics for a complex modality* (pp. 62–76). London: Jessica Kingsley Publishers.

Grohol, J. (2010). Lonely teens communicate more online. *Psych Central.* Retrieved on February 6, 2015 from http://psychcentral.com/blog/archives/2010/05/07/lonely-teens-communicate-more-online/

Malchiodi, C. (2013). Digital art therapy with hospitalized children. In *Art therapy and health care* (pp. 106–122). New York: Guilford Press.

Malchiodi, C. (1998). *The art therapy sourcebook.* CA: Lowell House.

Siegel, D. (2014). The essence of adolescence. In *Brainstorm.* Brunswick: Scribe Publications.

Social Media. (n.d.). In Wikipedia. Retrieved April 12, 2015 from http://en.wikipedia.org/wiki/Social_media

The Office of Adolescent Health, U.S. Department of Health and Human Services. (n.d.). Retrieved February 6, 2015 from http://www.hhs.gov/ash/oah/news/e-updates/eupdate-nov-2013.html

Biography

Jennifer Byxbee, MPS, ATR-BC, LCAT is a licensed, board-certified art therapist and creative arts therapies supervisor in New York City. Byxbee has worked as an art therapist for over ten years with children and adults in a variety of settings. Most recently, Byxbee spearheaded the creative arts therapy program at a large urban community health center. Her prior experience comprises of work at non-profits, at schools, and at community health centers, as well as at number of hospitals including Mount Sinai in New York City. In addition to art therapy Byxbee is trained in Gestalt therapy. She combines the two approaches with clients in her private practice in Manhattan.

Amanda Zucker, MPS, ATR-BC, LCAT is a registered art therapist who is board certified and licensed in New York. She is passionate about working with adolescents and with their families, and has done so in community centers, in schools, and in private practice over the last four years. Zucker has been committed to working with at-risk populations in urban areas for the last ten years, running mentoring programs in Minneapolis/Saint Paul, Minnesota and in Boston.

Part 2

MUSIC AND DRAMA THERAPIES

Chapter 7

PLAY MUSIC ON THE PILLOW WITH ME! DIGITAL AND MUSICAL "CO-CREATIVE TANGIBLES" IN EVERYDAY SETTINGS AND THEIR POTENTIAL HEALTH BENEFIT OF FAMILIES WITH A CHILD HAVING PHYSICAL OR MENTAL NEEDS

Karette Stensæth

Introduction

Imagine that objects in your home environment—a pillow, a carpet, or a toy—became musical and interactive. Do you think that they could offer new ways of playing and being together? The creative and interdisciplinary qualitative research project, RHYME, engages with such a question. It explores a new treatment paradigm based on collaborative, tangible, interactive Internet-based musical 'smart things' with multimedia capabilities, what we call "co-creative tangibles" (CCTs). By addressing the lack of health-promoting interactive and musical information and communication technology of families with children with disabilities, RHYME aims to reduce isolation and passivity and to promote health and well-being for them. In its finalizing rounds, the results from RHYME show that the technology appears to be valuable for inclusion, human interaction, and health promotion. The results are described in detail in the anthology, *Music, Health, Technology and Design* (2014a), which is edited by the present author, who is also one of the research participants in RHYME. The present chapter discusses the results deriving from the RHYME actions. To make some of the results more explicit, special attention is paid to how Petronella, with Down syndrome and her family explored the CCTs called the REFLECT. Theory from music therapy and disability studies, as well as from interaction design and informatics, create the background for the following research question addressed for the chapter: How can digital and musical CCTs lead to inclusion, human interaction and health promotion for families with a child with physical and mental needs?

Background

RHYME (www.rhyme.no) is a five-year interdisciplinary research project (2010–2015) financed by the Research Council of Norway through the VERDIKT program. The RHYME research team represents a collaboration among the fields of interaction design, tangible interaction, industrial design, universal design, and music and health that involves the Department of Design at the Oslo School of Architecture and Design, the Department of Informatics at the University of Oslo, and the Centre for Music and Health at the Norwegian Academy of Music. The project encompasses four empirical studies and three successive and iterative generations of CCTs. The REFLECT represents the second of the four generations of CCTs.

Ten families volunteered to participate. RHYME's user-oriented research incorporates their influence on the development of the prototypes in the project. The children with disabilities in the families range from 7 to 15 years old. Their mental ages range from 6 months to 7 years, while their physical handicaps range from being wheelchair dependent to being very mobile. These children vary considerably in terms of behavior style, from very quiet and anxious, to cheerful and rather active, the extreme outcomes relating to disability conditions, mostly those within the autistic spectrum. This applies to four of the children, and they have poor (or absent) verbal language and rigidity of movement. All of the children with disabilities become engaged in enjoyable activities when these activities are well facilitated for them. The Norwegian Social Science Data Services approved the RHYME project in February 2011, provided it would gather, secure, and store data according to the standards of ethics in Norwegian law.

Defining Kay Notions

To understand the background for a research project like RHYME, we need to understand some key notions. Inclusion relates to the wider and more overarching notion of *participation*. Before describing participation, we will draw attention to our society's use of the notion, *digital media*. After that, we will present perspectives on the combination of the notions, *health* and *music*.

Digital Media

Typical for the modern information society is our use of interactive and digital media. We sometimes call people who have the means to partake in this form of society, digital citizens. In qualifying as a digital citizen, a person generally must have extensive skills, knowledge, and access of using the Internet through computers, mobile phones, and web. Lack of access toward becoming a digital citizen can be a serious drawback, especially if it hinders social participation. The clinical psychologist Turkle, in her book, *Alone Together* (2011), argues that technology appeals to us mostly where we are most vulnerable in terms of our need to belong, and to feel part of something bigger. Because digital media creates an illusion of companionship without the actual presence (and demands) of it, they could in fact offer only a new form of isolation. While this may be true, if we cannot go backward, we might as well look ahead and ask together with the RHYME project: How can technology become a means of inclusion instead? How can we develop and design technology that hinders the spread of digitally enabled isolation and instead fosters new ways of participating in the digital society for everyone, including families where one member is illiterate, handicapped, or unable to adapt to the digital world? What does participation actually mean in this context?

Participation

Participation, in the everyday usage of the word, labels our interest in taking part in something. It might derive from the Latin *participare,* to share, impart, partake of, but it might also derive from the Latin *partem carpere*–that is, specifically to take something from someone (Myetmyology.com, 2008). The latter derivation connotes a certain dimension of power, which might explain the political applications of participation, as a motivating force for democracy, for example. As a noun, participation points to the act of sharing in the activities of a group, and/or the condition of having something in common with others (as fellows, partners, etc.).

The United Nations defines participation as a human right, but it remains unclear what impact this determination has on the reality faced by families with children with disabilities. Disability easily becomes the unavoidable result of modified participation due to a "defect" and "activity limitation." Normally, participation assigns several aspects: a person's preferences and interests; what he or she does, where, and with whom; and how much enjoyment and satisfaction she finds. For participation to be meaningful, it is crucial that she has a sense of choice or control over the activity. She also needs a supportive environment to facilitate her attention, a focus on the task rather than on the long-term consequences, a sense of challenge from the activity, and a sense of mastery over it. Therapists often refer to this as the "just right challenge."

The CanChild Centre for Childhood Disability Research distinguishes between two types of participation: (1) formal activities—that is, structured activities involving rules or goals that have a formally designated coach, leader, or instructor (e.g., music or art lessons, organized sports), and (2) informal activities—that is, activities with little or no planning that are often initiated by the person herself (reading, hanging out with friends, playing, watching TV, and talking on the phone). The center reports that children with disabilities often find the first type, the formal activities, most meaningful.

Other studies indicate that children with disabilities tend to engage in less varied leisure activities and in quieter recreational activities (Berg, 2009). In general, they participate in fewer social interactions, especially those of a spontaneous character. In addition, the participation level changes as children with disabilities move into adolescence, in that there are fewer activities that occur outside the home (Berg, 2009). These studies correlate with the results from the RHYME interviews where the parents tell that it is hard for them to provide proper stimulation for their children with disabilities in informal everyday activities. They feel that their children are in good hands in terms of activity and motivation as long as they are attending school and the activities are professionally provided for them. The parents fear the moment when their children have to leave school and have "nothing to do" all of a sudden.

Summarized, we could say that there seems to be a significant correlation between the severity of a person's disability and their social isolation, a tendency that is sometimes boosted by the digital society. Social isolation is a potential hazard for the children and their families in RHYME. To engage the children with disabilities in meaningful activities is very difficult for the families. This easily creates a problem that effects the family as a community. One mother of a girl with severe physical and mental handicaps in RHYME describes it this way: "At home we need things to do—together—things that are easily enjoyable and meaningful—over time!" (Stensæth, 2013, in the paragraph,Co-creation). The aim in the RHYME project is to design digital media that might empower vulnerable families' possibilities for social interaction. Before we can discuss if and how digital media can be a medium for health-promoting participation, we first need to ask: Why is the task, to engage in meaningful family activities, which may seem so easy for many of us, so difficult for families like those participating in RHYME? We will return to this question soon, which is after we have defined the overarching notions of health and music.

Health

What health is and how it is understood and interpreted, seems to have changed much over the last decade. The World Health Organization (WHO) changed their view on health in 2001, from considering it a "consequences of disease" classification (1980 version) to considering it a "component of health" classification (WHO, 2007). This more integrated understanding of health aligns with the salutogenetic health perspective, inspired by Antonovsky (1987), which sees (mental) health as a personal experience and as an on-oing process rather than as a biomedical state. Factors that support and promote well-being are essential in this perspective, for example, a sense of confidence in the fundamental coherence of the world.

Music therapists, at least in Scandinavia, support this view of health (Trondalen & Bonde, 2012). They even claim that there is a close link between music and health (Ruud, 2014; Stige, 2012). Even Ruud (2014) asserts that health, rather than a fixed state, should be regarded as a fluid state that can be influenced, for example, through meaningful music experiences such as music listening, singing in a choir, or playing in a band. Ruud calls for an experiential focus where music becomes a way to mobilize oneself toward a better quality of life. Additionally, Ruud refers to the philosopher Nordenfelt, who points to the fact that most holistic theories of health have been concerned with health as a feeling of well-being and even as a capacity for action or, in the case of poor health, as a state of suffering or a lack of ability to act (Ruud, 2014.). In these cases, there is a strong conceptual connection between the state of well-being and the ability to act (Nordenfelt, 1991; Ruud, 2014). It is therefore basic, as pointed out by one of the mothers before, that the families in RHYME to experience enjoyable collaboration that can lead to health promotion must first find ways to act together.

Music

In the context of RHYME, music has a particular position. If we draw the lines from Ruud (2014), we could say that music becomes a capacity for action and a practice that engages subjective feelings and the experience of participation. Andersson and Cappelen (2014), one of the designers in RHYME, claims that the main creative and collaborative doings in RHYME are playing, listening, exploring, composing, and improvisation. The music sociologist Small's (1998) notion of "musicking" is particularly evocative in this regard, precisely because it emphasizes music as action and as a doing: "To music is to take part, in any capacity, in a musical performance, whether by performing, by listening, by rehearsing or practicing, by providing material for performance (what is called composing), or by dancing" (Small, 1998, p. 8). For Small, musicking is an active means of relating to–and participating in–the rest of the world: The act of musicking establishes, in the place where it is happening, a set of relationships, and it is in those relationships that the meaning of the act lies.

The notion of "health musicking" combines health and musicking, and is one that appears frequently in the field of music and health and music therapy (Bonde, 2011; Stensæth, 2013; Stige, 2012). Health musicking creates a valuable perspective of the main aims in RHYME: While the last part of the notion, musicking, refers to Small's (1998) descriptions, the first part refers to those factors that support human health and well-being, rather than those that cause disease or illness. Health, in this regard, becomes almost a quality of human interaction and co-existence engagement (Halstead, 2013) and a health-performing practice (Ruud, 2010).

Eventually, in RHYME, the musical doings are embedded in the notion of health musicking: It incorporates the family's need *to do* (action) *something* (activities) *meaningful* (intentional) together:

> This is an ecological aim in that it implies the process of continuously promoting health while also preventing poor health. It also implies a strengthening of agency and mastery, as well as the creation of embodied, sensory and empowering interactions with both the tangibles and other people. (Stensæth, 2013, in the paragraph conclusion)

This way, the CCTs, by creating a field for musical and interactive co-creation, could represent a way to experience the feeling of being part of something meaningful and larger. In RHYME, the co-creation between the CCTS and the family members is seen as a resource that builds social capital and family bonds, and is therefore something that could hinder social isolation. Let us now see how these CCTs are designed to approach RHYME's goals.

The Co-Creative Tangibles

The CCTs are deliberately designed to be flexible, both in terms of the physical appearance of the artifact and the behavior of the system (Gaver, Beaver, & Benford, 2003; Stensæth, Holore, & Herstad, 2014). In a classic computer system, one expects a predictable, consistent relationship between user input and computer system output. In the RHYME prototypes, a certain amount of unpredictability (and computer agency) is built into the system, which is very different from what one would tolerate from, say, an accounting system. The RHYME designers in their development of the interactive and musical aspects, have emphasized the following qualities in the CCTs (Cappelen & Andersson, 2014, p. 17):

1. Continually evoking interest and positive emotions relevant to diverse users' interpretation of the tangibles and the situation
2. Dynamically offering the users many roles to take, many musicking actions to make, and many ways to express themselves
3. Offering the users aesthetically consistent responses and building relevant cross-media expectations and challenges over time and space, consistent with their character
4. Offering the users many relations to make: to people, to things, to experiences, to events and to places

The first empirical study in the RHYME project was of the CCTs called ORFI, the second was of WAVE, the third of REFLECT, and the fourth of POLLY. From the RHYME experiments (which we call "actions"), the designers have moved from one action to the other, making changes and development based on the previous action, weekly user surveys, on observations, and on multidisciplinary discussions. All of the sessions were video recorded from several angels to capture as much as possible of the situations (see Stensæth & Ruud, 2014). In the following section we shall look closer at the CCTs called REFLECT and soon we will describe how Petronella and her family played with this media.

The REFLECT

The REFLECT consists of a lumber-like soft object, shaped as an abstract glowing head with a trunk or an arm. Its embedded sensors, such as touchable glowing stars, and its speakers and lighting, makes it possible for the user to create dynamic music and light experiences. The REFLECT has a RFID-reader at the end of its trunk. RFID is an acronym for Radio-Frequency Identification, which relies upon small electronic devices that consist of a computer chip and an antenna. Like the magnetic strip on the back of a credit card, the RFID device provides a unique identifier for that object. With the help of the RFID-reader the user can select music tunes by choosing RFID-tagged Scene cards looking like CD covers, and dynamically change the music by interacting with the tagged objects (see Fig. 1):

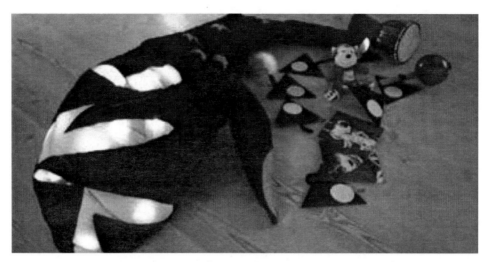

Figure 1. REFLECT. (Photo taken by Birgitta Cappelen.)

In Figure 1, we see the REFLECT's lumber-like soft "whale" in black and white in front. Around it is the RFID-tagged Scene cards and some small acoustic musical instruments. The REFLECT is designed to offer the users a multitude of ways in which to interact and to regulate their emotions and actions. They can select the kind of music they like, by varying the volume level and by choosing among many objects to play with in order to take part in the musical activities. The users can further dynamically manipulate, distort, and add effects to the sound samples while interacting with touch and bend sensors playing with the REFLECT. They can play with the REFLECT on the floor, hold it in their arms, or over their shoulders while dancing, but the users can also carry it over their shoulder playing it like a soft glowing guitar.

The software in REFLECT is written in the object-oriented programming language SuperCollider (SuperCollider 1996) and is running on an iPod Touch. The hardware is a mixture of custom-built circuits for sensors and light, and standard mobile phone technology such as a portable speaker and a battery pack. This makes the platform self-sufficient and wireless and offers high-quality sound experiences compared to current instruments and assistive music technology.

The REFLECT is built in an attempt to join together input and ideas from workshops, from user studies, and from other user inputs, in order to realize a mobile computer platform. To sum up, the REFLECT technology includes the following input and output devices:

- iPhone/iPod (as a computer)
- RHYME Device card to control sensors and actuators
- RFID reader to make musical choices
- 5 velvet star-shaped soft-touch sensors to play and to manipulate sound dynamically
- 2 bend sensors to play and to manipulate sound dynamically
- RHYME LED control card
- 24 LEDs that are integrated in the textile communicate interaction response and to provide rhythmic visual pulses
- Speaker

Additionally, REFLECT includes the following technology:

- SuperCollider as the musical programming language (real-time sound synthesis)
- Arduino as the programming language to control the jDevice card
- 6 musical scenes
- 50 RFID tags with associated physical objects and dynamic sounds

The musical scenes included six different kinds of music excerpts that were programmed into REFLECT at the time of this family's interaction with it, namely, the songs, *Mamma Mia, Gimme Gimme, Disco, Kaptein Sabeltann, Dyrene i Afrika,* and *Fairytale.* Benny Andersson and Björn Ulvaeus wrote the songs *Mamma Mia* and *Gimme, Gimme* while ABBA performed them. The Norwegian composers Terje Formoe wrote *Kaptein Sabeltann,* while Thorbjørn Egner wrote *Dyrene i Afrika,* and both of these songs are renowned Norwegian children's songs. *Fairytale* is the Norwegian 2009 Eurovison Song Contest winner written and performed by Alexander Rybak. The families in RHYME had told the research team that for the time being, these songs were of special interest to their children with disabilities.

Presenting Petronella and her Family

The family in focus is happy and loving and includes Petronella, her parents, and two older siblings. Petronella is a fun girl who likes to explore objects around her but also keeps everything in order. She is 15 years old, has Down syndrome, and she speaks in 2- to 3-word sentences and uses some sign language to communicate as well. Next to baking and cooking, she loves music and dancing the most, and as we shall see, ABBA in particular. She is sociable with one person at a time (whether young or old), but can be shy in groups. When compared to normal development, her cognitive level is below 5 years of age.

Petronella and her family seemed to enjoy the REFLECT very much during the actions where this media was tested. This chapter will discuss the findings from the second time Petronella came to the testing of the REFLECT. This time she came together with her mother and her grandmother. When they came to the room where the REFLECT was made ready for them, they were told that there were no rules and that they could approach the CCTs as they liked. They were alone in the room and stayed in it for over forty-five minutes. The session was video-recorded, from which a narrative was written based on the observations of the material.

After their exploration of the REFLECT, the mother and the grandmother were interviewed by one of the members from the RHYME research team. This person asked them how they experience REFLECT; if it "worked well" for them as a family or not–and whether they had any suggestions for improving REFLECT. They were also asked if and how they imagined that the REFLECT could create meaningful co-creation for them as a family and if this in turn could promote well-being for them as a family.

The Results

In the following, a narrative of a video observation of the family's exploring with the REFLECT is presented. After that, a short summary of the main findings in the narrative and in the interview is described. The narrative and the summary are almost identical as to the same passages from Stensæth, (2014a):

The Narrative of the Video Observation

Petronella and her mother enter the music room, followed closely by the grandmother. The three of them find a room with a sofa and with a large carpet where some of the toy-like objects are. There is a basket filled with more objects on one corner of the carpet. Petronella goes toward the objects on the carpet. The mother follows her, and the grandmother takes a seat on the sofa nearby. The mother sits down on the floor, close to the grandmother and in front of Petronella.

Petronella remembers what to do from the last time with the RE-FLECT–she picks up the (laminated) photo and holds it in front of the thing that resembles the shape of a "whale." Immediately, a loop of the song *Kaptein Sabeltann* starts to play. Petronella smiles and moves her body from side to side, as if dancing. The mother and the grandmother smile too.

Petronella does this over and over again while the mother and the grandmother watch and comment upon what Petronella is doing. Then the mother picks up the maracas from the floor and plays along.

The grandmother picks up a small drum and taps it a little.

Petronella changes the music to ABBA's *Gimme, Gimme,* then tries *Dyrene i Africa,* both of which are played in small melodic loops. Petronella grabs the mother's maracas and tries to accompany the music rhythmically.

Petronella continues to explore other musical scenes.

When Petronella finds *Mamma Mia,* the whole song plays. Petronella stands up.

She picks up the 'whale' and pulls its strap around her neck and starts to play on it as if it were a rock guitar. Petronella is very enthusiastic and happy, and she starts dancing to her own playing. The mother gets up and starts to dance as well. Petronella looks at her mother and dances while holding the "whale," as if she is pretending to be a rock star on stage.

The grandmother smiles and plays the drum from the sofa to accompany their dancing. The mother and Petronella dance while singing the whole *Mamma Mia* song together.

The grandmother puts the drum away.

The mother and Petronella move toward each other while dancing and singing *Mamma Mia.* They seem to negotiate with their bodies, not with words, to choreograph the dance.

Both of them smile.

They are having fun and Petronella is very excited.

The sound is loud.

The grandmother resigns herself and leans back on the sofa and watches Petronella and her mother silently. It starts to get too much for her, and the grandmother tells them to turn down the volume. The mother does not know how to do this and asks for help from the assistant from the research group outside the room.

Petronella picks up another photo and changes the musical scene to *Fairytale.*

The music is not as loud any more.

The mother starts to talk to the grandmother about REFLECT.

Petronella sings.

Then the grandmother and the mother sit on the sofa and look at Petronella without saying anything. Petronella sits on the floor and listens to the music while singing along.

Petronella then leans back and lies down on the floor and picks up another toylike object and cuddles it.

Petronella relaxes.

The grandmother asks for a break and says she wants to leave the room.

Short Summary of the Main Findings in the Narrative and in the Interview

The narrative describes a family having fun and enjoying themselves while exploring the REFLECT. Obviously, the child is very physically engaged, especially when she hears *Mamma Mia* and starts to dance. During the time they spend in the room, the family moves through various moods together in their musicking, from curious and exploratory, to energized and motivated, to calm and relaxed at the end. The narrative also describes how the family members relate differently to the process of exploring: the child takes the lead and the mother and the grandmother mostly follow along, perhaps in the interests of recognizing and supporting the child's initiative. Their interaction becomes more mutual later on, first when they all play music on the REFLECT together and afterward when the child and the mother share the initiative in the choreography of their dance.

In the interview, the mother and the grandmother stress the importance of having objects and toys at home that inspire them to interact and to have fun together. They also ask for items that can activate Petronella on her own. They explain that, in her playing and exploring, Petronella is very dependent on other family members to become activated and to keep her interest up, but that they do not always have the time and energy to help her. Petronella's mother stresses that she wants objects that will allow Petronella to learn and to develop. Ideally, she says, the REFLECT should be programmed so that Petronella's abiding interest in music and in dance will lead her to other types of stimulation, especially those that could enhance her speech and cognitive development. The interview reveals that the mother also lamented this REFLECT-inspired dancing, because they often do that sort of thing at home already, and they do not need any more of it, as the mother puts it. The grandmother says that the REFLECT works well because it matches Petronella's musical interests and desire to dance. The results lead us into the discussion, which brings us back to the initial research question: How can digital and musical CCTs lead to inclusion, human interaction, and health promotion for families with a child with physical and mental needs?

Discussion

The results are both promising and challenging. Obviously, there is a lot of co-creation going on between Petronella, her mother, and her grandmother and the REFLECT, and they all seem to be vitalized in varying degrees. In this regard, the results from this family's co-creation with the REFLECT correlate with other RHYME results in that the CCTs seem to promote *vitalization* among the users (Andersson & Cappelen, 2014; Andersson,

Cappelen, & Olofsson, 2014; Eide, 2014; Ruud, 2014; Stensæth, 2013, 2014a, 2014b; Stensæth, Holone, & Hevstad, 2014; Stensæth & Ruud, 2014). Basically, vitalization refers to the physical stimulation of movement and basic senses like hearing, sight, touch, and the kinesthetic, proprioceptive and vestibular senses. It also encompasses mental stimulation through its promotion of a sense of mastery as well as the strengthening of a sense of agency for the whole family. More important, vitalization relates to the feeling of having fun, both by oneself and in the company of others.

Petronella's is vitalized the most. She moves through different modes of emotions, from being physically active, moving around, and dancing before she relaxes in the end while listening quietly to the music (see the previous narrative). Furthermore, she manages, to some degree, to engage her mother and her grandmother in her interaction with the REFLECT. Vitalization this way becomes basic to any other results regarding inclusion, human interaction, and health promotion deriving from the co-creation between Petronella, her family and the REFLECT. Their vitalization is joined through intimacy and through the shared cultivation of memorable and joyful experiences. We could say that their vitalization shows some *potential* ways for building companionship and for strengthening of the family as a microcommunity and that the REFLECT for them, hosts several possibilities for health musicking.

Looking closer, we find that each one of them has unique requirements and expectations. Petronella, from exploring other CCTs before, expects the media to improvise with her. She has other expectations from the REFLECT, than what she has from other objects (e.g., instruments and toys or computer games). Probably, to engage Petronella's voice more, it would have been a good idea to include a microphone in the platform. The RHYME experiments before had shown that the microphone would allow her to interact with the media and with the musical selections differently through speaking and singing. A microphone element could this way have engaged the co-creation more totally perhaps.

The mother has other requirements. She says that for REFLECT to be most useful to them as a family, it should not compete with other fun activities, such as DVDs, PCs, and picture books, which Petronella already finds very appealing. Rather, the REFLECT should engage Petronella and her family differently than these activities. The mother also sought meaningful solo activities for Petronella. In the interview, she says that her daughter takes little initiative to involve herself in leisure activities (Stensæth, 2014a). The grandmother does not agree with the mother (who is her daughter) and replies that she thinks it is good that the objects (the REFLECT) engage Petronella exactly the way she likes the most. She cannot join Petronella in her exploring very long, though, because she tires, so probably the placing of the platform should allow her to walk away and to listen to the activity from a distance.

Obviously, and for many understandable reasons, the way in which the three family members relate to the REFLECT varies. So does the degree of their involvement. This aspect rephrases the question from before: Why is it so difficult for families like those participating in RHYME to find–to quote the one of the RHYME mothers again "things to do–together–things that are easily enjoyable and meaningful–over time"? (Stensæth, 2013, in the paragraph Co-creation) It is clearly difficult for them to find *one music* and *one activity* that are "right" for all of them at once. What Petronella finds interesting and fun to do and to listen to, is different from what the mother and the grandmother want. When Petronella wants to listen to ABBA, the mother wants to listen to classical music, and the grandmother, no music at all. Petronella wants to dance, the mother does not (but joins in more or less willingly), and the grandmother prefers to watch and wants to resign after some time. It seems that to stay within an interesting "here-and-now" for all of them at the same time, is the biggest challenge. The task is complex, and we need to look for several explanations to understand it.

Music and the Complex 'Sameness of Experience'

One explanation is found in the way in which they relate to music. It is perhaps helpful to remind us of what Ansdell (2013), the music therapist, says: To understand the ways in which music helps is also to understand how we relate to it, step into it, love it, share it–and how it still remains central to human flourishing (as cited in Stige, Ansdell, Elefant and Pavlicevic, 2013). We must, in other words, explore the what, why and how of music's meaningfulness in tandem with the REFLECT platform for each individual in turn, with a particular focus on Petronella.

This family member's interest in music is very different. To adapt the programming of REFLECT to fit the musical desires of the family members, we should probably customize the music selections by including both familiar and unfamiliar songs. Even more so, it seems like the three of them are seeking different types of musical experiences. In this respect, it is meaningful to remind us of the musicologist Keil (1995) who talks of the "sameness of experience" in music. Keil explains that people use music to form their own idioculture. People who are formed by different types of music experience the same music differently. Petronella experiences ABBA's music differently from her mother and from her grandmother. To her, ABBA means dancing. To the mother, who is 55, ABBA means something else. She was a teenager when ABBA was most popular, and who knows, perhaps ABBA reminds her of a special event back then? The sociologist DeNora (2009) thinks that music as a temporal medium, frames "situated memories": "Music moves through time, it is a temporal medium. This is the first reason why it is a powerful *aide-mémoire*. Like an article of clothing or an aroma, music is part of the material and aesthetic environment in which it was once playing, in which the past, now an artifact of memory and its constitution, was once a present" (pp. 66–67).

It is not just the choice of music that hinders the sameness of experience for Petronella and for her family. Another reason why this type of "conflict" occurs is that their personal interests and life worlds are fundamentally incompatible. In their case, the conditions that hinder the cultivation of a sameness of experiences go beyond simple intentions or preferences connected to the music. Petronella, for example, faces the world in a manner that is different from, and in a way narrower than, the rest of the family. She enjoys doing the same activities over and over again. This exhausts the other family members and makes it difficult for them to establish an ongoing interaction with her. In the interview, the mother confirms the challenges associated with her daughter's limited ability to sustain interest in other than a few favorite activities for a prolonged duration: "Petronella normally explores for five minutes . . . then she returns to the familiar," she says (Stensæth, 2014a, p. 108). It is hard for her to keep Petronella from doing the same activity over and over again, which is how the mother experiences Petronella's dancing (or "disco," as she calls it).

Here we need to remember that Petronella's cognitive level is around five years. Although she looks much older and in some ways behaves as an older child, we cannot always expect more from her than of another 5-year-old. The musicologist Vestad (2013), whose research is on children and on their engagement with music, finds that young children's ways of relating to music is best framed as "strategies of participating." Young children manifest a diverse set of strategies for participating through music. She lists the following strategies as the most prominent: doing, integrating, singing, moving, playing, listening, and playing. Petronella applies some of these strategies while inviting participation from her family members. By exploring the REFLECT and playing *Mamma Mia,* over and over again, she invites her mother to dance and to sing along with her. When she moves around and "plays guitar" with the trunk of the REFLECT, she underlines her desire to engage her family to join her in this type of musicking. Because her family responds to her dancing invitations by joining in, dancing has become a precious and memorable family activity for her. The grandmother confirms this fact in the interview when she says: "What is most fun for her [Petronella]

. . . that is, when she moves and is happy . . . and when mummy joins in and dances with her, it is most amusing for her!" (Stensæth, 2014a, p. 107).

Their co-creation involves different degrees of attitude and interest among the three family members. Yet, although they do not share existing intentions or interact in the sense of "experiencing sameness," they do, however, manage to coact in a consequential fashion. They therefore seem to realize a moment of "co-musicking," so to speak, becoming active and having fun simultaneously. To respond to the overall research question addressed in this chapter, we might ask: How do the results from this family's co-creation correlate with other RHYME results?

Other RHYME Results

The results from the case study correlate well with the other RHYME results, and particularly as regards to vitalization. Many of the participants find the CCTs fascinating and fun to explore and many of them see great potential in having such media at home. Not all of them respond as positively as Petronella and her family, and for some of them one generation of CCTs functions better than others.

The fact that the technology has the potential to be programmed to suit a given child's personal profile to some extent, CCTs like the REFLECT, vastly exceeds manual musical instruments and traditional toys in its interactivity. In this sense, the media provides other possibilities for musical co-creation than traditional musical instruments do. Andersson (2010), the sound designer in RHYME, explains that through interactive composing, and by creating dynamically changeable algorithms in the computer programs, he can transform the musical artifacts from simple intermediaries into "smart" technical and musical actors (Cappelen & Andersson, 2014). This aspect, that the media acts and improvises, is something that the children and the families find especially fascinating. The REFLECT, for instance, adapts and changes in relation to Petronella's actions. When she chose ABBA's *Mamma Mia* with the RFID-tagged Scene card, she can still dynamically manipulate, distort, and add effects to this sound sample while interacting with touch and bend sensors on the trunk (or the "whale," as she calls it). This way, the REFLECT is not simply an instrument or a neutral tool that gives the same response to the same stimuli. Instead, it acts on its own, enters into dialogue, imitates and answers her while she interacts with it and makes the musical variations. As we have seen before, Petronella knows this and expects the REFLECT to behave this way.

Of course, it is difficult to devise design solutions during RHYME prototype development that can accommodate every family technically, musically, and materially and to match all of the sensorial desires of the children with disabilities. The participating families offer valuable suggestions in the interviews, and together with the RHYME team (Cappelen & Andersson, 2014; Eide, 2014; Ruud, 2014; Stensæth, 2013, 2014b; Stensæth, Holone, & Herstad, 2014; Stensæth & Ruud, 2014) they find that some aspects are crucial for the media to give more, easier, and different interaction and shared musicking possibilities for many users with many types of different needs and requests. For instance, it is important that the media responds in sound and light close to the interaction place (Cappelen & Andersson, 2014; Stensæth, 2014b). By bringing the sound source closer, the users get more direct responses of their actions, which will not only make it easier for them to understand the CCTs' responses to their actions, but also stimulate actions and motivation more directly. The creators of the CCTs admit that this task is a complex design challenge regarding wireless objects, object size and weight, sensor qualities, sound quality, and wireless sound transmission. For these reasons, they believe it is wise to build future prototypes on smartphone technologies, since they can offer a very compact package of wireless technology, sensors, battery, and sound transmission.

It also important to enable the users to experience possibilities for more sensory and cross–media interaction (Cappelen & Andersson, 2014; Stensæth & Ruud, 2014). One family request is to develop a prototype that will engage their hyperactive child's gross motor skills, not just their fine motor skills. In order to allow the child to use his or her whole body–climbing, rolling, dancing, jumping, and so on–the CCTs have to be very solid and be able to tolerate rough treatment according to the parents. Stensæth and Ruud (2014) find that the ORFI engage the children at a gross motor level but that it needs to be sturdier to tolerate drooling and "wild" play.

The parents of two children with poorly developed sensory capacities have a different perspective. They propose that the design of the CCTs should incorporate powerful vibration to physically arouse them and to help them to become mentally 'accessible' to the outside world's impulses, impressions, and interactions. When introducing the vibration element in the WAVE prototype (see Stensæth, 2014a), it shows some promising potentials for a family with a boy afflicted with severe and multiple handicaps. Unfortunately, however, it turns out that the vibration element is not strong enough and therefore had a limited effect.

Media that stimulates many senses and interacts in a various ways–but which can also operate in one way at the time–will probably engage users who are "hard" to get interested. In order to stimulate their senses and their bodies, which is something we know from music therapy, is particularly vital for people with severe disabilities; it is, for example, a good idea to include vibration responses in the media and to build the objects with fabrics that gives very different and strong tactile stimulation.

Having learned from the case with Petronella and with her family, having explored the REFLECT in this chapter, we will work further with voice input as a base for the musicking experience, as it is of vital importance (Andersson & Cappelen, 2014; Stensæth, 2014b). Most children love the microphone and enjoy hearing their voices. Have we not all pretended to be rock stars singing into the toothbrush in front of the mirror in the bathroom?

In the last generation of CCTs built for the RHYME project, the Polly World and the designers try to meet all of the demands, suggestions, and wishes from the users and from the experts related to the three earlier generations of CCTs. On the RHYME website, they suggest focusing the media improvement on

- Dynamic and interactive change of microphone input in mobile in the CCTs, so that the users can continuously change their singing while interacting with diverse sensors of the wireless tangibles.
- Closer and more intimate and embodied relation to the video projection, compared to traditional wall projection, TV, and computer screens.
- Better sound quality in the mobile tangibles, regarding both sound frequency, range, and volume.
- More varied musical choices and tunes (to expand the self-regulating possibilities), regarding forms of musical interaction (musicking), and type of music and sound experiences (music tunes, genres, and soundscapes), so that the users can easily handle and choose music, music-related activity and intensity level.
- More robust transparent textile surfaces, since light is an important response dimension both in the interactive surfaces and part of the whole audiovisual experience.
- Better touch sensor solutions, both regarding interaction possibilities and surface qualities like color, softness, light response, responsiveness, and durability.
- More engaging and sensorial stimulating surfaces, to engage and motivate interaction with non-computer surfaces to gain a more fluent tactile, sensorial, and interactive (computer-based) experience.
- Easier grips and more possibilities to handle input sensors like microphone and bend sensors.
- Possibility for the user to include their own belongings into the musical experience and to make their own belongings sing along and expand the self-regulating possibilities.
- Easier battery charging of the mobile tangibles, so that the users easily can do it themselves.

- Easier start and stop of the system, so that the users themselves can handle it.
- Movable tangibles, so that the CCTs can be moved, installed and stored rather easily.
- Social media functionality for distributed interaction on smartphones and on tablets over the Internet (http://rhyme.no/?p=3227, 2015-04-05)

To summarize, the RHYME project shows promising results regarding health promotion depending on their affordances and to the degree that the users manage to appropriate these (Ruud, 2014). To suit the range of unique needs and requests, the media needs to be flexible. It should, in fact, allow each family to program it in their own way. This way, the media can generate qualitative and meaningful "here-and-now experiences" for them; either they are actively participating in the same activity or relating to the media (or other people in the room) simultaneously, but with different intentions and levels of activity.

Conclusion

This chapter asks: How can digital and musical CCTs lead to inclusion, human interaction, and health promotion for families with a child suffering from physical and mental needs? The background is the interdisciplinary research project, RHYME, where special attention has been given to Petronella and her family.

The health potentials depend on the degree to which the interaction between the family members and the media lead to vitalization. When the media engages the users creatively and aesthetically to explore through their basic senses like hearing, sight, tactile senses, kinesthetic sense, proprioceptive sense, and vestibular sense, they are easily aroused both bodily and mentally. From this, their sense of agency is strengthened too. At its best, the media can enhance the family members' feelings of bonding and belonging.

RHYME contributes to the promotion of participation in a very important life area—the home setting. The case with Petronella, her family, and the REFLECT, shows that the media represents a useful tool in their aesthetic home environment, one that has the potential to enhance the quality of life in the family. When doing so, the REFLECT clearly represents a means of deliverance from the problems of everyday life just by allowing the family to be in a better mood. For the future designers of such digital technology, it is important to know that unique and flexible programming is something they need to consider. A more individualized approach for each of the children with disabilities may ensure more transparency, better directions, and more predictable structures.

To facilitate the building of new relationships between (musical and interactive) objects and people, which this author thinks is an interesting focus for both music therapy and musical interaction design, media like the CCTs show the potential to change the way in which people see themselves in relation to themselves, to one another, and to the community of which they are a part (e.g. Stensæth, 2013). By developing digital media to engage people in their micro communities such as the home, can be the first step toward inclusion and social participation in the larger community.

REFERENCES

Andersson, A.-P., & Cappelen, B. (2014). Vocal and tangible interaction in RHYME. In K. Stensæth (Ed.), *Music, health, technology and design* (Vol. 7, pp. 21–38). Oslo: NMH-publications, Series from the Centre for Music and Health.

Andersson, A.-P., Cappelen, B., & Olofsson, F. (2014, 30 June–4 July 2014). *Designing sound for recreation and well-being.* Paper presented at the (NIME) International Conference on New Interfaces for Musical Expression, Goldsmiths, University of London.

Antonovsky, A. (1987). *Unravelling the mystery of health–How people manage stress and stay well.* San Francisco: Jossey-Bass.

Berg, M. (2009). Hva er deltagelse for barn som har en funksjonshemming? [What is participation for a child who has a disability?]. *Ergoterapeuten, 1*(09), 1–5.

Bonde, L. O. (2011). Health music(k)ing-music therapy or music and health? A model, eight empirical examples and some personal reflections. *Music and Arts in Action (Special Issue: Health Promotion and Wellness), 3*(2), 12–140.

Cappelen, B., & Andersson, A.-P. (2014). Designing four generations of Musicking Tangibles. In K. Stensæth (Ed.), *Music, health, technology and design* (Vol. 7, pp. 1–20). Oslo: NMH-publications, Series from the Centre for Music and Health.

DeNora, T. (2009). *Music in everyday life.* Cambridge, MA: Cambridge University Press.

Eide, I. B. (2014). 'FIELD AND AGENT': Health and characteristic dualities in the co-creative, interacive and musical tangibles in the RHYME project *Music, health, technology and design* (Vol. 7, pp. 119–140). Oslo: NMH-publications, Series from the Centre for Music and Health.

Gaver, W.W., Beaver, J., & Benford, S. (2003). *Ambiguity as a resource for design.* Paper presented at the CHI '03. SIGCHI Conference on Human Factors in Computing Systems, ACM, New York.

Globes. (n.d.). Carpe et colligere. Retrieved May 5, 2017 from https//globescom /la/en/carpeetcolligere

Halstead, J. (2013). "It just makes you feel really good": A narrative and reflection on the affordances of musical fandom across life course. In L. O. Bonde, E. Ruud, M. S. Skånland, & G. Trondalen (Eds.), *Musical life stories. Narratives on health musicking* (Vol. 5, pp. 75–95). Oslo: NMH-publications, Series from the Centre for Music and Health.

Keil, C. (1995). The theory of participatory discrepancies: A progress report. *Ethnomusicology, 3*(1), 1–20.

Nordenfelt, L. (1991). *Hälsa och värde* [Health and Values]. Stockholm: Bokförlaget Thales.

Ruud, E. (2010). *Music therapy: A perspective from the humanities.* Gilsum, NH: Barcelona Publishers.

Ruud, E. (2014). Health affordances in the RHYME artefacts. In K. Stensæth (Ed.), *Music, health, technology and design* (Vol. 7, pp. 141–156). Oslo: NMH-publications, Series from the Centre for Music and Health.

Small, C. (1998). *Musicking. The meanings of performing and listening.* Hanover, NH: Wesleyan University Press.

Stensæth, K. (2013). "Musical co-creation"? Exploring health-promoting potentials on the use of musical and interactive tangibles for families with children with disabilities. Open Access article at International Studies on Health and Well-being, 8/2013 (*Special Issue: Music, Health and Well-being*): http://www.ncbi.nlm.nih.gov/pmc/articles/PMC3740601/

Stensæth, K. (2014a). 'Come sing, dance and relax with me!' Exploring interactive health musicking between a girl with disabilities and her family playing with 'REFLECT'. In K. Stensæth (Ed.), *Music, health, technology and design* (Vol. 7, pp. 97–118). Oslo: NMH-publications, Series from the Centre for Music and Health.

Stensæth, K. (2014b). Potentials and challenges in interactive and musical collaborations involving children with disparate disabilities. A comparison study of how Petronella, with Down syndrome, and Dylan, with autism, interact with the musical and interactive tangible 'WAVE.' In K. Stensæth (Ed.), *Music, health, technology and design* (Vol. 7, pp. 67–96). Oslo: NMH-publications, Series from the Centre for Music and Health.

Stensæth, K., Holone, H., & Herstad, J. (2014a). PARTICIPATION: A combined perspective on the concept from the fields of informatics and music and health. In K. Stensæth (Ed.), *Music, health, technology and design* (Vol. 2014:7, pp. 157–186). Oslo: NMH-publications, Series from the Centre for Music and Health.

Stensæth, K., & Ruud, E. (2014b). An interactive technology for health: New possibilities for the field of music and health and for music therapy? A case study of two children with disabilities playing with 'ORFI'. In K. Stensæth (Ed.), *Music, health, technology and design* (Vol. 7, pp. 39–66). Oslo: NMH-publications, Series from the Centre for Music and Health.

Stige, B. (2012). Health musicking: A perspective on music and health as action and performance. In R. MacDonald, G. Kreutz, & L. Mitchell (Eds.), *Music, health, and wellbeing* (pp. 183–196). Oxford, England: Oxford University Press.

Stige, B., Ansdell, G., Elefant, C., Pavlicevic, M. (2010). *Where music helps: Community music therapy in action and reflection.* London, England: Ashgate Publishing, Ltd.

Turkle, S. (2011) *Alone together: Why we expect more from technology and less from each other.* New York: Basic Books.

Trondalen, G., & Bonde, L.O. (2012). In R. MacDonald, G. Kreutz, & L. Mitchell (Eds.), *Music, health, and wellbeing* (pp. 40–64). Oxford, England: Oxford University Press.

Vestad, I. L. (2013) Barns bruk av fonogrammer. Om konstituering av musikalsk mening I barnekulturelt perspektiv. [Children's use of phonograms. About the constitution of musical meaning in the perspective of child culture]. PhD thesis. Oslo: University of Oslo.

WHO. (2007). *International classification of functioning, disability and health-children and youth (ICF-CY)*. Geneva: World Health Organisation.

Biography

Karette Stensæth is an associate professor and coordinator of the Centre for Research in Music and Health at the Academy of Music in Oslo. She has worked as a music therapist for over twenty years, mostly in special education with children and youths with complex needs. Stensæth finished her PhD in music therapy (on improvization) in 2008. In 2015, she finished her Post Doc in the interdisciplinary research project, RHYME (www.rhyme.no) about interactive and musical technology and its application in the everyday life of families with a child with severe disabilities. Stensæth has edited five books (with the sixth in progress) in the area of music and health and music therapy. One of these is from 2014, and is called *Music, Health, Technology and Design.* She is now working on a book for Barcelona Publishers (U.S.) called *Responsiveness in Music Therapy Improvisation. A Perspective inspired by Mikhail Bakhtin* (Stensæth, 2017, in progress). Stensæth is active as a reviewer. She teaches and supervises students on all levels (bachelor's, master's, and PhD). Stensæth's publication list is long, and she presents her work at National and International congresses.

Chapter 8

THE ROLE OF TECHNOLOGY IN A SINGING THERAPY WORKSHOP

LUCIA CASAL DE LA FUENTE

Introduction

A rt therapy is an increasing field of study in the care and preservation of quality of life (Magee et al., 2011; Mihailidis et al., 2010); and "speech and voice impairment have significant impact on quality of life measures" (Shih et al., 2012, p. 548). These are just some reasons that fuel our interest and that are needed in conducting our research into the possibilities of voice-work, and specifically, of the singing voice, for our clients' welfare.

It is not new that rehabilitative approaches based on music were, and are used, in therapy interventions with people with speech and language impairments (Wan, Demaine, Zipse, Norton, & Schlaug, 2010). Research affirms that "musically based voice and speech therapy has been underexplored as a potentially useful method of rehabilitation" (Shih et al., 2012, p. 548). The literature has confirmed many benefits that come from voicework and singing (Spielman, Borod, & Ramig, 2003). For example, training vocal loudness appears to have benefits on other physiological voice parameters such as articulation (Sapir, Spielman, Ramig, Story, & Fox, 2007). Intonation and other important functions such as facial expression (Spielman, Borod, & Ramig, 2003) and swallowing, show promise.

Looking at our main interest in voicework employed to use in therapy, we can define singing therapy as the practice of singing activities, generally with the purpose of improving or imaintaining the quality of people's lives. Next, we will list some of the benefits of singing voice practice that research has confirmed: singing . . .

- • . . . aids anxiety and emotionalism; with physical and mental disorders, having positive results towards enriching both (inter-intra)personal and professional relationships (de Fonzo, 2012).
- • . . . activates the limbic system, whose connections to various subcortical networks are involved in the control of vocal intensity (Sapir, Ramig, & Fox, 2011).
- • . . . impacts the complete integration and coordination of the respiratory, phonatory, and articulation facets of communication, because when singing, syllables and words are articulated slower than when speaking (Schlaug, Marchina, & Norton, 2008).
- • . . . promotes and strengthens aspects of voice and speech production, favors louder voice production more than regular speech does, helps people assimilate to develop and train respiratory processes; and improves intonation, timing, and speech rates—when singing songs with pitch and tempo or range variability, and so forth (Haneishi, 2001).

Key issues related to these facts are the inner vibrations or oscillations produced when singing (de Fonzo, 2012), which reduces physical and psychological tension, which are usually an added element to the aforementioned circumstances.

It seems that to sing, it is enough to use our natural instrument—the voice. To learn how to improve its use, different materials and resources are needed because they enrich, complement, and help in understanding both the processes of teaching and learning. One of the most helpful tools to use in singing lessons or in singing therapy sessions is technology (both in its narrow and in its broad sense[1]), which allow us to get the best out of the sessions or out of the lessons. For example, a mirror—here understood as technology in its broad sense—let us see our bodies while practicing vocal technique; and musical instrument digital interface devices—here considered as technology in its narrow sense- are of service with people who are otherwise difficult to engage (Hunt, Kirk, & Neighbour, 2004). Therefore, it is not just the fact that technology improves and/or facilitates the development of the sessions (both for the teacher-therapist and for the student-user), but it is a catchy element through which we can rekindle people to get engaged into the proposed activities as a motivating and attracting component.

At this point, it is important to remark the origin of the technologies which we are working with—we should not confuse the different perspectives. It is not the same to use (any kind of) technology for doing therapy than cre-

---

1. We will go deep into the difference between technology in its broad and narrow sense in the section of this chapter called, "Technology in Our Creative Approach."

ating a specific technology to do therapy. In this sense, Mihailidis et al. (2010) distinguish between technologies that have been developed specifically as art therapy tools, and technologies used "as part of the art therapy process" (Mihailidis et al., 2010, p. 294). Our case is the second—we used technologies in our singing therapy sessions, but these technologies have not been prepared or created with the purpose to be used just in singing therapy.

There has been not much research in the use of technology in therapies linked to the arts. We can point out Wolf (2007) and Mihailidis et al., 2010–who did research about digital photography and about video respectively, reached very positive results. Yet, not many technologies have been developed with the same or with similar aims.

In this chapter, I will be showing the process of the singing therapy experience that was carried out with adults with intellectual disabilities at Down Compostela Foundation (DC).[2] The objectives of this workshop were:

- In regards to the users, I introduce them to vocal technique knowledge throughout singing exercises as a support for their daily speech therapy sessions. In other words, I provide them with a different approach.
- In regards to the *research,* I want to know to what extent the users were able to follow the planned tasks to extract some useful guidelines that could adjust the directions on instructional and assessment decisions for the design of a more complete singing workshop, especially paying attention to the means of technology.

I will explain some examples of the activities while focusing on the use of technology, which is indispensable for this kind of workshops.

Special Population: PwID[3]

The Universal Declaration of Human Rights states that everybody is entitled to all rights. In Europe, the most emblematic instruments of formal support of this level are the European Convention of Human Rights and the European Social Charter, both belonging to the Council of Europe. The institutions in charge of the protection of these rights are the European Court of Human Rights and the European Committee of Social Rights. However, vulnerable groups see many of these human rights broken with too much assiduity. Therefore, we should work along these lines as we must go on trying to help them:

---

2. http://www.downcompostela.org/. Down Compostela Foundation, in Santiago de Compostela (Galiza, Spain). Henceforth, DC.
3. People with intellectual disabilities; henceforth, PwID.

- • . . . to develop their qualities and personal skills of life.
- • . . . to accomplish more and more their inclusion to society and their lives independently, through three different procedures:
- • . . . in their educational approaches.
- • . . . in their policies.
- • . . . in their day-to-day practices.

The workshop presented here can be classified into the third subcategory, as it has been thought as a creative approach to replace, change, modify, or complement day-to-day practices. The II Action Plan for People with Down Syndrome in Spain for the period 2009–2013 (Down España, 2008) lays the foundation of the gears of this workshop because it promotes the right and the duty to participate in social life, increases autonomy, and promotes social competence. This is what we generally tried, in some manner, with the interventions in our singing therapy sessions.

Lots of texts in European countries (see Waddington & Lawson, 2009) express the concern and commitment that Europe shows for vulnerable groups. People with intellectual disabilities make up about 1% of the population of Europe and, thanks to research, they may expect to live longer lives and to live and work in their own communities (Walsh, Kerr & van Schrojenstein, 2003).According to the American Psychiatric Association (APA, 2013; as cited in Crowe, Salazar, Kertcher, & LaSalle, 2015) PwID have deficits in intellectual functions, such as reasoning, problem solving, planning, abstract thinking, judgment, academic learning, and learning from experience; deficits in adaptive functioning that result in the failure to meet developmental and sociocultural standards for personal independence and for social responsibility; and the onset of intellectual and adaptive deficits during the developmental period.

We believe that to help PwID so that they are more and more independent, and to maintain or to make them improve their daily lives, participation is a determining key. Among the aims that art therapy intervention follows, one of the most noted—and because it is a therapy itself—is to improve or to keep quality of life by dint of the encouragement of self-sufficiency through participation in artistic and creative activities that have therapeutic goals. Harlan (1990), Karp, Paillard-Borg, Wang, Silverstein, Winblad and Fratiglioni (2006), and Waller (2002) testify to this for the case of dementia. We are sure that we can extrapolate these ways to proceed for PwID; in fact, we are working in this line.

The sample of this experience belonged to the group of adults II of DC. It was composed of 13 participants: 6 women and 7 men in early adulthood. They were attending DC in the morning, since they had already finished their academic studies in ordinary schools and in their pre-professional practices. Given that the selection of the participants depended on the possibility to have access to them (Gravetter & Forzano, 2015), we used a convenience sampling method.

Rationale

This chapter may be of interest to students, to educators, and to therapists, and other creative practitioners because we explain the logical sequence to work on vocal technique to implement in the educational or therapy field, with neither singing nor musical goals in a strict manner, but with educational and therapy purposes. Speech therapy programs tend to be too intensive or may not engage enough to sustain a long-term commitment (Shih et al., 2012). Organized singing groups may provide an "effective alternative to standard therapies" or "complementary therapy to improve speech" (Shih et al., 2012, p. 549). Likewise, we consider singing as a support for speech therapy, with the aim to not to make it a routine, but to offer another way to work on it. In addition, as one of the most important aspects of this work, this chapter is focused on the essential role of technology,[4] as a tool at the service of our pedagogical activities. In fact, recent efforts incorporate telepractice and software-based training programs to help to maximize delivery of therapy (Constantinescu, Theodoros, Russell, Ward, Wilson, & Wootton, 2011).

The supervision on the role of technology in every session followed a qualitative methodology. The data collection techniques were observation and analysis of the use of those technologies. Their critical use and utility and the participants and personnel's of DC attitude toward technology, including verbal and nonverbal communication, were collected. The interviews with professionals of DC were very helpful on clarifying our doubts. We have positively received their professional opinions and suggestions toward our own development on the topics, such as opportunities and weaknesses on the use of gadgets and technologies in each session.

Our Creative Approach

We will present this creative approach through Diagram 1 and Table 1. We will explain its contents from bottom (individual and group singing) to top (vocal hygiene habits explanation), since the logic sequence of voicework is easier and more convenient to understand this way. So, in order to be ready to properly sing individually, or in group, it is recommended to have

---

4. Considering technology as our main source that supports and facilitates our work.

our voices warmed up in an appropriate way as it is essential to our vocal folds' health. This is a kind of training or gymnastics that let our folds (specifically) and vocal apparatus–and even complete body–to be sufficiently warm.

It is also necessary to practice breathing exercises first. If we do not have control on the inhaled and exhaled air, we will find difficulty controlling our voices (Casal, 2013). The more we experiment with our air's regulation, the more we manage our voices' projection.

All of these three first parts of our approach belong to a chain, as illustrated in Figure 1, and this sequence starts with relaxation exercises. Feeling our mind and body relaxed is the first step to be able to properly breathe (see Table 1).

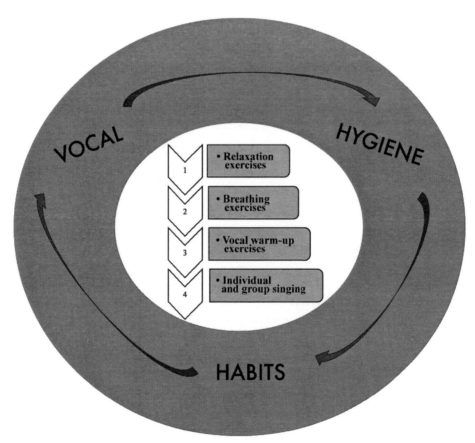

Figure 1. The logic of vocal technique and singing voicework. Source: Own elaboration.

- The more control we have on our body and on our mind (relaxation), the more control we have on our own breathing processes, and so, on our air (inhalation-exhalation phases).
- The more control we have on dominating the exhaled and inhaled air, the more control we have on projecting our both speaking and singing voice.
- The more control we have on projecting our voices the way we want, the more ability we have on mastering speaking and singing voice dynamics.

Table 1
Activities, Aims, and Examples of the Singing Therapy Workshop

Activity	Aims	Example
Vocal hygiene habits explanation	- To favor the acquisition of skills linked to vocal and hygiene care. - To foster a basic knowledge on the needs of our vocal folds and vocal apparatus. - To reveal fake beliefs about vocal care.	- With the help of a presentation, some vocal hygiene habits were explained: one each slide it was possible to see the rule written and an image that helped to remember the rule.
Relaxation activities	--To make the users become aware of their breathing when relaxing. - To have them discover how their bodies feel when practicing relaxation.	- To work imaginative relaxation with visualizations: lying on mats, faceup, with the help of soothing background music. - Tension-distension exercises, to watch mandalas, etc.
Breathing activities	- To make the users conscious about the right breathing process to internalize them.	- To blow a candle. - Various inhalation-retention-exhalation exercises.
Vocal warm-up exercises	- To facilitate the users to find, explore, emit, and hear their voices in a proper way.	- To tune arpeggios, up and down, along different scales. - To imitate different sounds.
Individual and group singing	- To get to identify and recognize voices: their own one and that of others. - To be able both to sing individually and as a group.	- To sing in unison. - To use images and gestures as a support to remember the lyrics.

Source: Own elaboration

The vocal habits we have when using our voices (either singing or speaking voice) are also crucial; that is why the vocal hygiene habits explanation is, broadly, a cross-cutting issue, and specifically, a management technique for individuals with voice disorders (Behlau & Oliveira, 2009). As you can see, it is a chain; hence, we follow this succession of activities in this specific order. Figure 1 is a support of what we have already explained and illustrates what we call, "the logic of vocal technique and singing voicework."

The experience we are writing about, regarding this creative workshop we are explaining in this chapter, was composed of five different types of activities, which aims were:

Technology in Our Creative Approach

Technology can be defined at a basic level as "the process by which humans modify nature to meet their needs and wants" (Selwyn, 2011, p. 6). The *technologies* shown in Table 2 are considered as such because they are not utilized just to sustain forms of life (Nye, 2007), but also to enhance and to improve existing forms of living–and of *doing*. In the therapy sphere, technology is a commonly applied tool "across the lifespan, from neonatal to elderly population" (Magee et al., 2011, p. 147). We speak about technology under a tridimensional conception. It deals with connecting ICTs[5] with their associated social contexts, joining together three components (Lievrouw & Livingstone, 2002):

- Technological artifacts and devices: technology itself and how it is designed and made.
- Activities and practices: what people do with technologies, including human interactions matters, organization and uses [digital] identity, and cultural practices.
- Contexts: social agreements and forms of organization that underlie the use of technologies, involving institutions, social structures, and cultures.

If we center this definition in the field of education, we should add to every of these three points the postscript with educational aims and in educational settings. Following Selwyn (2011), there is a general and basic categorization for technology: technology in a narrow sense and technology in a broad sense. Table 2 shows the different types of technology used in the diverse activities of the workshop presented in this chapter, divided into the two

---

5. Information Communication Technologies.

basic kinds of technology, in accordance with the categorization in the previous section.

Table 2
Activities and Technologies Used

Activity	Broad Sense of Technology	Narrow Sense of Technology
Vocal hygiene habits explanation	Mats	Computer, projector, PowerPoint presentation
Relaxation activities	Mats, mirror	Computer, projector, speakers, Windows Media Players, videos
Breathing activities	Mats, mirror, candles, lighter	
Breathing activities	Mats, mirror, candles, lighter	
Vocal warm-up exercises	Mirror	Keyboard
Individual and group singing	Mirror	Computer, projector, Windows Photo Viewer, pictures, speakers, Windows Media Player, audio tracks

Source: Own elaboration

Sharpening more technologies in their narrow sense, we will classify the used ones taking as a frame of reference the classification that Selwyn offers in his book, as a mentor to pursue in the field of technology education. He classifies digital technology (Selwyn, 2011, pp. 13–14):

1. Computing hardware; systems and devices (e.g., desktop PCs, laptop computers, tablet computers, interactive whiteboards, simulation systems, and immersive environments);
2. Personal computing devices (such as mobile phones, "smart" phones, personal digital assistants, and mp3 players);
3. Audiovisual devices (e.g., digital radio, digital television, digital photography, and digital video);
4. Games consoles and handheld games and machines;

5. 'Content-free' computer software packages (such as word processors, and spreadsheets);
6. "Content-related" computer software packages (e.g., simulation programs, and tutorial packages);
7. Worldwide web content, services, and applications (not the least, e.g., web-pages and web-based services);
8. Other Internet applications such as email and "voice-over internet protocol" (e.g., Skype and other web-based telephone services).

Table 3 displays the technologies in their narrow sense used in our workshop and classified in accordance with the listing in the previous section. This list is divided into eight categories; therefore, in Table 3 you will see a number– from 1 to 8–that matches one of the subdivisions directly overhead. The kind of technology is set in parentheses.

Before finishing this section, we would like to point out that both in Table 2 and Table 3 we just focused on the technologies used for this workshop. Albeit, in voicework, in vocal technique, and in singing therapy sessions, we can use many other technologies not detailed here.

Conclusion

Technology is considered a clinical tool[6] for practicing creative arts therapies, and its potential is recognized to enhance art therapists' abilities (Mihailidis et al., 2010) to reach target groups to work with. Our work confirms it and conceives the use of technology as a very important means on the teaching-learning processes for both of the agents involved:

Table 3
Activities, Digital Technologies Used, and Their Classification

Activity[7]	Digital Technology Used	Classification
Vocal hygiene habits explanation	• Computer and projector • PowerPoint presentation	• 1 (hardware) • 5 (software to elaborate and to show presentations)

continued

6. A tool for therapy and not a game for leisure (see Mihailidis et al., 2010, p. 293).
7. Breathing exercises are missing because we did not use any digital technology or technology in its narrow sense. To do this activity, we just used the so considered technologies in their broad sense.

Table 3–*Continued*

Activity	Digital Technology Used	Classification
Relaxation activities	• Computer, projector, and speakers • Videos • Windows Media Player	• 1 (hardware) • 3 (digital video) and 7 (video from the worldwide web) • 5 (software to play videos)
Vocal hygiene habits explanation	• Computer and projector • PowerPoint presentation	• 1 (hardware) • 5 (software to elaborate and to show presentations)
Relaxation activities	• Computer, projector, and speakers • Videos • Windows Media Player	• 1 (hardware) • 3 (digital video) and 7 (video from the worldwide web) • 5 (software to play videos)
Vocal warm-up exercises	• Keyboard	• 1 (hardware)
Individual and group singing	• Computer, projector, and spakers • Windows Photo Viewer • Pictures • Windows Media Player • Audio tracks	• 1 (hardware) • 5 (software to see pictures) • 3 (digital photography taken on purpose for this activity) • 5 (software to play audios) • 3 (digital audio) and 7 (audio from the wordlwide web)

Source: Own elaboration

- *The users.* The fact that users were able to watch mandalas or images projected on a wall was very motivational[8] for them, because it is a more attractive way to get in touch with knowledge, thus learning environments are more striking. It reinforced learning consolidation (Dale, 1969) since this way the information reaches them straight through different channels: video, audio, image . . . (sight, hearing . . .). What is more, with regards to image, Magee et al. (2011) state that "conceptual learning can be difficult without visual information" (Magee et al., p. 149).

---

8. Magee et al. (2011) consider that incorporating devices in music therapy can be motivating.

- *The singing therapist.* Technology let the therapeutic interventions flourish in a more efficient way. The fact of using an audio (e.g., a song the users should learn) or some candles (to do breathing exercises) means to give some space and pause to the singing therapist. In the first case, we avoid the singing therapist repeating the song again and again, to the point where he or she feels its voice tired (even if it is extremely positive and recommendable–and necessary–to work with live voice). In the second case, technology is a means with and/or through which we can practice something specific (e.g., breathing exercises), but not only using our bodies (the most primitive instrument) but any other items, that incite participation. This idea is also supported by Magee et al. (2011), since these items are external to our bodies and, therefore, they raise curiosity to interact with them and to try them.

In the introduction of the chapter we distinguished between two main uses of technology in therapy:

- As *part* of a therapy process (technologies thought and created for doing therapy).
- As a *support* for the therapy process (technologies not created with therapy purposes, but used in therapy).

Magee et al. (2011) conceive that technology-assistive devices reinforces broader program goals. So we do. Although we would like to insist on the fact that the technologies on which this text is focused are not "technologies for art therapy" by themselves, because they have not been designed neither for their use in art therapy specifically, nor for therapy in general. That is why they cannot be considered "art technologies," but they are an irreplaceable means that facilitate and enhance the proposed activities, as well as helping in engaging the groups that we are working with into the activities. Some other research went further in the role of technology in art therapy. One example is the study by Mihailidis et al. (2010), in which they have developed three prototypes of potential art therapy technologies on the basis of a previous study on the needs, practices, and ideas about technology, felt by creative arts therapists.

After finishing the sessions, we came to the conclusion that technologies are essential in singing therapy activities. It is true that the users in this experience just manipulated technologies in its broad sense, the *"forgotten"*[9] ones

---

9. Technologies in their broad sense here are considered as the "forgotten" ones because technology is generally "thought" as any item that can be plugged in: devices, systems, or equipment.

(or pre-digital technologies, so-called by Selwyn, 2011, p. 13). For future research, we contemplate these ideas, without forgetting ethical considerations:[10]

- To bring the users prominence in manipulating all kinds of technology themselves.
- To do full and pre-planned supervision, and try different intensities and frequencies of therapy (Shih, 2012); and maybe with different populations (Mihailidis, 2010).

The last consideration would be to develop a specific technology to work on singing therapy, if needed: we should not have to use or create technology if we do not really need it. We think this kind of decision should be based on authentic needs. So, if needed, a good start on it could be:

- To look into the prior conceptions, perceived needs, and real practices of singing therapists.
- To study this information and to try to know if there is some point in which we can help through *inventing* a "new and future technology," either software, devices, or contents. At this point, it is essential to contrast the perceived needs and the real needs, which are frequently not the same, and which are many times mixed up. Yet, it would be optimal if this technology was serviceable for using with different populations, and not only with PwID.

The option of "co-creation" that Mihailidis et al. (2010, p. 299) speak of, is based on the fact that both art therapists and users interact together, using the device to "create" art. They are being ambitious and making sure that the final technology will answer to both the needs and the desires of users and therapists. Users' voices should be considered and heard as well (Parrilla, 2010), to get more complete information on which to base the design of that *idealized technology.*

Acknowledgments

I would like to thank the supervisor of the work realized, Dr. María A. Muñoz Cadavid, for having cheered me up and for having believed in me in such a superb way; and the Down Compostela Foundation, for letting me enter the institution and do my research work with total freedom, confi-

---

10. Parrilla (2010) sets out some ethical considerations to take into account when doing research.

dence, and respect. Thank you very much for the acknowledgment and help. I would like to thank Mirella de Fonzo for inspiring me on singing therapy studies; and Almudena Alonso as well for the help on technology education issues.

REFERENCES

Behlau, M., & Oliveira, G. (2009). Vocal hygiene for the voice professional. *Current Opinion in Otolaryngology & Head and Neck Surgery, 17*(3), 149-154. doi: 10.1097/MOO.0b013e32832af105

Casal de la Fuente, L. (2013). Los vocalizos en la introducción al trabajo de la voz cantada: Una experiencia con adultos con discapacidad intelectual. *Journal for Educators, Teachers and Trainers, 5*(1), 55–67.

Constantinescu, G., Theodoros, D., Russell, T., Ward, E., Wilson, S., & Wootton, R. (2011). Treating disordered speech and voice in Parkinson's disease online: A randomized controlled non?inferiority trial. *International Journal of Language & Communication Disorders, 46*(1), 1–16. doi: 10.3109/13682822.2010.484848

Crowe, T. K., Salazar Sedillo, J., Kertcher, E. F., & LaSalle, J. H. (2015). Time and space use of adults with intellectual disabilities. *The Open Journal of Occupational Therapy, 3*(2), 2. doi:10.15453/2168-6408.1124

Dale, E. (1969). *Audio-visual methods in teaching.* New York: Holt, Rinehart and Winston.

de Fonzo, M. (2012). *Canta che ti passa.* Roma: Sovera.

Down España (2008). *II Plan de Acción para las personas con Síndrome de Down en España 2009-2013.* Retrieved from http://goo.gl/8D2fvN

Gravetter, F., & Forzano, L. A. (2015). *Research methods for the behavioral sciences.* Stamfort, CT: Cengage Learning.

Haneishi, E. (2001). Effects of a music therapy voice protocol on speech intelligibility, vocal acoustic measures, and mood of individuals with Parkinson's disease. *Journal of Music Therapy, 38*(4), 273–290. doi:10.1093/jmt/38.4.273

Harlan, J. (1990). Beyond the patient to the person-promoting aspects of autonomous functioning in individuals with mild to moderate dementia. *American Journal of Art Therapy, 28*(4), 99–105.

Hunt, A., Kirk, R., & Neighbour, M. (2004). Multiple media interfaces for music therapy. *IEEE MultiMedia, 11*(3), 50–58. doi:10.1109/MMUL.2004.12

Karp, A., Paillard-Borg, S., Wang, H. X., Silverstein, M., Winblad, B., & Fratiglioni, L. (2006). Mental, physical and social components in leisure activities equally contribute to decrease dementia risk. *Dementia and Geriatric Cognitive Disorders, 21*(2), 65–73. doi:10.1159/000089919

Lievrouw, L. A., & Livingstone, S. (Eds.). (2002). *Handbook of new media: Social shaping and consequences of ICTs.* London: Sage.

Magee, W. L., Bertolami, M., Kubicek, L., LaJoie, M., Martino, L., Sankowski, A., & Zigo, J. B. (2011). Using music technology in music therapy with populations across the life span in medical and educational programs. *Music and Medicine, 3*(3), 146–153. doi:10.1177/1943862111403005

Mihailidis, A., Blunsden, S., Boger, J., Richards, B., Zutis, K., Young, L., & Hoey, J. (2010). Towards the development of a technology for art therapy and dementia: Definition of needs and design constraints. *The Arts in Psychotherapy, 37*(4), 293–300. doi:10.1016/j.aip.2010.05.004

Nye, D. (2007). *Technology matters: Questions to live with.* Cambridge: MIT Press.

Parrilla Latas, Á. (2010). Ética para una investigación inclusiva. *Revista de educación inclusiva, 3*(1), 165–174.

Sapir, S., Ramig, L. O., & Fox, C. M. (2011). Intensive voice treatment in Parkinson's disease: Lee Silverman voice treatment. *Expert Review of Neurotherapeutics, 11*(6), 815–830. doi:10.1586/ern.11.43

Sapir, S., Spielman, J. L., Ramig, L. O., Story, B. H., & Fox, C. (2007). Effects of intensive voice treatment (the Lee Silverman Voice Treatment [LSVT]) on vowel articulation in dysarthric individuals with idiopathic Parkinson disease: Acoustic and perceptual findings. *Journal of Speech, Language, and Hearing Research, 50*(4), 899–912. doi:10.1044/1092-4388(2007/064)

Schlaug, G., Marchina, S., & Norton, A. (2008). From singing to speaking: Why singing may lead to recovery of expressive language function in patients with Broca's aphasia. *Music Perception, 25*(4), 315. doi:10.1525/MP.2008.25.4.315

Selwyn, N. (2011). *Education and technology: Key issues and debates.* New York: Bloomsbury.

Shih, L. C., Piel, J., Warren, A., Kraics, L., Silver, A., Vanderhorst, V., Simon, David K., & Tarsy, D. (2012). Singing in groups for Parkinson's disease (SING-PD): A pilot study of group singing therapy for PD-related voice/speech disorders. *Parkinsonism & Related Disorders, 18*(5), 548–552. doi:10.1016/j.parkreldis .2012.02.009

Spielman, J. L., Borod, J. C., & Ramig, L. O. (2003). The effects of intensive voice treatment on facial expressiveness in Parkinson disease: Preliminary data. *Cognitive and Behavioral Neurology, 16*(3), 177–188.

Waddington, L., & Lawson, A. (2009). *Disability and non-discrimination law in the European Union. An analysis of disability discrimination law within and beyond the employment field.* Luxembourg: Publications Office of the European Union. Retrieved from http://goo.gl/aXgJ5q

Waller, D. (2002). The difficulty of being. In D. Waller (Ed.), *Arts therapies and progressive illness.* London: Routledge.

Walsh, P. N., Kerr, M., & van Schrojenstein Lantman-De Valk, H. M. J. (2003). Health indicators for people with intellectual disabilities: A European perspective. *The European Journal of Public Health, 13*(suppl 1), 47–50. doi:10.1093/eurpub /13.suppl_1.47

Wan, C. Y., Demaine, K., Zipse, L., Norton, A., & Schlaug, G. (2010). From music making to speaking: engaging the mirror neuron system in autism. *Brain Research Bulletin, 82*(3), 161–168. doi:10.1016/j.brainresbull.2010.04.010

Biographies

I have been working with vulnerable groups in the Down Compostela Foundation, and in the Galician Autism Federation. In the academic year, 2013– 2014, I taught the subject, "Special Education" in the Degree on Psychopedagogy; and in 2014–2015 taught the subjects, "Curriculum Design and Development," "ICT: Use and Improvement Processes," and "Inclusive School and Special Educational Needs," all in the Childhood Education Degree. I taught as well this last subject in 2015-2016, and I will do it again in the next academic year. I have been doing research in Università degli Studi di Milano-Bicocca and in CAG Padre Piamarta, implementing a singing and vocal technique workshop; and so did I on singing therapy and Parkinson in Bosco in Città (a residence for elderly people) in Milan (2013), in collaboration with the Centro di Neurocanto (Brugherio, Italy). I have also done research at Masaryk University, and worked on curriculum development at Mateřídouška Školka in Brno (Czech Republic, 2014). In 2015, I was granted by the Spanish Ministry of Economy and Competitiveness a scholarship to do my first case study for my PhD at Universidad Nacional de La Plata, within the Research Group on Vocal Technique. The second one was done in 2016, thanks to financial support of the Galician Fundación Barrié. I attended the Special Research Program at University College London with Prof. Graham Welch, an expert on singing pedagogy and children. In the same year, I did as well a research stay at UNIRIO (Brazil), as a visiting researcher and as a teacher, offering vocal technique classes and collaborating in research projects and music education initiatives focused on vulnerable children.

Lucía Casal dela Fuente is a psychopedagogue specializing in therapy and training programs. She did research on singing therapy in Italy and on teaching practices in the Czech Republic. Her doctoral thesis focuses on singing didactics in childhood education and it is supervised by Dr. Miguel Zabalza and Dr. Carol Gillanders. To collect her data, she did research stays in Argentina and in the United Kingdom. She has teaching experience in music and vocal technique courses in diverse countries. She currently works at the University of Santiago de Compostela as a researcher and as a teacher in the Department of Pedagogy and Didactics, thanks to funding from the Spanish Ministry of Economy and Competitiveness. She has presented diverse research papers in international conferences, as The Neurosciences and Music-V (Dijon, 2014), the European Conference on Educational Research (Porto, 2014), the 25th Conference EECERA (Barcelona, 2015), and the ABEM Congress on Music Education (Rio de Janeiro, 2016). She is a reviewer in some journals and takes part in different scientific committees, and she is an editor in the Journal RELAdEI (*Latin American Journal on Early Childhood Education*).

Chapter 9

ACTION ACROSS THE DISTANCE WITH TELEMEDICINE: THE THERAPEUTIC SPIRAL MODEL TO TREAT TAUMA–ONLINE

KATE HUDGINS

Introduction

This chapter begins with an overall description of the state-of-the-art of what is now called telemedicine (Bashur & Shannon, 2009; Shabde, 2009), a term that encompasses all forms of administering long distance global health care using electronic communication in lieu of an on-site presence in local settings. The author details advantages and concerns about using electronic formats even as advances keep evolving in terms of what is relevant to mental health practice (Khetrapal, 2015; Miyazaki, Igras, Liu, & Ohyanagi, 2012). The Therapeutic Spiral Model (TSM) is then presented to treat trauma and post-traumatic stress disorder (PTSD) using clinically modified psychodrama (in Hudgins, 2002, 2007b; Hudgins & Toscani, 2013). As a model of experiential change in the global community (Hudgins, in press, 2007b, 2015, 2013), TSM was challenged to respond to requests for long-distance learning through training, supervision, and personal growth consultations following on-site workshops in over thirty countries. This chapter provides composite case examples of using TSM across current electronic communications platforms, including text, phone, one-to-one and group video-conferencing, online teaching, and social media. Unique to the literature, TSM presents the use of clinically modified action methods of classical psychodrama to treat trauma and to train providers across the distance of time and space using electronic methods communication for training, teaching, supervision, and personal growth.

Background

My mother picked up the phone to call the nurse to schedule the home visit for the doctor who was coming for a home follow-up appointment after my tonsillectomy in 1959. Using the then, state-of-the-art electronic communications available, my mother used a device, the telephone, to connect with a medical health provider at a distance, if only in the same town. Here is telemedicine in action in its long-ago form. Smartphones contain the power of a computer at your fingertips. Seismic shifts are occurring in the provision of global mental health care due to the exponential increases in both the need for services and in the technological development to meet those needs in new and different ways.

After briefly describing the therapeutic spiral model to treat PTSD in the global community and its research (Hudgins, in press, 2002, 2007, 2007b; Hudgins & Toscani, 2013), this chapter adds to the literature on mental health and on telemedicine by providing composite case examples. TSM shows how telemedicine has been used to train professionals to treat trauma with online courses and with videoconferences for individual and group supervision. This chapter also demonstrates the use of direct intervention with PTSD and eating disorders, using clinically modified classical psychodrama and Gestalt therapy interventions (Hudgins, 2007a, 2007b) even across time and space.

Telemedicine and Mental Health

Telemedicine is an important development in global mental health as it increases the reach of services being provided through the use of electronic communications from the transfer of documents to real time face-to-face videoconferencing, and more (Khetrapal, 2015; Miyazaki, Igras, Liu & Ohyanagi, 2012; Neufeld & Case, 2013). Training, education, and supervision, as well as personal consultation for therapy, coaching, and professional development, are now being offered around the world by some of the best experts in their fields through TED Talks, webinars, Youtube videos, videoconferences, and online teaching. Yet, research on best practices seem to be always trying to catch up with the exponential demand for these and other global health services.

Research

Most of the outcome research using telemedicine in global health shows promising results, especially with a vanguard of nurse practitioners and care workers (Hailey, Roine, Ohinamaa, & Dennett, 2011; Hunkeler, 2000).

Meanwhile, a number of therapeutic protocols have been developed for in-house electronic home care provided by social workers and by other mental health professionals to provide interventions in rural areas around the United States via telephone, email, and videoconferences (Bennett-Levy & Perry, 2009; Griffiths, Blignault, & Yellowlees, 2006). A few studies directly address the provision of psychological services via telemedicine with cognitive-behavioral therapy models for PTSD (Gros, Yoder, Tuerk, Lozano, & Acierno, 2011), obsessive-compulsive disorder (Himle et al., 2006), bulimia nervosa (Mitchell et al., 2008), and depression (Nelson, Barnard, & Cain, 2006).

However, there remains many questions about licensing across state and global boundaries, as well as concerns about the quality of services and about their regulation (Novotney, 2011). Advances in technology are rapidly changing the practice of psychotherapy (DeAngelis, 2012; Fatehi, Armfield, Dimitrijevic, & Gray, 2015). Psychotherapists now offer educational and clinical resources around the world by telephone and via the Internet by e-mail, chat rooms, blog posts, websites, and interactive audio and video technology. At the moment, most of it is unregulated. Recommendations for effective legal and ethical practice are still being made to assist practitioners and clients alike using these technologies to provide mental services safely. Licensing boards are developing guidelines for practice, although in most cases there are, as of yet, no binding decisions (Wicklund, 2016).

An Interesting Note

While many other theories of psychotherapy and behavioral change have always advocated one-on-one contact in a private, confidential room with just therapist and client, classical psychodrama has always been connected with the goal to reach humankind (Moreno, 1953). In the early 1940s, Moreno, the pioneer of psychodrama, was very interested in using radio, film, and later television, in creating mass psychodrama experiences, already envisaging a future where psychodrama was done through electronic media. He produced a psychodramatic film in collaboration with S. Bates, which was presented at the meeting of the American Psychiatric Association in Washington, DC, 1935 (Moreno, 1964). He made additional films during these years, demonstrating the power of psychodrama. Sergio Guimaraes, a psychodramatist and trauma worker with UNICEF in South America, produced a series of Youtube interviews of Zerka T. Moreno, the mother of psychodrama. Here is a link to one of the final videotapes between Zerka T. Moreno and Sergio Guirmelliz, a psychodramatist from South America and a longtime friend and colleague. This video is very touching. https://www/youtube.com/watch?v=LuehSrite_/

Another bastion of psychodrama training and patient work was St. Elizabeth's Hospital in Washington, DC, from the 1940s though the end of the twentieth century (Buchanan, in press). Here too, psychodrama was already involved with using electronic communication to spread the wealth of knowledge to reach the world. James Enneis, MD, head of the psychodrama section for many decades, received an Emmy from the National Capital Chesapeake Bay Chapter in the late 1960s for a televised psychodrama conducted at St. Elizabeth's Hospital–titled, "The Shattered Mind."

As Dale Richard Buchanan (personal communication, November 28, 2016), the next head of the psychodrama section stated: "In the early 1970s I routinely used videotaping with a group of geriatric long-term inpatients to provide feedback to the group members. I recall one member who wondered how the camera made her disappear–she insisted that she was not sitting between two other group members but that we had substituted some 'old' lady to sit in her chair." Thus, the stage was set for the process I will demonstrate in the next section of creativity weaving together TSM psychodrama and telemedicine to produce a tool that is greater than either or its two parts.

Most recently, his son Jonathon (2014), wrote a book demonstrating how many of Moreno's ideas were actually the core foundation of what has now become social media. So, while it may seem to be an odd juxtaposition to use electronic media to conduct experiential sessions, there is a long history of it in the psychodrama world of creativity in action. As you will see, four primary theories and concepts of classical psychodrama help build a bridge for TSM action methods with trauma via telemedicine.

The Therapeutic Spiral Model

I turn on my computer, and like my mother decades ago, but in the different roles of clinical psychologist and TSM psychodrama trainer, I reach out to professionals, colleagues, students, and clients alike, across the distance. In my case, it just happens to be halfway around the world some days. Most mornings, no matter where my TSM work brings me to train and to teach, I start my mornings with a half hour of texting to people using TSM for professional supervision or for personal consulting. Over a cup of coffee, I sit and connect with folks around the world with just a brief message back and forth, but one that anchors in TSM for the day. At least one morning a week, I have a Skype session with someone in China at 8:00 a.m. my time, and 8:00 p.m. their time, followed by 2–4 videoconferences a day for personal growth and supervision in the global mental health community working with trauma. Sitting in my home office, a small corner of my family room, I connect with people in both Western and Eastern countries where TSM has been presented, helping improve the sustainability of their in-person learning with following up connections via telemedicine.

The Therapeutic Spiral Model (Hudgins, in press, 2002, 2007b; Hudgins & Toscani, 2013) is an evidence-based system of clinically modified psychodrama and Gestalt therapy integrating research on the neurobiology of trauma and attachment with action methods. An extensive review of TSM can be found in other books (Hudgins, 2002; Hudgins, Culbertson, & Hug, 2009; Hudgins & Toscani, 2013; Kellermann & Hudgins, 2000). While much has been written about TSM in the past twenty-five years, only a few references detail work using electronic media, for example with supervision for new eating disorder therapists (Hudgins, 2008) and examples of global health initiatives with PTSD in other chapters (Hudgins, 2007). In other theoretical writings (Hudgins, 2013, 2015), TSM is presented as a model of healing energy that connects people across cultures and languages with real-life workshops and practice, thus presaging the use of TSM with telemedicine.

However, research has been conducted in face-to-face individual therapy sessions on one of the main TSM clinical action intervention modules called the containing double (CD), which showed significant decreases in dissociation, general PTSD symptoms, anxiety, and depression over just three sessions (Hudgins & Drucker, 2000; Hudgins, Drucker, & Metcalf, 1998). TSM has also been shown to provide increases in self-efficacy and decreases in anxiety and depression in community workers following 911 (Hudgins, Culbertson, & Hug, 2009). In a cross-cultural study, Lai (2013) used TSM with mothers and daughters in a long-term outpatient program in Taipei, Taiwan, demonstrating individual and family changes with six months of treatment. Perry, Saby, Wenos, Hudgins, and Baller (2016) demonstrated the TSM weekend protocol as a success in increasing self-esteem and in decreasing symptoms of PTSD with female veterans from the wars in the Middle East.

TSM uses Terr's (1991) definition of trauma as "an external blow or series of blows rendering the person temporarily helpless and breaking past ordinary coping and defensive operations" (p. 12). All good theories of the treatment of trauma now follow Herman (1992) three-stage model of strengths, working through, and integration. As we know from recent advances in neurobiology (Cozolino, 2016), trauma work must always begin with self-regulation before advancing to the work of piecing together dissociated affects and fragmented memories, so that true integration can happen. It is this clear guide that TSM provides to experiential methods of change through the TSIRA using simple role theory terms rather for easy understanding across cultures, populations, and settings.

In the previous literature on TSM, the main focus has been on the theory of TSM and on the specific roles and action interventions that make up the clinical map or the trauma survivor's intrapsychic role atoms (TSIRA; Hudgins & Toscani, 2013). This chapter briefly mentions four classical psychodrama theories and concepts that are streamlined to promote the weaving of electronic methods of communications via humans and computers.

Classical Psychodrama

Classical psychodrama developed by J. L. Moreno, his wife, and colleague Zerka T. Moreno (1969) always saw the goal of therapeutic treatment to be to reach all of humankind (Moreno, 1953), thus envisaging a world where persons are connected throughout the world via action methods. Corey (2008) states that classical psychodrama is unique in its goal of experiential change to increase spontaneity and creativity in order to develop new roles in the present moment. Spontaneity itself is defined as an adequate response to a new situation or to a novel response to an old behavior, making it an ideal match to the new challenges of telemedicine and communication across distances. Several core concepts are relevant in today's ever-expanding world of technological marvels and challenges in global health. They will now be discussed as they can relate to telemedicine and to TSM trauma work:

- Spontaneity and creativity theory
- Tele and sociometry
- Surplus reality
- Role theory

These psychodramatic guidelines are particularly important in today's world where the impact of trauma is all around us. If we are lucky enough to not be directly affected by violence on our doorstep, it now booms out at us through the television, computer, and smartphones all around us. In turn, it is now our chance to use the very same communication methods for healing and change. Thus, psychodrama's theory of spontaneity and creativity both embraces the evolution of technology as just mentioned with J. L. Moreno's early interest in radio, films, and TV, as well as has the concretization of spontaneity as the curative agent of all change. As you will see in the following examples, this directly impacts both the content and process of TSM sessions online or in person. Together, these three theories and principles of self-organization and interpersonal connections inform how I have conducted TSM via text, phone, videoconferences, online courses, and social media postings.

Spontaneity and Creativity Theory

The first and most important contribution that psychodrama makes to the evolution of global mental health and telemedicine is this emphasis on spontaneity and on creativity as the curative guide for all therapeutic interactions. In his 1953 seminal book, *Who Shall Survive?*, J. L. Moreno stated that only the spontaneous shall survive. This axiom is being concretized in the field of telemedicine. Creativity is flourishing at such an exponential rate, that one must rely on spontaneity in order to keep up with ever-changing technology. In fact, DeAngelis (2012) states that the bar has risen in the provision of psychological services using technology. Not only does the provider need educational credentials and training in the fields of mental health practice, but they must also learn to be proficient in different methods of communication that are ever changing.

After her husband's death, Zerka Moreno, wife and codeveloper of classical psychodrama, continued to develop and to spread psychodrama worldwide, bringing together many cultures under the banner of spontaneity and creativity as curative for today's ills. Decades of her research are gathered and shared in a book by Moreno, Horvatin, and Shreiber (2006), showing the Morenos' early dedication to research to prove that the changes they saw in people with psychodrama, were true and replicable (Moreno & Moreno, 1969). Stadler, Wieser, and Kirk (2016) demonstrate psychodrama's effectiveness across settings, populations, languages, and cultures.

One of the additions of TSM to the classical psychodrama and trauma literature is that it provides the operational definition of a spontaneous state of learning through the enactment or concretization of the prescriptive (RX) roles that are the beginning of the clinical map to address trauma in all situations using action methods (Hudgins, in press, 2002, 2007b). More recently, the writings on TSM show the connection to the impact of TSM across the distance (Hudgins, 2013, 2015). The case examples now show how these and the rest of trauma-based and transformative roles of the TSIRA are utilized via videoconferencing for supervision and for personal consultations.

Like many issues about creativity, my use of telemedicine to conduct TSM trauma work in the global mental health community to create experiential change for trauma, was born of necessity. Since 2004, I have been working firsthand in Mainland China to help build the first generation of university mental health centers. Following a three-month sabbatical in 2008 at Hua Qiao University in Quanzhou, China, I was asked by Prof. Zhao Bingjie to conduct ongoing monthly group supervision sessions, as well as individual sessions for supervision to provide sustainability of experiential skills training, case development, and further teaching on diagnosis (Personal communication, September 2008). Skype had been used at the university for several years and thus they had all of the electronic equipment needed, even for group supervision, where a standing panoramic camera and multiple microphones are used. As time developed, I became comfortable with this way of communication. TSM embraced the electronic medium as just another office, another place to do experiential work, using my own spontaneity and creativity in each setting.

Tele and Sociometry

The second important classical psychodrama concept that matches the new world of technology is that of *tele,* which is an original psychodrama term that means reciprocal connections among persons across the distance. Kellermann (1979) summarizes the concept of tele as a relationship where people can communicate with each other at a distance. They can be in contact from afar, and can send messages at a feeling level, much like the rotary phone was first able to do. Thus, you can immediately see the connection between the early tenets of psychodrama and its evolution with TSM into the realm of telemedicine.

Early in the development of psychodrama, J. L. Moreno (1921) spoke of humans as beings as having unconscious, unknown connections across the cosmos through the actual essence of spontaneity and creativity. Psychodrama was actually at first a new theology, where he saw a world where we are all connected to an internal source of constant renewal and then connected to each other in creativity. He taught and researched the sociometry of people as they were naturally drawn together and apart as they helped create—or destroy—functional groups or communities (J. L. Moreno, 1953). His son Jonathon has written about how his father's work on sociometry serves as the earliest foundation of what we call, the social media (J. D. Moreno, 2014).

In TSM, tele and sociometry are used naturally in all-live workshops and builds a basis of interpersonal connection for anyone who chooses to contract for ongoing training, supervision, or personal growth, using telemedicine for sustainability. In fact, my experience has shown that it is best to combine in-person meetings with telemedicine for the best results with TSM, especially since it is a model of addressing trauma and attachment wounds from any cause. Most people come to either quarterly or biannual workshops to renew the interpersonal connection. This provides us with a physiological template of the felt experience of being together. In turn, the body-based cues can then be used later to help promote connection when communicating via text, phone, or videoconferences as you will see in the next section.

Surplus Reality

The third contribution of classical psychodrama that informs TSM and telemedicine, is the concept of surplus reality. Moreno, Blomkvist, and Rützel (2000) describe surplus reality as the internal experience that goes on continuously in every person's body, mind, heart, and spirit, much of which is out of conscious awareness until we begin to pay attention. In psychodrama, this is expressed externally by concretizing the internal experience through roles, dialogues, dramas, and techniques of psychodrama. For example, at any given moment, someone can give an ongoing soliloquy about their internal awareness of movements, thoughts, feelings, defenses, and other manifestations of self-organization and interpersonal experiencing in the here and now. All psychodrama techniques (Moreno & Moreno, 1969) were created to externalize and to concretize this internal reality so that is becomes tangible in the supervision or in the personal growth session.

While Zerka and J. L. Moreno brought an awareness of the cosmic connections of all human beings, and created the seminal system of experiential methods of change, TSM has always had a more modest clinical goal. That is, to make all action and expressive art therapy modalities safe for persons who have been traumatized using advances in clinical psychology to support changes in practice. As for surplus reality, TSM concretizes safe trauma therapy using clinically modified psychodrama and Gestalt therapy guided by the clinical map we have called the trauma survivor's intrapychic role atom for all action methods, whether in person or online (Hudgins, in press; Hudgins & Toscani, 2013).

Since surplus reality can be concretized through the use of imagination, pen and paper, drawings, objects, and empty chairs, it is ideally suited to bridge the communication gap across time and space via telemedicine. Using concretize objects, rather than abstract language while working in the digital and visual world, helps communicate thoughts, feelings, and behaviors in ways that words alone could not. TSM psychodrama is not just about analyzing a problem caused by trauma, but is most importantly, about providing the surplus reality for change to occur. As you will see in the next section, this is easy to do via text and videoconferencing.

Role Theory

A final psychodrama concept that benefits telemedicine is that people's behavior is classified in role theory terms rather than in medical or psychological diagnoses, which may or may not go across country or culture. Roles describe clusters of thoughts, feelings, and behaviors. They are user-friendly because they describe behaviors that everyone knows. It does not require a strong grasp of current psychological thought, or even familiarity with a particular language, to talk to people about their relationships as mother, father, aunt, uncle husband, wife, grandparents, teacher, doctor, musician, artist, daughter, or son.

Blatner (2000) and Corey (2008) both promote the use of role theory as a core foundation of both psychodramatic theory and practice and states that it provides a bridge for communication that goes across status, gender, culture, and language, even more important as telemedicine expands the borders of communication. Simple role terms are easily understood across cultures and languages, though how these roles are defined in healthy functioning certainly varies by culture (Hudgins, 2013). Now, this chapter examines how role theory provides the language for the innovative clinical map of TSM to guide all action interventions, regardless of the method of communication.

The Clinical Role Map of TSM: The TSIRA

One of the greatest contributions of TSM to the psychodrama and trauma literature has been the definition of spontaneity provided by role theory (Hudgins & Toscani, 2013). As stage 1 of trauma treatment, TSM creates the seven prescriptive roles that teach mindfulness, build resilience, and provide self-regulation, thus establishing a state of spontaneous learning. Stage 2 consists of the trauma-based roles that show the internalization of trauma using the TSM trauma triangle for identification and for change in trauma patterns. The final stage creates new meanings for the future and provides integration and transformation. After a brief description, you will see how this clinical map informs and help provide guidance to the safe use of TSM via telemedicine.

Prescriptive Roles

Stage 1 of TSM is to install the seven RX roles that are needed for cognitive clarity, emotional self-regulation, and connections to others. TSM creates the role of the observing ego (OE) at the beginning of any session with the use of inspirational cards that have both words for the meaning making part of the brain, and images for the creative, feeling, relationship part of the brain. People pick cards and connect to each other. Next, they increase their active experiencing of restoration, resilience, and safety with others through establishing roles of strengths. Finally, containment and self-regulation is provided by several action interventions that are easily learned in a single weekend training or in a personal growth workshop. The TSIRA's RX roles can be assessed and developed through paper and pen, dialogue, or interactive action tools such as doubling, role, reversing, and an empty chair, which can easily be done in person or via electronic communication. More in-depth TSM dramas are best done in person, via a workshop, a private team, or individual in-person sessions.

Trauma-based Roles

It is here with stage 2 trauma work, that more questions begin to come into the use of telemedicine for trauma repair. While mental health stabilization has been researched to some small degree in these studies, there is little research on direct trauma intervention using telemedicine at this time. While we are still waiting on research, the TSIRA can guide the use of action methods to help accurately label the internalization of trauma using the TSM trauma triangle in telemedicine, just as it does in face-to-face transactions.

TSM provides a simple pen and paper test that can be presented in person or via electronic formats, or in a combination of both. TSM teaches the usual roles of victim and perpetrator that are mentioned in the trauma literature, but it presents its own innovation of the role of abandoning authority as crucial to change. Furthermore, TSM proposes that trauma would never happen if there was an appropriate authority available to provide the necessary safety when violence or natural disaster occur. When there is no authority, the person internalizes a sense of worthlessness and self-abandonment, which must be addressed directly to prevent some of the worse aftereffects of trauma. The following examples show that it is possible to use action methods via videoconferencing with the sufficient clinical guidelines that the TSIRA provides.

Transformative Roles

Like the RX roles that establish psychological stability following trauma, there is less risk of focusing on developing the roles of transformation from the TSIRA, whether in person or via telemedicine. Over the years of development, TSM found that there are roles that naturally evolved out of the spontaneous interaction of the RX and trauma-based roles, such as the sleeping-awakening child and the good parents that are demonstrated in this chapter. While these initially came out of the here and now, direct interpersonal experiences, TSM is now able to transmit these same roles through text, audio, and visual communications that rely on a different kind of spontaneity that includes humans and computers.

Case Examples

The ding-dong of the old-fashioned doorbell sounds and I know that the person I have a ZOOM session with has arrived in my virtual office. It is a pleasant sound. As I click online, there is a sense of a door being opened, and inviting the other person into an office that is as near as their elbow; yet, far away—often on another continent, in another country, or in another state in the United States. Whereas the ringing of a rotary phone belongs in my childhood, today's world is peppered with sighs, beeps, chimes, and music. Some sounds are of my choosing on my iPhone, others at the whim of the electronic application I am using for the myriad of ways I use to communicate with people across both physical and psychological distance.

As a general protocol, TSM is primarily used after having met the person in real life. Most often, someone attends a TSM personal growth or training workshop and then seeks further consultation. Occasionally, I have a referral from a friend or from a professional colleague of someone who is certified in TSM in another country. I have found that for people who are doing ongoing personal growth or certification supervision work, that striving for a quarterly or biannual in person connection provides the needed opportunity to experience each other face-to-face. This interpersonal experience helps anchor the actual embodied presence of each other into our relationship, so that we can draw on it when we are physically apart. Later, these bodily felt experiences can be used to connect to the same sensations, images, and feelings of safety, nurturance, comfort, empowerment, and choice using imagination, concretization, or role plays via the electronic platforms of text, voice, video, and beyond.

In this next section, you will see composite case examples of the weaving together of the TSM clinical map via electronic media for personal growth and for professional development for trauma workers in the global community. Texting, phone conversations, video-conferences, online courses, and social media are all presented, knowing that even by the time this book is published, that there will be still further innovations in the ways in which people communicate and connect across distance.

Texting: Simple Connection on a Daily Basis

Texting is one of the most rapidly evolving methods of electronic communication. It can be used for simple events like scheduling or communicating logistical information, or can be a main source of connection between people in many roles, mother to child, husband to wife, worker to boss, trainer to student, provider to client, and so forth. I have incorporated it into my work as an American board-certified trainer, educator, and practitioner of psychodrama, sociometry, and group psychotherapy (Hicks, 2016) for daily connections with colleagues, trainees, and clients alike. Texts can be used not only for scheduling or information, but also as a way to communicate information quickly, almost instantly, between professionals. I have also used it to increase connection and stability to counteract some of the distance created by videoconferencing and by my travel schedule.

My morning starts out and my day ends with at least a dozen texts to persons around the world who are colleagues, trainees, and clients. Most are simple responses to time-sensitive questions, but each and every day I send and receive texts from people who are doing long-term TSM work for personal growth and for certification supervision with me via telemedicine. For personal growth work, I offer daily text contact when they are doing trauma work so that they can feel connected across the distance. It is a way to increase the stability of the attachment because it is done in a regular and consistent pattern that is dependable. They can draw upon a simple text for support in the everyday world. It can be a morning hello or a wish of support for a good day. An evening kiss on the forehead is often shown with emoticons. Most people report it being a simple, yet, profound reminder that they have the power to change their lives each and every day. Examples of morning texts now demonstrate their usefulness in personal and training consultation, as well as in collegial contact.

For Personal Consultation Clients

Dr. Kate: Thinking of u this AM as I start my day. Hope u can connect to grounding and stability today through taking deep breaths.

Client 1: Thanks. I just took 3 deep breaths like we do when we start our Skype sessions and feel ready for the day. Have a good day! (Emoticon of a heart.)

Dr. Kate: Morning here. Night 2U. Hope ur day has had moments of "good enough" and that u could find connections u enjoyed throughout your day. (Emoticon of a sunset since it is nighttime in Asia.)

Client 2 (in Asia, a 12-hour time difference): Xie xie ne, thank you. OK have a good day. Thanks for checking in. I am good.

Dr. Kate: Sure. Can u share the memory of one connection u made 2day that actually helped u feel better?

Client 2: At the university I had lunch with a colleague. I don't usually do that, but I thought about what u tell me about reaching out and so I did. It was nice to have a friend to share lunch with today. I think I will do it again.

Dr. Kate: Great. Great! I hope you can have good dreams and a good sleep.

For a Trainee in the International Certification Program in Trauma Therapy

Dr. Kate: Just sending you support to use the TSM inspirational animal cards with your clients today to establish the OE role for each of your sessions. The more you use it, the easier it gets to move into action.

Social worker in USA: Thanks for the encouragement. I am just getting ready to go into the inpatient trauma and addictions group and teach them the OE for the first time. I know this is an important role, especially to teach addicts. I like using the cards.

Dr. Kate: Enjoy and let me know how it goes! (Smiley face emoticon.)

For Collegial Communication

Dr. Kate to another clinical psychologist, Dr. Enid, who sees her individual Skype client for in-person couples therapy in the UK: Good morning. I am copying u last night's check in from our client w her permission. She is still struggling to be present to her body and her feelings as she gets stuck up in her head as we know. I hope this gives u info for your couples session tmr.

Dr. Enid: Just got home. Thanks for the info. It is good we can communicate so quickly so that we can work together to support her to come into her feelings and out of her head. Will let you know how it goes after CT tmr.

As you can see, it can be a quick method of encouraging a workshop participant to try out a new skill, such as the simple one of establishing the OE through the TSM animal cards, or a quick communication with a colleague. While texting has become ubiquitous, I have found that it helps clients maintain a sense of connection, especially when I am traveling. While I am in the taxi going to my hotel, I will quickly send a number of texts to people who might otherwise be concerned for me, whether real or projected. I have found that being able to text a person who I have safely landed after a fifteen-hour plane ride, can make all the difference in people feeling abandoned . . . whether they are my family or my professional relationships.

A note of caution here is that the norm for texting is that it is casual and done immediately, that there are few filters in what is said, and that it is a useful tool for short communication. It often uses acronyms and emoticons created especially for this platform of communication. However, as a global mental health professional, there is always the responsibility to recognize that this new form of instant communication still invokes the need for thoughtful responses and for the ability to think how your text will be received before sending it. As a friend of mine often reminds me—restraint of words as a proverb, has evolved into restraint of pen, typing, or texting.

Phone: The Old Standby Evolved

The smartphone I hold today, the size of a grocery shopping list, is far different from the standard black, heavy, cord connected rotary phone that we had when I was growing up. Yet, it remains an important fallback tool that is very important when using videoconferencing, which cannot always be counted on to be stable, especially across physical and cultural differences in the provision of services. As DeAngelis (2012) reminds us, there is a need to be competent in the technology that affects the psychological quality of services provided via the internet, and this is one I take seriously.

An important part of the protocol I teach to clients and to trainees when first setting up communication via Skype, Zoom, or other online platforms, is to make sure we also have a way to connect via the phone. If the person has an iPhone like I do, we set up FaceTime as a backup to disrupted Internet connections. If not, I ask them to get an international calling card so that they can call me on my phone if we are cut off. This is an important structure to help contain disruptions in the sessions, especially if important information or feelings are coming up when the internet cuts off. Ideally, the provider has an international calling plan that can always be used for emergencies without a costly charge so that you are literally "only a phone call away." With the advent of FaceTime and its Android equivalents, a phone call can now provide face to face contact so that you can ask a pending question or complete a disrupted videoconference.

A question that is raised is the element of physical visual distance and how different it is to be on FaceTime or on other video chats than it is to be sitting in a room face-to-face with someone. If eighteen inches is supposed to be the ideal distance for eye contact to foster attachment (Cozolino, 2014, 2016), then what does it do to literally be "up in the face" of the person you are communicating with via video phones and computers? As the review of the literature shows, there is no research on such clinical and neurobiological questions; yet, it is important to remain aware of what has been thought of as gospel in terms of attachment as we are now experiencing communication channels that both expand and constrict distance telescopically via telemedicine. Before you used to get a medical report face-to-face with a physician; most likely in United States, you get it via an electronic chart you access on the Internet by yourself. Yet, on your smartphone, you can be much closer than you would ever be in real life, interesting questions to be answered as time goes on, I am sure.

I was doing a long-term TSM consultation with a young woman who had a combined eating disorder that fluctuated between restrictive anorexic eating and compulsive binge overeating for several years before seeking services. She was referred by a family member and had attended a Woman's Salon, a small group workshop I conduct quarterly in my home in the United States. As you can imagine, issues of body dysmorphia, inaccurate mirroring of the physical self, and lack of emotional attunement to her wants and needs, were primary symptoms from the start of care. Because she did not have an Internet connection in her apartment, we resorted to using Face-Time (FT) for our weekly sessions. What this meant was that I would be able to see every eyelash, every tear, every micro-facial movement of a defense coming on. It also meant she could see the same in me.

As part of our initial assessment and consultation planning, I brought up how familiar she was with this form of communication in her work and in her personal life, and asked her about her experience with this form of communication. She was very forthcoming saying that she has to use it for work all the time as part of her job in human relations, but that she almost always hates it and worries that someone will see that she is not perfect. I then asked her how she thought it would work to use FT as a method to connect when she has so much anxiety about it. This was our conversation.

Dr. Kate: Hmmmm . . . seems like you are very familiar with FaceTime and other methods of visual communication via videophone and computer . . . and that you are uncomfortable with it?

Client 3: Yes, I am always anxious, thinking maybe I didn't check my teeth to make sure no food got caught in them over lunch; maybe my mascara has smudged. It is really awful actually.

Dr. Kate: Yes, I have used FT for a few years now, years where I have aged beyond sixty years old. It is, at times, a bit startling to see myself in this way, so close, so upfront. Yet, at my age, I know that while my looks served me well in my life, what I look like is not as important as what I think or what I feel. I wonder how I can communicate that to you via this difficult form of connection.

Client 3: Starts to cry, which we can both see very closely. Tears are streaming down her face and she is looking down at her hands, which I cannot see.

Dr. Kate: I am going to move into a body double (BD) role with you. I am moving my phone so you are no longer looking at me but I am beside you. I am an internal voice that supports you as I sit beside you. (Turns phone so they are both looking off into a distance and can see each other side by side.) You know the role from the workshop. I will speak in the first person as your healthy body, and you repeat what I say in your own words if it's useful and if not, you correct it in whatever way is possible for you.

Client 3: OK. (and cries some more)

Dr. Kate as BD: I can take a deep breath. (BD does audible breathing through the earphones.) I can feel my back against the chair. I can see that I am in my room. I can . . . take . . . a . . . slow . . . deep . . . breath.

Client 3: Responds with an autonomic response of a deep breath . . . yes, I can take a deep breath. I can slow myself down just a bit. But I am so unhappy. I hate myself so much! I am so ugly!

BD: I am going to continue to take deep breaths and feel my body in the room in this moment. My body is OK. I am in it. I can feel my heart beating, my breath, and my bottom on the chair. In this moment, I am okay and my body is okay.

Client 3: Yes . . . okay . . . I can feel that I am okay right now but then you are no longer looking at me on the phone!

BD: I would like to keep this feeling of being okay in my body and still be able to turn and look at Kate as we begin our healing journey together. I really believe she won't judge me. And hey, I can judge her if I want! (A gentle laugh.)

Client 3: Yes . . . okay . . . alright, I would like to do that and you are right. I see you and your imperfections just as you see mine. And I would never think to use them against you, so maybe I don't have to always use them against myself.

Dr. Kate returns to her role as a consultant and faces her client face to face again on their computers: Well, there you go . . . we found at least one way we can use FT without having to be face to face at all times. We now know it works to use the body double to shift the focus from such direct eye contact, face contact really . . . there is a reason it is called face time . . . to shift it so we are on the same side of the judgment and are not there judging each other. In fact, we both have to step up to the plate and be honest as much as possible . . . because if we are not . . . the face will say so! What do you think?

Client 3: Well, since I have to use FT all the time anyway, I guess this just gives us real life experience of how it works for me. Pretty awful I see! I would like to become more comfortable in my skin . . . but also with this way of connecting to others that I interact with on a regular basis. Looks like it might be a plus!

As you can see here, the discussion and use of this method of visual and auditory communication and connection actually augmented the use of action intervention with a videoconference via smartphone. The demonstration also shows how easily one of the RX roles of TSM, the BD, allowed the client to feel supported rather than scrutinized, and connected rather than facing judgment. Having participated in the TSM Women's Salon she was able to draw on her body memory of this role that was used throughout the weekend, and to accept the action intervention easily and with gratitude.

One-on-One Videoconference: The Home Visit

One of the great benefits of doing personal consultation or supervision online using videoconferencing platforms such as Skype and Zoom, is that it is like doing a "home visit" as a mental health provider, trainer, or educator. As the research shows, this form of electronic connection is highly effective in providing support for increasing numbers of mental health conditions via telemedicine. I find that seeing the person in their home setting always provides a more vulnerable, more real picture of what day-to-day life is like, than if they came all dressed up for a therapy or supervision hour in a physical office. For example, I have seen people in their pajamas, trying to sneak a drink in while doing addiction work, or yelling at their children as they run around wild during the session.

Initial Consult

As just mentioned, most people who contract with me for consultation services via telemedicine, have already met me in person and had at least a weekend experience with TSM. When they ask for follow up consultation for training, for education, for supervision, or for personal growth, I tell them how I work with text, smartphones, and the platforms of Skype or Zoom to use TSM in action methods across electronic communication. Most people are familiar with online communication formats, and in many cases, have more knowledge about such things than I do. We set up a visual, face-to-face, one-on-one online consultation for 1.5 hours to discuss goals and the suitability of using electronic platforms to do so.

In addition to standard intake information or training planning, I also reserve part of our first session online to discuss and to experience how we might work together in this electronic world as just described with FT. When interviewing a potential client for personal consultation or a supervisee via the Internet, I always demonstrate and use action methods during the initial consult to determine if we can work together over the distance.

Client Assessment

With a client in Vietnam who was a referral from a professor at a university who I had not met, I was able to establish an immediate and strong connection by asking him to imagine that he had a pile of brightly colored scarves beside him on the floor and to pick one that represented our connection. After a moment's hesitancy, he looked down at the floor and said he found one.

Dr. Kate: Hold the scarf up please (moving her hands in the movement she wants) and tell me what it looks like. Tell me what color our connection is to you as we start working via Zoom.

Client 4: I see a neon yellow scarf. It is vivid and alive. I see this as the connection between us. It is like a sunshine. A sunrise sets at different times for you, but it always rises.

Dr. Kate: Great. Take one end of it and throw the other end to me through the computer. Then let's play with it. You pull me and I'll pull you; we can skip rope; we can push and pull. You guide what we do.

Director's Soliloquy: I am use this imagination exercise for three clinical reasons. The first is to warm up the client to action methods. In between this first session and the next, I asked him to buy different materials to use in the session, with some being brightly colored like strength, and others dark like trauma. The second is to let the client use his imagination, largely located in the right brain that is about emotions and relationship, to increase the impact of our connection with each other across the distance, especially since we had not met in person. The third is to assess the client's attachment style with the visual push-pull between us.

Individualized Training Plan for International Certification

During an initial supervision session, I also test out how much we can use action methods via the Internet. For example, during the initial individualized training plan for persons entering the TSI International Certification in Trauma Therapy (TSM, 2016: see www.drkatehudgins.com), I will ask them to use the TSM OE cards to concretize a witness role to their year-long plan for training and supervision. Then, as we talk about what they want out of their year of training, I ask them to pick objects to represent them and to place them on their desk, or wherever they are, when we are speaking. Often, there is a spontaneous order that emerges when they choose and place the objects on the "stage" of their desk. If not, I ask them to arrange them to indicate what they want to be high on the priority list. With a new trainee, a female psychiatrist from the Middle East:

Dr. Kate: I hear you have many goals for your level 1 training in TSM. You want to learn how to install the RX roles. You want to learn how to provide safety and containment. And you want to be able to direct psychodramas for children who have been affected by the war as your ultimate goal. You have so much excitement and spontaneity today. I would like to use that energy to see how we can work in action today and in the future. Please pick out items in the room that represent each of your goals. Don't think about it so much as let yourself be intuitively drawn to the colors, the shapes, and the textures of the things you have around you in your home.

Middle Eastern Trainee: I so enjoyed your presentation at the international conference and am glad to be working with you even though we live so far apart. I like that we can meet once a month and I can continue to learn even though I am not sure when I will see you again in person. I see a samovar sitting on my mother's table in the other room. Let me go get it.

Dr. Kate: Give a soliloquy out loud as you walk to get it so that I can still hear you from the computer.

Middle Eastern Trainee: Ah . . . I also see my notebook sitting on the dining room table; I will bring that as well. I am looking around seeing this old house, which I have lived in with my family for twenty-five years. I am seeing both the old and new are coming together in my life. This is exciting for me, my family, and my community.

Dr. Kate: You had three goals; pick one more object and bring them back to where I can see you in the computer. Use the desk in front of your computer as though it were a mini-psychodrama stage. Put all three objects there, in whatever places they seem right in relation to you and to each other.

Middle Eastern Trainee: The samovar is in the middle of my desk. It is my goal to learn TSM trauma work for my family and my community. The notebook looks at it and takes notes on what works and what I can use in my work as a psychiatrist in Egypt. Interestingly, the finally object I picked up was a picture of myself as a kid that my mother keeps on the shelf. In it, I am only four years old, holding the hand of my grandfather, looking up at him with big bright eyes of wonder. I think this is myself as I look beyond the rubble around me right now in my country and connect with you and others that live in another world where there is still wonder (she starts to cry gently).

Dr. Kate: Ah . . . Rihanna . . . it is good you can see and feel the meaning of why you are committing to a training program that includes distance learning and supervision. It shows the depth of the work we can do even when we are not sitting in the same room together. Can you remember the feeling of my hand as I shook yours at the conference? The hug we had at the end of the presentation?

Middle Eastern Trainee: Yes, I can actually smell the ginger perfume you had on that day and remember how connected I felt, through what you call tele. I think we can use that to work in this way.

One interesting difference in doing an international home visit is learning about different cultures. As you can see with this psychiatrist learning TSM work in Egypt, there is wealth sitting in the home of someone who only has a few personal belongings. Often the ones that are kept, are in fact, exactly those that can bring hope for the future, whether a childhood photo or a family samovar. After an experiential session such as this one, the objects used retain a sense of energy from the positive representation they concretized, and thus continue to foster connection between videoconferences.

When working in China teaching my first online course, my interpreter's mother was visiting during the spring holiday. Since her apartment was so small, the mother would walk in and out of the scene as she interpreted for me, sitting in my home in the United States. An American woman showed her open boundaries when doing online supervision with me from her home, while her adolescent son could hear everything she was saying. In both cases, this provided a teaching opportunity about confidentiality when using videoconferencing from their home to mine. Obviously, these are some of the areas of discovery that still need attention as telemedicine continues to be used so that safety, especially with trauma work, can still be maintained via electronic formats.

Ongoing Individual Consultation

During the last eight years of practice, I have worked with persons in the United States, Canada, the United Kingdom, China, Egypt, and Taiwan using electronic videoconferencing for ongoing personal development and for individual and group supervision. I have also served as a consultant on many trauma cases around the world in the thirty countries in which TSM has been introduced since first starting to use telecommunications in 2008. Here, a client example details the building of the RX roles, while the demonstration of the TSM trauma triangle is done with a trainee in the TSI International Certification Program in Trauma Therapy (ABE standards, 2016; TSM standards, 2016).

Individual Consultation with a Woman with Anorexia in Asia: The RX Roles

About five years ago, at a TSM personal growth workshop in a large Asian city, I was introduced to a young woman by a professor trained in TSM. Yan-Ting later emailed and asked if I would work with her on the Zoom application and platform. She said she wanted help with her anorexia because there was no adequate treatment in her hometown, despite the fact that it was an international hub of commerce and trade. After an initial consult, we contracted for weekly ZOOM sessions, each for an hour and a half in order to make the most use of action interventions. The treatment planned included twice yearly sessions when I was working in her city during the following year.

During the first two months of electronic consultation, we focused on the RX roles to give her a foundation of clearly seeing herself as she built her residence and increased her self-regulation. Then, we used the TSM trauma triangle to look at the internalization of an eating disorder voice, and finally anchored in new narratives for her future through the roles of her healthy body and connected relationships. Here, I present an example of how I used the interactive electronic media when it seemed to have a "mind of its own" during the establishment of the RX roles. As an integrated therapeutic tool, the actual medium became a tool for action change.

Dr. Kate (Skype Session 5): It is good to connect with you again today. Thanks as always for seeing me at night your time and morning my time. It is after dinner there now, so I am wondering how you have been doing with building the strengths to really accept that you have an eating disorder that disrupts your life.

Client 5: I have really been trying to accept that what you tell me is true . . . that what I call healthy eating, is in fact, anorexic restriction. I know I contracted with you because I know, at some level, that I am anorexic and need help, but it is just so hard to believe. I just feel so fat and ugly when I look in the mirror. I know you and my teacher are worried about me.

Dr. Kate: Yes, we both are worried. Because of that, I'd like to suggest that today, you role reverse with your teacher. Rather than tell me what she says, I'd like you to be her and to speak to yourself in the empty chair.

Director's soliloquy: I ask her to stand behind the chair she was sitting at in front of her computer and desk. I ask her to pick an object that reminds her of her teacher and she chooses a stone that is smooth, beautiful, and connected to nature. As she holds it, I direct her to speak to the client part of her in the chair.

Dr. Kate: Dr. . . . please talk to Yan-ting in the chair. Tell her about your concerns and why you even suggested she start seeing me for help.

Client 5 in role reversal as her teacher: Yan-ting, I really want to help you. I see you unhappy, not eating, and having trouble with your school-work. That worries me. Our families have known each other for almost twenty years now and you know I have watched you grow up. It seems like you are stuck for the past year or more. Please accept that you are anorexic and that how you eat is not actually healthy. There must be reasons for that and Kate can help you figure out what they are and makes changes, so you can get on with your life again.

Dr. Kate: Great, now role reverse back and what do you say to your teacher?

Client 5 as Self: Teacher . . . you are right. You have known me for a long time, so I trust you. I'd like to be able to accept that I am. . . .

ZOOM cut off here and she could not finish her sentence. I waited to see if she would call back per the protocol I give persons working with me via videoconferencing. She immediately called back.

Dr. Kate: Oh, sorry I lost you . . . what were you saying to your teacher?

Client: That I am an anor . . . ZOOM cut off again and again she called back immediately.

Client: Alright, alright, I am an anorexic; now don't cut off on my computer anymore!

We had a good laugh at the computer problems together, which created a bonding moment at a difficult time of truly accepting her anorexic eating. It was a masterful blending of using this electronic platform, not just as the method of communication, but actually as an action intervention. It was an assessment of her commitment to consultation and personal growth that she did immediately call back twice as per the protocol for when video conferences get disrupted. Knowing that she wanted to share this new acceptance with me and was determined enough to get through the electronic challenges, even at a highly emotional moment, was a moment to celebrate. As we laughed, we felt our bodies celebrate across time and space.

Consultation with a Trainee: The TSM Triangle

After persons attend a TSI training in the United States or around the world, where courses are offered, they can apply to the International Certification Program in Trauma Therapy and contract to receive monthly face-to-face, real time, video supervision as part of the requirements (TSM, 2016). You saw how TSM action tools could be used to assist with this initial individualized training program. Here is an example of how one of the TSM clinical action interventions, the TSM trauma triangle, can be used to assist in helping a new therapist sort out issues of his own countertransference, while on Zoom. This example is taken from the Western world where students are usually both in TSI training (TSM, 2016; see www.drkatehudgins .com), as well as studying for national certification with the American Board of Examiners in Psychodrama, Sociometry, and Group Psychotherapy (ABE, 2016).

Canadian Trainee: Kate, I want to learn how to use the TSM trauma triangle to sort out my feelings toward one of the clients you have been following for the last six months of my TSM and psychodrama training. After the workshop, I have used it several times with clients and everyone has found it very helpful. Can we use it for me?

Dr. Kate: Of course. Do you have some ideas about how you are caught in the trauma pattern of victim, perpetrator, or abandoning authority roles?

Can you get a piece of paper and draw the triangle and put each of these roles at one point on the triangle? Then fill in thoughts, feelings, and behaviors you have in relation to your client.

The trainee draws a quick triangle and immediately writes down the words that belong to each of the roles. He is angry at himself and at the client from the perpetrator role, feeling like a victim in response to the client's rage, and wanting to avoid, to distance, and to cancel sessions is like abandoning authority. All are there quickly written on paper, leaving us with a chance to put it further into action for the Skype session.

Dr. Kate: Great. So now, pick three objects in your home office there, one for each role and place them on your desk in front of you. Make it bigger than the one that you drew on the paper.

The trainee picks up a Raggedy Anne doll for the victim role and places her slumped over, with her head down. He picks up a dragon-puppet for the perpetrator role. Eventually, he uses his agenda book for abandoning authority. When he has these all lined up, I ask him to role reverse with the role of his choice and to speak to himself in the empty chair inside the triangle.

Trainee from perpetrator role: You really should be ashamed of yourself being angry with the client. It is not her fault that she was abused and is transferring her anger from her grandfather onto you. You know that! What is wrong with you?

Dr. Kate: Role reverse to the part that answers that question. Is it the victim or abandoning authority?

Trainee: Moves to victim role and says: You are right. I feel like a failure. As a man, she particularly makes me feel guilty and helpless. I really don't even want to see her again.

Dr. Kate: Role reverse to the abandoning authority role now as you want to leave.

Trainee: Stops and says. I really don't want to abandon her. I care about her and her recovery deeply. I just need some help with how to deal with this stage of the TSM trauma work when we are directly working with the trauma from the past . . . and all the feelings that are coming up!

Dr. Kate: Did you just see what happened? You just spontaneously walked off of the TSM trauma triangle by claiming your truth. That you don't want to abandon her or yourself. You are not a bad therapist or a failure. You are just learning to deal with this stage of long-term consultation with people with PTSD. It is good to ask for help. That is a strength. Now, we can plan out some ideas for how to get her off the trauma triangle so that she will stop throwing all of her feelings from the past onto you.

Group Supervision

It was, in fact, the need for continuous training and supervision at Hua Qiao University's Counseling and Mental Health Center in Quanzhou, China that really started my use of Skype as an online platform. Following the intensive three-month in person training and supervision in 2008, I conducted group supervision for the following year online. We conducted this as "live supervision" with people role playing students who were their clients at the center. Other staff members took on the RX roles of body or containing doubles and strength for each other. An early, real life example follows, which also demonstrates the use of an interpreter with videoconferencing and action methods using TSM.

Connection with Interpreter via Skype

Interpreter: Hello Teacher Kate. We are almost ready for you. We have to finish getting the cameras set up so you can see the whole room.

Dr. Kate: Thank you and please start the interpretation even as they are starting up. I'd like to say: Notice your warm up as you physically move the chairs in the consulting room. Let yourself remember me being there in person just a few months ago. Put an empty chair there for me. You are not only setting up cameras and arranging chairs, you are creating a supportive space for your learning. (Interpreter gives these directions to the small group in the room.) (More noises of setting up.)

Dr. Kate: As you are getting ready to sit down, pick up an OE card that will help you let yourself learn new information, open your hearts, and connect to each other. As you sit down, share with someone else on the staff. (Waits while this is done.)

Professor Zhao Bingjie: We are ready now. I would like to present my client, a student who was referred to the center because he is writing suicidal notes on his papers and on his We Chat social account to friends. We all know the history of this student. He is a junior and comes from a high-status family in a different province. His grades are not good and his parents are concerned what he plans to do when he graduates. The school is worried he is serious about suicide and wants us to do everything we can to stop that from happening.

Dr. Kate: Thank you, xie xie ne. Thank you, Zhao lao shi. I hear that this is an important student to you and to the staff here. I would like to start by asking each staff member to share the one word on their TSM Animal Cards they are using for their OE. I want to ask them how this quality will help you and others to see the case with spontaneity and with creativity.

Mr. Huang, senior psychologist: I picked the big cat and the word says Leap. I always feel like my learning takes a big leap whenever we come together to discuss our cases and to learn more about how to help our students.

Ms. Wang, senior psychologist: I picked the two kittens that are cutting in the frying pan and the word is trust. I feel we have to trust our intuition with how to help this boy and his family, not just to follow rules from the university related to suicide prevention. I want us to trust each other as well.

Mr. Liu, a new staff member: I chose the elephant and wisdom. I want to bring the wisdom of thinking to this case. We need to think about how to help him and have a plan that takes into consideration everything. Staff members continue to share.

Dr. Kate: Great. Now, we have the strength of wisdom, trust, leaps into learning, as well as other observations from our OE cards. Imagine someone standing behind you putting their hand on your shoulder. Who is it that gives you this message about learning? Who gives you the encouragement to trust, learn, leap, and gain wisdom?

Director's Soliloquy: Using imagery helps to concretize the internal surplus reality of the OE role and helps connect it to attachment figures. Taking it interpersonally is important because learning difficulties often occur due to pressure from the culture, tradition, parents, and teachers in China.

Dr. Kate: Okay. Now share with us the role that came up for you. The roles of grandmother, Western teacher, an older sister, and a younger brother all brought the interpersonal experience of a new legacy in the surplus reality of imagination. Each person said one sentence as this interpersonal support and we could easily feel the increase in restoration, curiosity, and connection over the waves of time and space in the here and now.

I then have Zhao role play the student. Wang plays the mental health center's staff psychologist and helps the boy to pick an OE card to see his school difficulties without shaming or blaming himself. As Zhao plays the client, she demonstrates his obsessive behavior. He cannot choose a card, so the therapist asks him to just randomly choose one and to see what the message is. The therapist in the client role is surprised when the card is that of a mama bear and a cub with the word nurture on it. In the role play, Zhao feels the depth of the client's longing for nurturance and care to break up long historical patterns of perfectionism, high expectations, and physical discipline. She role reverses back to herself and there is a brief group discussion on using both the OE and then a role reversal with someone who has been nurturing or kind to him in school over the years.

Online Courses

At the time of this chapter, I have only recently taught my first online course. It spontaneously happened when my organizer in Xiamen, China, Rebecca Chang of the organization called Present, asked me if I would like to teach a course on TSM psychodrama and trauma . . . in two weeks! Responding as I always have when there is a call for TSM work I can meet, I said yes and we experimented in action about how this would work. Using the ZOOM platform for group videoconferencing, we were determined from the beginning, to not only teach via lecture and seminar, but also through action methods since TSM is always an experiential method of change. With Rebecca Zhang, owner of Present and a certified team member in TSM, as my interpreter, we taught twelve weeks of an online course where we presented powerpoints, pen and paper tools, role reversals, role plays, and ultimately an assessment of one student's TSIRA in action. While there is still much to be learned in this new format for me, it promises to combine the best of written, audio, and visual communication not only for training, but for personal growth and trauma healing.

Social Media

Like with online courses, social media such as Facebook, Instagram, Linkedin, We Chat, and other applications around the world, are fairly new to me to use in any structured way using the TSIRA. I have used them for communicating information about upcoming workshops and we have a TSM newsletter that goes out via email, once a quarter that provides teaching notes and stories about TSI community members around the world. I look forward to learning more about this intriguing form of social networking, that as J. D. Moreno (2014) says, was first started by his father, J. L. Moreno, in the early 1930s as just described. You can reach me at my Facebook page at Therapeutic Spiral Model in the Western world, and via We Chat at DrKateTSM in Asia.

Conclusion

As we conclude our time together in one of the original means of telecommunication . . . the written word . . . I want to once again anchor in the classical psychodrama concepts that guide all TSM theory and practice, but never more so than when using the new and ever-evolving technology of interpersonal communication using electronics and other methods still to come. It is clear that spontaneity and creativity are demanded at all times when using instantaneous audio and visual communications that can both start and drop out unexpectedly. As we build the roles of resilience and self-regulation through the RX roles in TSM, this chapter concludes with the suggestion of the role of IT experts both in surplus reality and in protocols for using TSM via electronic communication across states, countries, and cultures. Most of all, we can return to Moreno's concept of tele and how we can meet across the distance now more than ever. We can remember that only the spontaneous shall survive and that TSM psychodrama brings all of this together to form creative solutions to the old trauma patterns that continue to disrupt individuals, families, societies, and cultures in the global community.

This chapter has presented what will no doubt turn out to be only the first publication on TSM psychodrama and telemedicine. It brings to light both the possibilities for experiential methods in the electronic world, as well as some of the questions that remain. One of the most frequently asked questions of me is how I can ethically practice around the world as a clinical psychologist. I have to say, this is another time that psychodrama's roots as a worldwide view of training, education, and personal development has supported my work with TSM. Legally and ethically, I am an American board-certified Trainer, Educator and Practitioner of Psychodrama, Sociometry, and Group Psychotherapy with a Ph.D. in clinical psychology. I am nationally certified through the body of the American Board of Examiners in Psychodrama, Sociometry, and Group Psychotherapy (Hicks, 2016; see www.psychodramacertification.org). More recently, this national certification has become international in its efforts to regulate the development of psychodrama in Asia and around the world. I am also the co-developer of TSM (Hudgins, in press, 2002; Hudgins & Toscani, 2013) and run the TSI International Certification in Trauma Therapy (TSM, 2016) as a global health initiative (Hudgins, in press).

As you saw, psychodrama not only provided theories and concepts to guide the use of TSM methods through telemedicine, but its forward-looking regulatory structures provide guidelines for ethical practice across states, countries, cultures, and languages. It is my hope that the composite case examples will show you that the electronic world can actually serve as a powerful enhancer of therapeutic intervention, where one piggy backs on the other. When both the provider and the client learn to exercise their muscles of spontaneity to tackle the difficulties of these new technologies, creativity is enhanced, rather than disrupted. Technology now creates new and vibrant ways to provide "live" supervision, whether in one-to-one contact or small groups through videoconferences. Additionally, TSM with large groups is often transmitted as a video after a presentation to a student body or to a professional conference using various electronic platforms.

In many ways, this chapter brings up more questions than it answers about how to safely provide services via telemedicine, especially as neurobiology and attachment is concerned. However, the TSIRA continues to enlighten all trauma practice with action methods, no matter where the setting is, providing clinical safety and guidance. In moments of confusion, using a new medium for communication, you can always fall back and determine whether you are operating from your RX roles or have stepped back onto the TSM trauma triangle. In this way, the TSIRA directs all trainers, supervisions, and practitioners of TSM, as we continue to expand the model to reach beyond the current boundaries of time and space using our spontaneity and creativity. Most importantly, TSM psychodrama provides the spring board for you to use your own creativity to responsibly use the ever-expanding tools of communication to help heal trauma in the world, and to train others to do so.

REFERENCES

American Board of Examiners in Psychodrama, Sociometry, and Group Psychotherapy approved training programs: Training program resource. Retrieved October 20, 2016 from https://www.uclartsandhealing.net/view_trainingprogram .aspx?rid=15

Bashshur, R., & Shannon, G. W. (2009). *History of telemedicine: Evolution, context, and transformation.* New Rochelle:

Bennett-Levy, J., & Perry, H. (2009). The promise of online cognitive behavioural therapy training for rural and remote mental health professionals. *Australasian Psychiatry, 17*(S1). Retrieved October 20, 2016 from doi:10.1080/1039856090 2948126

Blatner, A. (2000). *Foundations of psychodrama: History, theory, and practice.* New York: Springer Publishing Company.

Buchanan, D. R. (in press). Forty years of psychodrama training at St. Elizabeths Hospital. In *Journal of Psychodrama, Sociometry and Group Psychotherapy.*

Corey, G. (2008). Psychodrama in Groups. In *Theory and practice of group counselling* (7th ed., pp. 185–215). Belmont, CA: Brooks-Cole-Thomas Learning.

Cozolino, L. J. (2014). The neuroscience of human relationships (2nd ed.). New York: W .W. Norton & Company.

Cozolino, L. J. (2016). *Why therapy works: Using our minds to change our brains.* New York: W.W. Norton & Company.

DeAngelis, T. (2012). *Practicing distance therapy, legally and ethically. Psychology is developing guidelines for practitioners in this rapidly changing area.* Retrieved November 20, 2016, from http://apa.org/monitor/2012/03/virtual.aspx

Fatehi, F., Armfield, N. R., Dimitrijevic, M., & Gray, L. C. (2015). Technical aspects of clinical videoconferencing: A large scale review of the literature. *Journal of*

Telemedicine and Telecare, 21(3), 160–166. Retrieved September 19, 2016 from doi:10.1177/1357633x15571999

Griffiths, L., Blignault, I., & Yellowlees, P. (2006). Telemedicine as a means of delivering cognitive-behavioural therapy to rural and remote mental health clients. *Journal of Telemedicine and Telecare, 12*(3), 136–140. Retrieved September 19, 2016 from doi:10.1258/135763306776738567

Gros, D. F., Yoder, M., Tuerk, P. W., Lozano, B. E., & Acierno, R. (2011). Exposure therapy for PTSD delivered to veterans via telehealth: Predictors of treatment completion and outcome and comparison to treatment delivered in person. *Behavior Therapy, 42*(2), 276–283.

Hailey, D., Roine, R., Ohinmaa, A., & Dennett, L. (2011). Evidence of benefit from telerehabilitation in routine care: A systematic review. *Journal of Telemedicine and Telecare, 17*(6), 281–287. Retrieved September 19, 2016 from doi:10.1258/jtt.2011.101208

Hick, A. (2016). *Choosing the right people to co-create with.* Workshop held January 23, 2016, North Los Angeles, CA.

Herman, J. L. (1992). *Trauma and recovery.* New York: Basic Books.

Himle, J. A., Fischer, D. J., Muroff, J. R., Etten, M. L., Lokers, L. M., Abelson, J. L., & Hanna, G. L. (2006). Videoconferencing-based cognitive-behavioral therapy for obsessive-compulsive disorder. *Behaviour Research and Therapy, 44*(12), 1821–1829. Retrieved September 19, 2016 from doi:10.1016/j.brat.2005.12.010

Hudgins, M. K. (2002). *Experiential treatment of PTSD: The therapeutic spiral model.* New York: Springer Publishing Company.

Hudgins, M. K. (2007a). Building a container with the creative arts: The therapeutic spiral model to heal post-traumatic stress in the global community. In S. Brooke (Ed.), *The use of creative therapies with sexual abuse survivors* (pp. 280–300). Springfield, IL: Charles C Thomas, Publisher.

Hudgins, M. K. (2007b). Clinical foundations of the therapeutic spiral mode: Theoretical orientations and principles of change. In C. Baim, J. Burmeister, & M. Maciel (Eds.), *Psychodrama: Advances in theory and practice* (pp. 175–188). London: Routledge Press.

Hudgins, M. K. (2008). Nourishing the young therapist: Action supervision with eating disordered clients using the therapeutic spiral model. In S. L. Brooke (Ed.), *The creative therapies with eating disorders* (pp. 254–262). Springfield, IL: Charles C Thomas, Publisher.

Hudgins, K. (2013). The spirit of trauma healing: The therapeutic spiral model. In S. B. Linden (Ed)., *The heart and soul of psychotherapy: A transpersonal approach through the arts* (pp. 361–271). Bloomington, IN: Trafford Publishing.

Hudgins, K. (2015). Spiral healing: A thread of energy and connection across cultures. In S. L. Brooke & C. E. Myers (Eds.), *Therapists creating a cultural tapestry: Using the creative therapies across cultures* (pp. 260–281). Springfield, IL: Charles C Thomas, Publisher.

Hudgins, K. (in press). PTSD unites the world: Prevention, intervention, and training in the therapeutic spiral model. In C. Stout & G. Wang (Eds.), *Why global health matters: Innovations and inspirations.* To be self-published.

Hudgins, M. K., & Drucker, K. (1998). The containing double as part of the thera-peutic spiral model for treating trauma survivors. *The International Journal of Action Methods, 51*(2), 63–74.

Hudgins, K., & Toscani, F. (Eds.). (2013). *Healing world trauma with the therapeutic spi-ral model: Stories from the front-lines.* London: Jessica Kingsley Publishers.

Hudgins, M. K., Culbertson, R., & Hug, E. (2009). *Action against trauma: A trainer's manual for community leaders following traumatic stress.* Charlottesville: University of Virginia, Foundation for the Humanities, Institute on Violence and Culture. www.lulu.com/action-against-trauma-a-trainers-manual/6009176. Accessed 5/20/12

Hudgins, M. K., Drucker, K., & Metcalf, K. (2000). The containing double: A clini-cally effective psychodrama intervention for PTSD. *The British Journal of Psychodrama and Sociodrama, 15, 1,* 58–77.

Hunkeler, E. M. (2000). Efficacy of nurse telehealth care and peer support in aug-menting treatment of depression in primary care. *Archives of Family Medicine, 9*(8), 700–708. Retrieved September 19, 2016 from doi:10.1001/archfami .9.8.700

Kellermann, P. F. (1979). Transference, counter-transference and tele. *Group Psychotherapy, Psychodrama and Sociometry, 32,* 1–12.

Kellermann, P. F., & Hudgins, M.K. (2000). (Eds.). *Psychodrama with trauma survivors: Acting out your pain.* London: Jessica Kingsley Publishers.

Khetrapal, A. (2015). *Telemedicine Benefits.* Retrieved November 20, 2016, from http://www.news-medical.net/health/Telemedicine-Benefits.aspx

Lai, N. W. (2013). A workshop using the therapeutic spiral model and art therapy with mothers and children affected by domestic violence in Taiwan. In K. Hudgins & F. Toscanin (Eds.), *Healing world trauma with the therapeutic spiral model: Stories from the front-lines* (pp. 226–240). London: Jessica Kingsley Pub-lishers.

Mitchell, J. E., Crosby, R. D., Wonderlich, S. A., Crow, S., Lancaster, K., Simonich, H., Myers, T. C. (2008). A randomized trial comparing the efficacy of cognitive–behavioral therapy for bulimia nervosa delivered via telemedicine versus face-to-face. *Behaviour Research and Therapy, 46*(5), 581–592. Retrieved September 19, 2016 from doi:10.1016/j.brat.2008.02.004

Miyazaki, M., Igras, E., Liu, L., & Ohyanagi, T. (2012). *Global Health through EHealth/ Telehealth.* EHealth and Remote Monitoring. Retrieved November 20, 2016 from doi:10.5772/47922

Moreno, J. D. (2014). *Impromptu man: J.L. Moreno and the origins of psychodrama, encounter culture, and the social network.* New York: Bellevue Literary Press.

Moreno, J. L. (1921). *Words of the father.* Beacon, NY: Beacon House Publishers.

Moreno, J. L. (1953). *Who shall survive? Foundations of sociometry, group psychotherapy and sociodrama.* Beacon, NY: Beacon House. WSS Index. ASGPP. Org, 5 July 2013. Web. 21 September, 2016

Moreno, J. L. (1964). *Psychodrama* (Vol. I, 3rd ed.). Beacon, NY: Beacon House Pub-lishing.

Moreno, J. L., & Moreno, Z. T. (1969). *Foundations of psychodrama* (Vol. 1I). Beacon, NY: Beacon House Press.

Moreno, Z. T., Blomkvist, L. D., & Rützel, E. (2000). *Psychodrama, surplus reality and the art of healing*. London: Routledge Press.

Moreno, Z. T., Horvatin, T., & Schreiber, E. (2006). *The quintessential Zerka: Writings by Zerka Toeman Moreno on psychodrama, sociometry and group psychotherapy*. London: Routledge Press.

Nelson, E., Barnard, M., & Cain, S. (2006). Feasibility of telemedicine intervention for childhood depression. *Counselling and Psychotherapy Research, 6*(3), 191–195. Retrieved September 19, 2016 from doi:10.1080/14733140600862303

Neufeld, J., & Case, R. (2013). Walk-in telemental health clinics: Improve access and efficiency: A 2-year follow-up analysis. *Telemedicine and E-Health, 19*(12), 938–941. Retrieved November 20, 2016 from doi:10.1089/tmj.2013.0076

Novotney, A. (2011). *A new emphasis on telehealth: How can psychologists stay ahead of the curve—and keep patients safe?* Retrieved November 16, 2016, from http://www.apa.org/monitor/2011/06/telehealth.aspx

Perry, R., Saby, K., Wenos, R., Hudgins, K., & Baller, M. (2016). Psychodrama intervention for female service members using the therapeutic spiral model. *The Journal of Psychodrama, Sociometry, and Group Psychotherapy, 64*(1), 11–23.

Stadler, C., Wieser, M., & Kirk, K. (Eds.). (2016). Psychodrama: Empirical research and science 2. *Psychodrama und Soziometrie, 15*(1). Retrieved November 19, 2016 from http://link.springer.com/journal/11620/15/1/suppl/page/1

Strehle, E. M., & Shabde, N. (2006). *One hundred years of telemedicine: Does this new technology have a place in paediatrics?* Retrieved November 16, 2016 from https://www.ncbi.nlm.nih.gov/pmc/articles/PMC2082971/

Terr, L. (1991). Childhood traumas: An outline and overview. *American Journal of Psychiatry, 148*(1), 10–20. doi:10.1176/ajp.148.1.10

Therapeutic Spiral International: *International certification training standards*. Retrieved November 30, 2016 from http://www.drkatehudgins.com

Wicklund, E. (2016). *On telehealth license portability, each state follows its own path*. Retrieved November 20, 2016, from http://mhealthintelligence.com/news/on -telehealth-license-portability-each-state-follows-its-own-path

Biography

Kate Hudgins, PhD, TEP, is an internationally recognized healer, consultant, author, and teacher who brings sensitivity, laughter, and deep healing to people and groups. She calls herself a blessed journeyer who has experienced the healing of her soul wounds. She describes herself as a psychospiritual practitioner, melding her rigorous study in clinical psychology with her seven years of work with an indigenous Mohawk teacher in the United States, learning from Asian masters of energy medicine for ten years, and her exposure to the traditions of Australian aboriginal elders, Buddhism, and other spiritual paths. She lives in Charlottesville, Va., with her husband and her beautiful husky dog, Spirit. For more on her work, please see her website: http://www.drkatehudgins.com

Chapter 10

ONLINE SOCIOMETRY
AND CREATIVE THERAPIES

Introduction

One of the big challenges facing all forms of therapy is how to utilize them through distance technologies. This chapter proposes a potentially exciting method that addresses both effective therapy and different technologies. Its potential lies in the knowledge that, while the method has a long-running history in the face-to-face, interpersonal realm, it has gone virtually undeveloped in online worlds. Yet, online interaction is where most of us increasingly find ourselves, both as private individuals and as professional practitioners.

The method is sociometry. It is a means of measuring the extent, and the intensity, of links that exist between individuals, dyads, and groups. This makes it ideal in online universes where, as with Facebook, with LinkedIn, or with any other form of digital interaction, connection is king. Sociometry measures the strength of the relationship–its explicit expression as well as its implicit, unconscious dimension. In short, it measures the strength of connections, both for the individual and for the collective of which an individual is part.

This chapter investigates the relationship of sociometry and digital interaction. It does so by outlining two aspects of sociometry as it applies particularly to online worlds. These aspects hold true regardless of whether online worlds are individual, dyadic, or collective, and whether they are mobilized through email, social media, instant messaging, web or mobile communication, or any other means.

The first aspect is sociometry's potential as a method of investigation and inquiry, one which can plot the distribution of likes, preferences, and often

169

hidden allegiances among any two or more individuals. Plotting provides diagrams and diagrams display visual information about a person's inner state of mind, or a network's clustering of affiliations. This has been extensively explored in face-to-face settings (Ridge, 2010), but has been almost entirely superseded in online worlds through digital analytics and network analysis, as I outline in the next section.

The second is the capacity of sociometry's parent body, psychodrama, to act as a therapeutic practice. As I will outline, this is not simply on behalf of the individual, but for the individual as in the collectives of which he or she is part. It is also to enhance the collective's broader social health in itself. Again, this has been developed extensively across the globe, over decades, where face-to-face settings are concerned (Dayton, 2005; Fonseca, 2015; Horvatin & Schreiber, 2006; Kellerman & Hudgins, 2000; Holmes, Kalp, & Watson, 2005; Williams, 1989). Yet, it is still in its infancy where online, virtual interaction is concerned. I will illustrate, using cases from supervision and healing, how these can be developed quickly and effectively.

Sociometry and Psychodrama

Sociometry is part of a larger therapeutic model: psychodrama. Psychodrama was created by Jacob Moreno, a younger contemporary of Freud's. From 1889 to 1974, he evolved it into a dynamic, eclectic set of practices that encompassed sociometry, sociodrama, role theory, and group psychotherapy (Ridge, 2010). At its heart, Moreno conceived psychodrama as a dynamic method of healing, not simply for individuals, but for society as a whole. As the twenty-year-old Moreno said, in his typically bracing way, to the fifty-six-year-old Freud in 1912:

> Well Dr. Freud, I start where you leave off. You meet people in the artificial setting of your office. I meet them on the streets and in their homes, in their natural settings. You analyze their dreams; I give them the courage to dream again. You analyze and tear them apart. I let them act out their conflicting roles and help them to put the parts back together again. (Moreno, 1989, p. 61)

Whether he was entirely accurate about Freud's method, Moreno's statement symbolizes the focus on the health of the social group; as he commented, his concern was the development of the "spontaneous, creative protagonist in the midst of a group" (Moreno 1989, p. 62). The statement also highlights Moreno's emphasis on meeting individuals in any setting and it became the heart of his sociometric exploration, carried out in schools, in hospitals, in informal groups, intraining settings, on stage, and in many other places (Moreno, 1953). Of course, in 1912, he could hardly have anticipated the rise of the Internet; yet, he was still remarkably prescient about technology. In this sense, he thought far more about the implications of technology than Freud. As he wrote in 1941,

> The technological devices which aroused man's deepest suspicion were the products of the printing press, the motion picture industry and, later, the radio; in other words, of the so-called "cultural conserves." Man, as an individual creator, was outwitted by the products of his own brain–his books, his films, his radio voice. He saw himself being more and more replaced by them. (p. 18)

He was equally sanguine about the destructive potential of the collectives which he was bent on investigating: Sociometric explorations reveal the hidden structures that provide the group with its form such as the alliances, the subgroups, the hidden beliefs, the forbidden agendas, and the ideological agreements, as well as the "stars" of the show.

A key method that Moreno created to study ties and connections was the sociogram. Remer (2008) notes that sociometry theory is focused on "measuring relationships, the purview of both social atom theory (longterm relationships and their development and maintenance over time) and sociometry (fluctuation of interpersonal connections over short periods)" (p. 390). It does so by identifying some criteria against which individual preferences can be measured. These can be simple or complex. As Remer puts it:

> for example, with whom we eat lunch; whom we marry; whom we sit next to in classes, receptions, and other meetings; whom we like and do not like (based on tele, warm-up, role reciprocity). Using both positive (choose/acceptance/attraction) and negative (not choose/rejection/repulsion) choices, the connections between people and the patterns of connections throughout groups are made manifest, explored, and influenced. (p. 390)

These choices can then be plotted and out of this emerges the sociogram (Fig. 1). The example given is Moreno's (1978 [1953], p. 133), investigating how informal power is distributed in a working-class setting: a steam laundry. As Moreno describes, one worker who is not the forewoman, has gained a surprising degree of influence to the extent that she, effectively, dominates this workplace rather than her formal boss. Of course, this is hardly uncommon in a typical workplace; what is remarkable here, is how clearly lines of interaction and influence can be delineated.

STRUCTURE OF A WORK GROUP–STEAM LAUNDRY

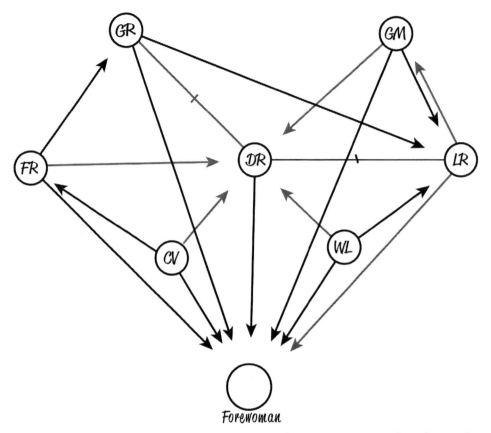

Figure 1. Structure of a work group-steam laundry (from Moreno, 1978 [1953], p. 133).

Remer's diagram, Figure 2, shows how sociograms are created and what symbols are used. As the sociograms illustrate, choices and cumulative likes and dislikes can be readily plotted to reveal how relational patterns cluster: who feels positive or negative toward others in a group; who is highly chosen (a sociometric "star") who is an isolate, and where pairs in a group exist. This is as true in Moreno's example from a steam laundry (see Fig. 1) as it is in Remer's diagram (see Fig. 2).

Sociograms can as easily be created with individuals. The one given in Figure 3 illustrates what Moreno describes as a social atom. An individual lies at the center of the atom, just like a nucleus, and significant others are arrayed at a closeness or at a distance that represents the positive or negative feelings they generate in the individual at the center. In this example, the links are be-

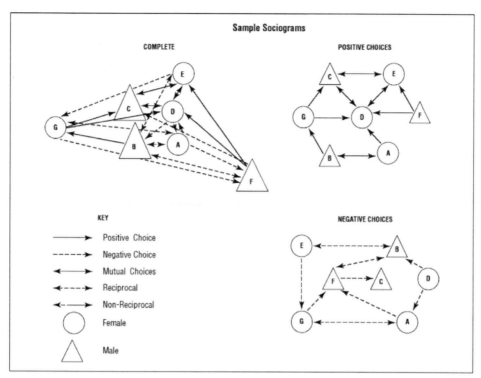

Figure 2. Creation of sociograms (from Remer, 2008, p. 291).

tween a reader and it represents the reader's fondness or indifference to a set of books he or she has read according to the books, distance from the author.

Whether it is the relationship to a book, as here, or to a set of people, a common starting point is to ask someone to locate themselves and then to place anyone, or anything, of significance in relation to them. In face-to-face settings, this can be undertaken on paper, by using other group members to represent those appearing in the sociogram, or by using objects or even small figures placed on a board. In each case, the sociogram can be enhanced by providing focusing questions that pick out the underlying criteria for an individual's choices—such as book preferences. More details can be generated by shifting which way the central individual faces by asking them to sculpt themselves or other figures to reveal the strength of underlying feelings and many other interventions.

From here, it is a small step to see how all of these methods can be easily translated to online sociograms. The added advantage online is that these diagrams can be shared, can be developed collaboratively, can be discussed, marked up, and commented on over distance. There is now a range of con-

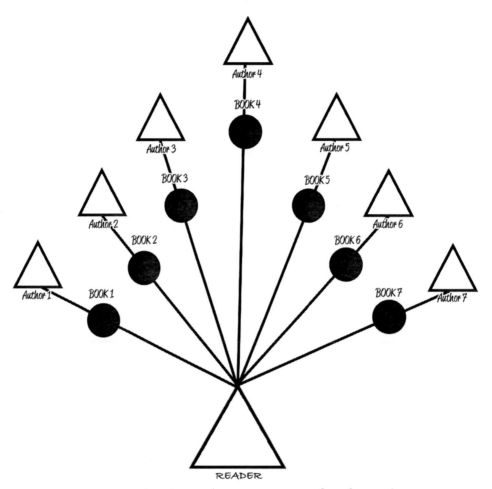

Figure 3. Social Atom (from Moreno, 1978 [1953], p. 147).

ferencing software, for example, ideally suited to just this (Weller, 2015). They can be constructed in 3D form through 3D software, or they can be utilized through video capture and screenshots, similar to professional sports team analysis (Davenport, 2014). They can also be generated dynamically through continuous real-time plotting that can be saved for later analysis. In each case, just as with face-to-face or analogue sociograms, they provide a reliable platform for therapeutic or reparative work.

Of course, this is only a small selection among a huge range of possibilities. Equally, these are face-to-face sociograms. These can readily be taken online as some sociometrists have done (Hale, 2006; Jones, n.d.). Whichever method is used, the implications of accurate measurement not just for psychodrama, but for any area of social science becomes clear, and a range of sociologists, social psychologists, anthropologists, and others, have not been slow to grasp this (Jones, 2006).

Alongside this has been the comprehensive development of network analysis across a large area of the social sciences. This has rapidly proliferated from a focus on social network analysis beginning in the 1930s among sociologists and anthropologists, to a variety of online applications. Borgatti, Brass, and Halgin (2014) and Watts (2004) are two extensive reviews. There has been a subsequent and massive development of network analysis that moves well beyond social networks to computer and network systems, to biological mapping, and to a diversity of other alternatives. For instance, Carley (2003) lists dynamic network analysis (DNA), a scientific field that brings together traditional social network analysis (SNA), link analysis (LA), and social simulation and multi-agent systems (MAS) within network science and network theory.

Equally, the emergence of the Internet and social media has vastly superseded not simply the measurement of interactions, but also the dynamic, moment-to-moment tracking of individual preferences. Since dynamic tracking often takes place in the commercial domain, for example by way of Google or Facebook, the opportunity to monetize these relationships, and on-sell the results to advertisers, is central to their business models. They utilize sophisticated mathematical tools that have become the cornerstones of social media and online data analysis (SocialGraphProject, 2010). The acceleration in the growth of "analytics" as they are often called, has been so startling, that it has led the commentator Fisher (2011) to ask, "will an analytics overload hurt social media?" She has in mind such technologies as Facebook Insights, Google Analytics, Web Analytics, Social Media Analytics, and infographics, let alone other search or social media tools such as Alexa, Compete, Quantcast, Google Trends for Websites, or Google Ad Planner, to name just a handful.

Sociometrists are unable to compete with these armies of analysts and their complex tools, they have not attempted this, which poses a dilemma where creative therapies are concerned. How can effective online work be undertaken when the tools of investigation needed to pinpoint and to diagnose therapeutic problems remain undeveloped? Before turning to individual and collective forms of intervention and therapy, it is worth outlining some strategies that are feasible and practical.

Sociometric Approaches to Online Investigation

One is simply to utilize, and to piggyback on, the sophisticated digital tools available online. Many of these are free and are readily available. Sites such as Webanalysis or mashable, for instance, list a variety of alternatives. Facebook has *Facebook Insight* which includes details such as the total number of comments or wall posts on your site; statistics on the gender and age of your fans; scores measuring how engaging your content is to Facebook users; how many times your page has been rated in the reviews application, and so forth—all of interest to sociometrists (Smallbiztrends, 2010). The second is to exclude, if only temporarily, some kinds of internet activity as incompatible with sociometry objectives. I am thinking, for example, of web marketing, which has, at best, a debatable relationship with spontaneity and with creativity in the forms that Moreno (1978 [1953]) has defined them.

A third solution is to acknowledge that sociometry, historically, has worked within relatively bounded worlds, if only because of the computing limitations that it was originally faced with. By comparison, the Internet and social media are effectively unbounded. Placing bounds on a sociometric investigation allows us to study the group or community we have selected without the danger of constant dissipation of the community with which we are working. This procedure still enables us to extrapolate our results, or to revisit our assumptions, at a later date. In addition, it is the way in which much online social network analysis already works (Catanese, De Meo, Ferraras, Fiumare, & Prouett, 2011; Liben-Nowell & Kleinberg, 2008).

A fourth solution is to consider social media such as Facebook not as a whole, but as a complex of communities and subgroups, each interacting with others. Seen this way, it allows us to identify, select, and engage particular networks or interactive communities rather than to confront one massive online population. It also has the advantage of drawing on an another sociometric principle. This is the implicit and instant quality of positive or negative tele. *Tele,* a term coined by Moreno, equates the instant, precognitive humans have to each other: similar, for example, to the look across a crowded room that instantly joined the medieval poet Dante to his Beatrice. This, in Morenean terms, is an example of positive tele where no words are spoken but where an instant bond is established between two people.

Fifth, and most importantly, the focus of sociometry differs, at root, to the aims of most social media. Moreno frequently emphasizes the role of sociometry (Moreno, 1978 [1953], pp. xxi, 118–120, 378), with its roots in religious and axiological planes (pp. xx–xxi). He emphasizes the quality of human relationships: their spontaneity, their creativity, and their strengthening of social relatedness. Sociometry measures this in order for us to expand and to enhance these capacities. Social media certainly encourages connectedness, and online tools measure their degree of effectiveness. Beyond this general goal, more specific objectives are either unstated or left over to individual social media forms. Google's well-known, aspiration, "don't be evil," is a celebrated case in point. However, this is a far cry from Moreno's (p. xxi) aims "to co-exist, co-create and co-produce" in the pursuit of an ideal community. As he put it (p. xxxiii), "The burning problem now, as it was then, is the combination of two variables, the healer and an adequate theory or method."

These orientations are the key to finding a useful and influential place for sociometry online. It enables us to keep Moreno's vision and method in mind whilst we engage with the social media world. This is despite the concerns over the massification of online users, the emotional contagion or algorithmic manipulation that social media sites can generate (Kramer, Guillory, & Hancock, 2014). Facebook, for example, is not a single entity but a nested population of intersecting, overlapping connections. These connections rely on the strength or weakness of individuals' tele and their criteria for choosing or rejecting others: they form the hidden links that create or that sustain online community. Knowing this, we can begin to engage or assist these networks by using the range of psychodrama tools already at our disposal. We can begin to double, mirror, or role reverse with them just as we might face-to-face in order to begin our engagement. We can act as auxiliaries, coaching, modeling, or role playing as required of us. All that differs in this activity is that it takes place online or through particular communication media. This can be by text, messaging, or chat forms, or through images, video, or audio exchanges by means of posting and downloads rather than face-to-face.

Working like this, we can identify a community, invite, or accept its invitation for an encounter and act as an ongoing auxiliary. This clarifies how little difference there is to between sociometry face-to-face and what can be practiced online. For instance, Facebook has as many different kinds of communities online as there are face-to-face. Online, we can find hugely different communities of interest: flower arrangers, photographers, space-gazers, foodies, or petrolheads, to name a very few. There are occupational communities numbering scientists, hairdressers, seismologists, professional philosophers, counselors, or master electricians among them (Ebizma, 2015, for example, gives current lists of social media sites). Each of the participants on Facebook, or on any form of social media, form affiliates with others on the basis of criteria identical to those identified for any form of sociometry.

From Sociometry to Online Intervention

To repeat Moreno (1978 [1953], p. xxi), "The burning problem now, as it was then, is the combination of two variables, the healer and an adequate theory or method." The value of a sociogram is that it reveals the weighting and clustering of emotional preferences, whether for an individual or between several members of a group. This, in turn, begins to reveal disharmonies, imbalances, or congruences, based on any given pattern of preferences displayed by the sociogram.

One way in which this can be explored, prior to therapeutic intervention, is by identifying what aspects of an individual are overdeveloped, absent, underdeveloped, or emerging. This is the domain of role theory, as it is known in psychodrama. As Moreno (1964, p. 153) expressed it, "Role can be defined as the actual and tangible forms which the self takes . . . the functioning form the individual assumes in reacting to a specific situation in which other persons or objects are involved." Such a definition at once, places individuals in relation to each other, so that a "role," an aspect of self, always emerges through interaction, even if it is a silent one, with others.

A therapeutic intervention does not necessarily require a knowledge of role theory. However, it is one highly effective way of defining "an adequate theory or method," as many of its practitioners have demonstrated (Clayton, 1982, 1994). Nor do interventions necessarily require a knowledge of psychodrama; the method can be used in conjunction with other approaches, such as CBT or Cognitive Behavioral Therapy (Colwell, 2010). What sociometry provides is evidence about the way components of a group, collective, dyad, or an individual psyche are functioning–whether an individual is beginning to fragment because of trauma or psychological pressures they are experiencing, or whether they are developing a new, embryonic capacity to function. The same applies with groups, or even with organizations (Blumberg & Hare, 1999). Sociometric analysis discloses whether these develop a cohesion and flexibility, even in complex systems, or whether a group or organizational climate is constantly undermined by clusters of subgroups and hidden allegiances based on suspicion and envy.

A key way in which all of this can be translated to online environments, is through the notion of relationship which, as noted, is central to the concept of sociometry. From here, with an understanding of the relationship between healer (usually known as the director or producer in psychodrama) and individuals, it is possible to develop highly sensitized means of intervention. Intervention, in psychodrama, is usually termed *production* since its organizing metaphor came originally via drama and the stage. Consequently, psychodrama, as an expressive method, deploys instruments of the drama: doubling, role reversal, "scenes" or sequences of action, soliloquys, asides, and many other methods (Blatner, 2000); yet, each of these techniques is premised on relational interactions.

For example, if we return to the sociogram of Moreno's steam room depicted earlier, the sociogram offers a wealth of potential interventions. In

Moreno's day, these would have been enacted face-to-face, but many of the same interventions could be produced online. Where the sociogram depicts the powerful informal influence of a worker rather than the formally appointed forewoman, it suggests further means of investigation. Did the sociogram display a constructive or dysfunctional workplace; were the alliances it portrayed implicit or explicit; were there specific moments where these relationships obstructed or assisted the work? If these individuals were still alive and could be contacted online, we could develop these questions with them and draw out an even more in-depth, more dynamic map of their relationships.

From investigative questions based on the plotted relationships, hypotheses about effective interventions can be readily generated. For instance, a psychodrama director might want to reproduce a salient moment when work production suffered because of these relationships; or to engage the forewoman's sense of self through her role system or by investigating in action exactly how weak or resilient her connections to her colleagues. Often, of course, these may be based on nonwork relationships from which the forewoman may be excluded: for example, among women who are married with children or who are single. Whatever the case, a sociometrist or psychodramatist will be interested in the formal and informal system of relations and how, for example, they create or impede lively, productive teamwork. In this context, the teamwork could as easily be online or globally distant: the same system of relations, whether these are between information technology specialists or regional managers, will apply. In turn, these provide openings for investigation and action.

In what follows, I will outline a variety of interventions. I will also emphasize that psychodrama methods can, in many cases, be translated into other therapeutic approaches. For instance, psychodrama is identical to other psychotherapies in identifying nonverbal cues, working with symbolic material, attending to signs of trauma, engaging with intergenerational dynamics, or engaging with powerful affect (Fonagy, Gergelvi, Juiist, & Target, 2002; Schore, 2003; van Meurs, Reef, Verhulst, & Van der Ende, 2009). As with many other modalities, there has been a trade in techniques: Moreno, for example, invented the empty chair method, but this is now a staple in Gestalt. Often differences reside in terminology and in practices. For example, psychotherapists frequently refer to family of origin where as psychodrama refers to the original social and cultural atom. Broadly speaking, the concepts are similar, with a close attention to family dynamics, but their working-out and enactment, may differ (Blatner, 2000).

In the next section, I illustrate how one simple concept of relationship functions as both a guide to intervention, and as a monitor to the verbal and nonverbal interactions that emerge from interventions. I do so by focusing on a particular distance case study with an individual as an illustration. The value of following the relationship in this context is to sustain a focus on how therapeutic or reparative work takes place regardless of medium. In other words, it demonstrates how one can move from face-to-face interactions to repeatable cycles of investigation, analysis, and intervention over distance.

Sociometry Over Distance: A Case Example

I begin with a sociogram generated by a client. From here, I will discuss how it can be translated into forms of broader psychotherapy engagement. I will also illustrate how this illuminates the role of multiple technologies in terms of the different modes of communication which take place between us.

Sarah is a client I initially saw face-to-face in my practice. However, she moved to another city and we agreed to continue weekly sessions using Skype. Sarah, in her mid-40s, came from a highly dysfunctional family. Although the eldest, she was bullied by her younger brothers who were indirectly supported by her father. He had also abused her as a child, while her mother was neglectful and self-absorbed, expecting Sarah to be available anytime she needed her. Sarah, herself, was a very able child and succeeded at school, although this only reinforced the envy and jealousy of her brothers. Her main source of support in these very difficult circumstances were aunts, but she saw them infrequently. While she recalls them with fondness, they were too distant to be readily available. She saw me initially to deal with her persistent depression, and because of the anxiety she was experiencing with a partner who had a life-threatening illness.

We could plot Sarah's relationships using either a genogram or a sociogram. The one displayed, however (see Fig. 4), depicts a sociogram she drew for me based on her current relationships.

This is illuminating for a number of reasons. First, it was completed when we were doing distance therapy; it was easy for her to complete and she could simply attach her rough sketch to an an email (which I have reproduced here using drawing software). Second, it shows her positive and negative feelings toward significant figures in her current social atom, with herself at the center. Each figure is also at a different distance from Sarah, showing her warmth or coldness toward them. It also includes plus and minus symbols indicating if she believes that the feeling is reciprocated. In other words, the sociogram instantly conveys considerable information through a simple sketch. In addition, it conveys the strength of a relationship regardless of time or space. For example, in terms of time, her father had long died when this was completed, and her mother was recently deceased. In terms

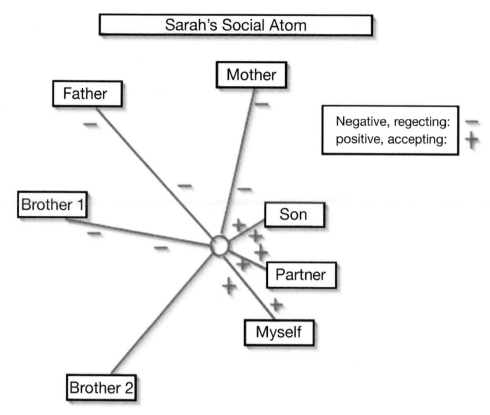

Figure 4. Sarah's Social Atom.

of space, only her partner was in the same city; even her son was continually on the move. Yet, we can immediately see how strong or distant each relationship is regardless of time or space; and online sociometry enhances this capacity since it works outside of the constraints of physical location. So, the sociogram represents continuing live feelings for past as well as for present figures. The sociogram could have been extended in numerous ways. One, for example, would be by asking Sarah to delineate the relationships between her father and mother; or between her parents and their other children, or between her siblings—information which was implicit in our conversations.

For Sarah, the sociogram was immediately therapeutic: she could concretize these relationships by sketching them. They became real in a new way for her and mobilized a capacity to think and to reflect on them symbolically. In effect, this promoted a process of mentalizing (Fonagy, Gengely, Jurish, & Tarseti, 2002). In addition, the simple, tangible image of the sociogram provided a form of stability for her.

In the distance work we were doing, it also provided me with further ways to intervene and to inquire. It also provided us with a shared, available resource that either of us could consult. I could ask about the strength of her connections to any figure in the sociogram. I could ask her to recall significant moments that crystalized these relationships. Or, I could ask her what it meant for her to cluster her partner, son, and myself so near to each other. Each of these questions opened up projections and transferences as it enabled me to ask, for example, what connection between her son and her father might be, or what parallels she saw between them, or what intergenerational transmission might have taken place. Her son, a young adult, had moved into a healing profession and it was easy to see that, as a child, he had responded to her unverbalized needs for comfort and for affection that was unavailable in her family of origin. Equally, he had chosen a profession that, in effect, promised to undo the kinds of wounds her family had inflicted on her.

As a therapist, I also received a new source of countertransferential information from the sociogram. What were my own responses to where I had been placed? This was next to her partner, which hinted at an erotic transference partly unavailable with him because of his illness. It was also as distantly opposite her father as was possible: so I could become more aware of an idealizing transference as the good father. I was already aware of her heavy burden of expectations on me: I was to be the healer who, perhaps magically, resolved all of the transferential longings she had experienced, but the sociogram helped confirm this.

And it is here that one significance of a distance sociogram becomes clear. Sarah was physically distant from me, despite the use of Skype, it minimized the nonverbal signifiers of empathy—the precise tones of voice, and our bodily presence in the same room, let alone the interruptions caused by Skype communication. In addition, there were fluctuations in connection, dropouts, delays, and frozen screens, or absent sound and vision. In a sense, I became a subtly unavailable figure because the technology constructed our relationship this way.

Inevitably, this has expressed itself: her disappointments and anger toward me came either directly through unaccountably missed sessions, through delays in connections, or through emotional dropouts, in effect. They became expressed more implicitly through the technology itself: at moments, the picture would freeze, or the sound would disappear, or both would go out of phase in ways which reproduced, indirectly, the charged nature of the emotional content between us.

In later sessions, her cat began to appear onscreen and, I hypothesized, became a self-object (Kohut, 1984) as it snuggled into her shoulder, replacing me at times as a warm, constant, soothing presence. Nonetheless, our relationship has endured and, in enduring, it has allowed her a slow mourning for what our therapeutic relationship could not replace in her early life. Through this, she has been able to develop the success that her early talent promised; her husband's illness has continued but they have jointly addressed and accommodated this. The work is not yet over, and a more recent sociogram might indicate how her figural relationships have since changed.

One other point is worth noting. This is how the relationship, and by extension the therapy, was carried and shaped by distance technologies. Prime among these was Skype, but there was also email. This not only carried Sarah's attachment to me but it acted, in the setting of appointment times, to sustain a background tempo of barely visible interaction. I was constantly aware; however, of responding quickly and consistently, since the replies themselves constituted a form of affective self-other regulation between Skype calls (Schore 2003). The same was true with short messaging service messaging which, on occasion, we also used. As with email, it formed a constant, slow pulse: a ticking-over the relationship and a reminder of my continuing presence even at distance. Placed against Sarah's early neglectful and sometimes intrusive mother, it formed a means of therapeutic repair.

Conclusion

This chapter has described a new use for an existing method: deploying sociometry in the context of digital technologies. What it illustrates is how a long-standing face-to-face approach can be readily translated not simply to online environments, but to a variety of relational contexts: individual, dyadic, and collective. As emphasised by Moreno, it is with the aim of relieving social and individual suffering rather than, as with digital analytics, interrogating social formations or network configurations. Sociometry, as developed by Moreno, also moves from a process of investigation, utilized primarily through sociograms, to a means of intervention and assistance. As the case example illustrates, sociograms can quickly reveal a wealth of emotional and dynamic information, not just about an individual, but about the family, social, or work systems of which they are part. Because of the key emphasis on relationship, this is as effectively carried out online and across distance as it is in person. Moreover, it alerts therapists to how these dynamics may become shaped by the very technologies that carry them. In short, sociometry suggests itself as a valuable and reliable method regardless of the therapeutic modality that employs it.

REFERENCES

Blatner A. (2000). *Foundations of psychodrama: History, theory, practice* (4th ed.). New York: Springer.

Blumberg, H., & Hare, P. (1999, Spring). Sociometry applied to organizational analysis: A review. *The International Journal of Action Methods, 52*(10), 55.

Borgatti, S. P., Brass, D. J., & Halgin, D. S. (2014). Social network research: Confusions, criticisms, and controversies. In D. J. Brass, G. Labianca, A. Mehra, D. S. Halgin, & S. P. Borgatti (Eds.), *Research in the sociology of organizations* (Vol. 40, pp. 1–33). Bradford, UK: Emerald Publishing.

Carley, K. (2003). Dynamic network analysis. In R. Breiger, K. Carley, & P. Philippa (Eds.), *Dynamic social network modeling and analysis: Workshop summary and papers* (pp. 133–145). National Research Council. Washington, DC.

Catanese, S., De Meo, P., Ferrara, E., Fiumara, G., & Provetti, A. (2011). *Crawling Facebook for social network analysis purposes.* Paper presented to the International Conference on Web Intelligence, Mining and Semantics, May 31.

Clayton, L. (1982). The use of the cultural atom to record personality change in individual psychotherapy. *Journal of Group Psychotherapy, Psychodrama and Sociometry, 35*(3), 111–117.

Clayton, M. (1994). Role theory and its application in clinical practice. In P. Holmes, M. Karp, & M. Watson (Eds.), *Innovations in theory and practice: Psychodrama since Moreno* (pp. 121–144). London: Routledge.

Colwell, J. (2010). *Integrating Morenian role theory and cognitive behaviour therapy with Babushka dolls: An example of healthy role development in individual counselling.* Thesis presented to the Board of Examiners of the Australian and New Zealand Psychodrama Association.

Davenport, T. H. (2014). Analytics in sports: The new science of winning, *International Institute for Analytics.* Retrieved from: http://www.sas.com/content/dam/SAS/en _us/doc/whitepaper2/iia-analytics-in-sports-106993.pdf

Dayton, T. (2005). *The Living Stage: A step-by-step guide to psychodrama, sociometry and experiential group therapy.* Deerfield Beach, FL: Health Communications.

Ebizma. (2015). Top 15 most popular social networking sites, June 2015. Retrieved from http://www.ebizmba.com/articles/social-networking-websites

Fisher, L. (2011). Will an analytics overload hurt social media? Retrieved from http://www.socialnomics.net/2011/06/07/10-wow-social-media-statistics/

Fonagy, P., Gergely, G., Jurist, E. L., & Target, M. (2002). *Affect regulation, mentalization and the development of the self.* New York: Other Press.

Fonseca, J. (2015). *Contemporary psychodrama: New approaches to theory and technique.* New York: Brunner-Routledge.

Hale, A. (2006). Sociometry: Expanding on the meaning of the term. International Sociometry Training Network. Retrieved from http://www.sociometry.net/odules.php?name=Content&pa=showpage&pid=20

Holmes, P., Karp, M., & Watson, M. (Eds.). (2005). *Psychodrama since Moreno: Innovations in theory and practice.* New York: Routledge.

Horvatin, T., & Schreiber, E. (2006). *The quintessential Zerka: Writings by Zerka Toeman More no on psychodrama, sociometry and group psychotherapy.* London: Routledge.

Jones, D. (2006). *Exploring social networks–The third entity in the dyad: The relationship.* Paper presented to the INSNA Conference, Vancouver, April. Retrieved from http://www.jones.org.nz

Jones, D. (n.d.). Sociometry–Making sense of the invisible dynamics in work groups. Retrieved from http://www.sociometry.co.nz/index.htm

Kellermann, P. F., & Hudgins, M. K. (Eds.). (2000). *Psychodrama with trauma survivors: Acting out your pain.* London: Jessica Kingsley Publishers.

Kohut, H. (1984). *How does analysis cure?* Chicago: University of Chicago Press.

Kramer, A., Guillory, J. E., & Hancock, J. T. (2014). Experimental evidence of massive-scale emotional contagion through social networks. *PNAS, 111*(24), 8788–8790.

Liben-N. D., & Kleinberg, J. (2008). Tracing information flow on a global scale using Internet chain-letter data. *PNAS, 105*(12): 4633–4638.

Moreno, J. L. (1934). *Who shall survive?* Washington, DC: Nervous and Mental Disease Publishing Co.

Moreno, J. L. (1941). Foundations of sociometry: An introduction. *Sociometry, 4*(1), 15–35.

Moreno, J. L. (1964). *Psychodrama first volume* (3rd ed.). Beacon, NY: Beacon House Inc.

Moreno, J. L. (1978 [1953]). *Who shall survive?* Beacon, NY: Beacon House Inc.

Psychodrama and sociometry. Retrieved from http://asgpp.org/pdf/Ridge%20Journal .pdf

Moreno, J. L. (1989). The autobiography of JL Moreno, MD (abridged). *Journal of Group Psychotherapy, Psychodrama, & Sociometry, 42*(1), 52.

Remer, R. (2008). Sociometry. *International Encyclopedia of the Social Sciences* (2nd ed.). MacMillan International, n.p. Retrieved from http://www.uky.edu/~rremer /sociometry/Sociometry.pdf

Ridge, R. (2010, May). A literature review of psychodrama. *Journal of Group Psychotherapy.* Retrieved on January 16, 1917 from http://asgpp.org/pdf/Ridge%20 Journal.pdf

Schore, A. (2003). *Affect dysregulation and disorders of the self.* New York: Norton.

Smallbiztrends. (2010). Getting your feet wet in facebook analytics. Retrieved from http://smallbiztrends.com/2010/08/getting-your-feet-wet-in-facebook-analytics .html

SocialGraphProject. (2010). The history of social network analysis. December 10. Retrieved from http://socialgraphproject.org/blog/2010/12/the-history-of -social-network-analysis/

van Meurs, I., Reef, J., Verhulst, F. D., & Van der Ende, J. (2009). Intergenerational transmission of child problem behaviors: A longitudinal, population-based study. *Journal of the American Academy of Child & Adolescent Psychiatry, 48*(2), 138–145.

Watts, D. (2004). The 'new' science of networks. *Annual Review of Sociology, 30,* 243–270.

Weller, N. (2015). The 15 best webinar software products from around the web. Elegant Themes Blog, January. Retrieved from https://www.elegantthemes.com/blog/resources/the-15-best-webinar-software-products-from-around-the-web

Williams, A. (1989). *The passionate technique: Strategic psychodrama with individuals, families, and groups.* New York: Tavistock/Routledge.

Biography

John Farnsworth, PhD is a registered psychotherapist with an extensive background in psychodrama. He works in private practice in Dunedin, Florida (http://www.555george.co.nz) and has published extensively in the fields of psychotherapy, psychodrama, sociology, and media studies. He is also associated with the University of Otago through its Media, Film and Communication Department and is a member of NZAP, AANZPA, and IARPP.

Chapter 11

UNPACKING SHAME AND HEALTHY SHAME: THERAPY ON THE PHONE OR INTERNET

SHEILA RUBIN

I begin this chapter about the Internet with the fact that my clients think I am a Luddite. I grew up with a wall phone telephone that, by definition, was attached to the wall. At most, we could stand a few feet from the wall, with a few inches of cord linking us to the phone. This was in a time even before answering machines. I came of age andstudied radio and television in college during a black-and-white portapack video machine that was heavy, where we actually spliced tape with our fingers—just before electronic news-gathering. Response time to a letter was a couple of days to a couple of weeks. I am fully aware that the words I am writing here will likely be out-moded as technology changes even before the book is out in the world. I have accepted the use of a smartphone into my private practice along with doing therapy over the phone or Skype if I have met the client at least once in person. I have come a long way!

Speed

Something has speeded up. Instant responses are expected. I am out of the office, but my clients know I have a cell phone. There is an expectation to respond to them instantly, and I have set a boundary that I respond dur-ing office hours only.

Communication with Clients via Email

I conduct group therapy and the bonding that happens during group therapy in my office leads people to begin to hear each other's stories. Each person slowly begins to trust that the other group members are truly present, listening to his or her story. At the end of each group or at some point in the middle, they ask for each other's email addresses and, with everyone's permission, I provide them. This is a way for group members to get support from each other between sessions. Facilitating this means of communication "grows" their resourcefulness and increases the number of people with whom they feel safe.

Who Wants Therapy over the Internet?

People who live far away, people who do not have time to drive to a therapist's office, and people who are shy, comprise the population of those who request therapy via the Internet. I use the word shy to describe people who may feel uncomfortable or even ashamed about what they want to talk about "in private." The Internet provides a safe venue in which shy people may feel safer about seeking help. In working with shy people, I use extra care to welcome them, to help them feel safe, and am aware of the fact that they may, at some point, reveal their shameful feelings.

Containment

I foster a sense of containment in the group that meets in person by beginning with sitting in a circle and by starting with a brief meditation and check-in period. Group members look around and feel familiar faces. I have learned what not to do in an initial meeting. In one of my newly formed groups, one client excitedly gave everyone her email and started communicating with group members in a way that did not foster mutual support, but that began to undermine it. In a manic-type response to some event in her life, an hour before the group was to begin, she would email the whole group. "I'm not coming to group tonight. I had a fight with my husband." People responded, "We'll miss you." That exchange was followed by another member's email: "I'm tired from flying, just got back to town. Need to take tonight off." What followed was a flurry of others sending the group emails; the third person sent an email, "I'm too tired to drive there. See you all next week." Then the next one came. "Don't feel like meeting tonight." The flurry of emails and responses built in a direction. That was not the direction I had intended. This caused splitting, as she was busy emailing to another group member rather than getting the support from the group where I had some containment and could offer better support. I learned to tell that client to contact me one-to-one if she was not going to class and to not contact the others until after the group was over.

Therapy on the Phone or Internet

On both the phone and the Internet, is how I work with individuals or couples. I find that I check more often for feelings that I might be able to sense when working face-to-face. I slow the pace down and tend to do more somatic work, asking clients to ground and to sense somatically for part of the session. I always ask at the end, "What are you taking from this session? What was helpful?" I also give homework after each session. For example, "Make a list of the coping skills from the session and put them on your calendar day by day, or take the powerful objects from this session and put them out in your room at home with a note by each to remind you what each part said to you today." Or, I suggest that they find an object to represent the shy part of their self that is afraid to speak and take the card we wrote today and put it next to it. I direct them to practice it in the mirror before they talk to their boss.

Concerns about Technology

What about when technology fails . . . when a person just revealed something that has been hidden and Skype freezes? In the middle of a session, a husband was telling his wife why he had trouble when she touched him. Suddenly, the screen froze and this tender moment was interrupted with my frantically trying to call them on Skype, which would not reconnect. I had to call them on my cell phone, the tender moment had passed and they were fighting again. I had to slow it down and gently find the words to tell them about the negative cycle their communication was in and how to do a repair to get out of it.

Shame is the rupture of the interpersonal bridge, says Kaufman (1974, 1992). Any disruption in connection with a significant other can disconnect the person from himself or herself, or the therapist, and activate the feeling of shame. What I realized was I had to let them know ahead of time the constraints and the benefits of using the phone or Skype for therapy. It will save them time coming to my office when they are in a difficult place in the relationship, but it may not be as contained as an in-person session. One couple was struggling with the husband having an online affair and the wife needing to see his phone to be reassured that he was not meeting the woman. I spoke slowly and carefully to them to get an agreement before we began to talk. "Because we are not face-to-face, I can't just interrupt you if there is shouting. I am going to do the session slowly and have you repeat what you hear the other person saying so that I can know you heard them and they can know that you heard them. We are going to take turns. Are you both in agreement? Because the phone is not a predictable medium, each of us is on a cell phone, if one of us gets disconnected for any reason we need to have a plan. Are each of you near a home or office line? If someone's line dies, we will momentarily stop the session and I will wait for the call from the person who was disconnected. Call me back on your office phone and I will use my phone to accept both calls."

Shame

Shame can be right there in the shadows. It is easy for misunderstanding. When I cannot see the emotion on clients' faces, I do not know what they are experiencing and truly expressing. In the book, *Shame and Pride* Nathanson (1992) explained that throughout life we are balancing between pride when we are seen in a good light, and shame when we make a mistake and are seen in a less than favorable light. Fosha (1992) later wrote that we would call this our "self at best" and our "self at worst." We strive to be seen as smart or clever or helpful, but when a mistake is made and something is unclear, suddenly the person is risking being exposed and seen as self at worst. This concept is helpful to remember as a client is sharing vulnerable revelations. I know from my own vulnerability how scary it can be to be exposed at the wrong time or without kindness and support.

Skype Therapy

I have done consultation for colleagues as well as therapy sessions on Skype. The good news is that Skype can serve as a bridge between family members who are not living within driving distance of one another. It can also get in the way of direct eye contact and physical contact that those family members long for. It proved to be very therapeutic for an elder client to see her grandchild over Skype, even though she believed it would not "do the trick." She had been hurting because her son did not call her as often after the baby came and that the other grandparent was invited and she was not. We role-played her talking to her son, but nothing shifted. She still felt left out, like something was wrong with her for not being chosen to spend time with the new family. We unpacked under all the feelings of anger toward her son for not insisting that his wife invite her at the same time as the other grandparents and under that was the feeling of shame. She felt ashamed to not be invited and fought with him on the phone when they did talk. I asked her to role-play talking to her son in a way that invited a solution instead of blaming him for her frustration. I invited her to role play the visit with the grandchild. She rocked back and forth. Finally, I suggested that she use Skype as a way to visit her grandchild. She told me that I did not understand. She wanted to pick her up and rock her in her lap in the rocking chair. I invited her to try just one phone visit on Skype with her son and grandchild. She sat in the rocking chair at her home and rocked. She was delighted to see her grandchild recognize his grammy over Skype. This experience fulfilled her longing to visit with her grandchild. There were many Skype visits thereafter. Her feelings of shame about being left out decreased and invites to visit increased.

Containment

Please note that I only do sessions remotely if I have met with the client in my office and we have developed a solid therapeutic container first. When the client is in my office, I can observe a range of nonverbal cues and get a sense of his or her energy. Over the phone, there are subtle cues I may miss. Here are ways in which I work with the absence of the visual modality. Because I am not seeing them, there are strategies I practice to contain the energy of the session and the pace of the session. Since the client is not seeing me, there are ways in which I want to structure the session to help them feel me where they are sitting.

Case Example of Phone Session

This client was feeling dark; her boyfriend was spending time with his ex-lover again instead of going on the date they had planned.

Client: He's still in the role of letting his ex-partner rely on him. I couldn't stop crying for hours. My emotions got all wacky or something. I see his side when he's helping his kids. But every act of his kindness is an act of affection toward his ex. One day its good between us, and the next day I feel ignored, neglected.

Therapist: How about if you choose something in your room to represent your feeling neglected and ignored?

Client: OK, this plant.

Therapist: Can you move it near you and look closer at it? And as you are looking at it, what does it say to you? What does it symbolize?

Client: You have to pay attention to a flower. You have to water it or it dies!

Therapist: So that is a very powerful symbol of needing to be tended and cared for.

(I wanted to pause and have her reflect on the importance of her attachment needs. She really wanted to just rush past them in the session. Choosing an object helped me direct the session to make space for that subject. The act of choosing something took her into another part of her brain where creativity was more open to her. Having a symbol can be a very powerful metaphor. Having it in front of her helped her to focus on it during the whole session). [You might add commentary in places; here, for example, I wanted you to explicitly see how her selection and answer helped you compensate for the absence of one-on-one perceptions. Indent your commentary and use brackets, as I've done here.]

Client: Yes! I want to be cared for. But when I feel this way, I don't feel like myself. It feels like I don't exist. It's too painful when he says he's coming over and then he cancels because he's with his ex-lover. Why am I punishing myself? I could go out and be in another relationship!

Therapist: So there is another part of you that does not want to be punished any more, that wants to find another relationship, one where the guy is choosing you instead of choosing his ex. Can you look around the room and find an object that represents this part of you? (This is another place where I wanted to pause the session and give her time to feel the power of what she just said. I want a symbol for that part so that we can talk to that part as well, maybe have a conversation with both of them.)

Client: This candle!

Therapist: Can you put the candle in front of you and look at it? What does it represent?

Client: (*Surprised*) There's a light in it! I can attract things . . . people! But I'm not ready to move on.

Therapist: Can you give each a voice? What does the flower say and what does the candle say to you? (The candle told her that she is bright inside when she is not so depressed worrying what is going on with this guy she is dating. It gives her inspiration to grow herself and to step out of the relationship to a real relationship where someone could really be available for her. As she was expressing this, another feeling showed up.)

Client: I feel deep anxiety.

Therapist: Where is the anxiety in your body?

Client: My diaphragm.

Therapist: Can you put some space around it and take some slow deep breaths?

Client: I'm not being logical. I should just leave him. But I don't want to leave him. He says kind things to me, offers to work it out. I really care about him. He's clear about his intention that he wants to be with me!

Therapist: There are a lot of conflicting feelings. (Because we are on the phone, I want to keep the connection and let her know that I am here and that I hear her.)

Client: I'm scared. Lonely.

Therapist: Yes, there's a part that's scared and lonely. (I want to support this part.)

Client: It's like a pouting child! (And it feels like she is putting down that part. It is like some part of her is shaming that part of her for wanting what she is wanting.)

Therapist: I wonder, I'm curious if there is some shame around that part.

Client: Yes.

Therapist: Can you look around and find an object to represent the part that comes out and shames you when you talk about your attachment needs?

Client: (*Apparently looking around her room for a few moments*) A hat.

Therapist: How does a hat represent shame?

Client: I put it on myself! I have a hard time asking him to meet my needs and I'm scared that they won't get met again. That he'll cancel plans with me again!

Therapist: Maybe the shame comes out to put you down for feeling what you are feeling?

Client: Yes. If I'd recognize those things, logically I would leave.

Therapist: That inner conflict is so painful. So one part of you shames you for having normal wants and needs from him and when you think he lies again or cancels plans, then that part shames you again for not leaving.

Client: He told me he couldn't have me over because he didn't want his neighbors to think I was a home wrecker because his ex just moved out. So now I feel shame for wanting to come to his house. It's been over six months we've been dating. So when is he going to tell people?

Therapist: How did you feel when he said that?

Client: Insecure! Nerves all over my body. On edge!

Therapist: What did the nerves say?

Client: Run!

Therapist: And what did you do when you felt that strong urge to run?

Client: I'm feeling shame about my feelings. He's good with his words, but his actions don't match. Then I feel shame for wanting to leave.

Therapist: I wonder if this current feeling of shame reminds you of anything that happened before in your life.

Client: I feel so much shame in this relationship. It reminds me of my last relationship.

Therapist: The one where the guy was hiding his porn addiction and hiding his other lovers?

Client: Yes. That was terrible. But I want to give this guy more opportunity, more time to show me that he can make the life for us he is always promising. I want to give him the benefit of my doubts. I want this relationship to work.

Therapist: Of course you want this relationship to work. Can you turn to the plant that represents your needs? What does the plant say?

Client: The plant says, "You're making yourself suffer!"

Therapist: What does the hat say?

Client: It says that I'm ashamed of my feelings. I'm embarrassed that I want him to visit me instead of his kids. That's terrible.

Therapist: What does the candle say?

Client: It says that I don't need to shame myself for my feelings. I have light inside me. I need to remember. (I wanted her to stop here and to reflect and to work to understand if maybe there is something here for her to be shameful for. That would be a form of healthy shame.)

Therapist: Sometimes, shame can pull a person out of her deep insecurity by cutting off the life force or the light. Sometimes, there is healthy shame that tells a person that there is something he or she doing or another person is doing that is actually shameful, that *should* be shameful. And there might be helpful information here if this is healthy shame. Healthy shame can help a person make new decisions or understand things in a different way. Here is some homework to do before our next session. I ask her to get out her journal at the end of the session and ask, "What did you get from this session?" Please write it down. And please write down some of these questions. Please do some journal writing to answer these questions:

- What does the plant say?
- What does the candle say?
- What does the hat say about how you shame yourself?
- Listen to the shame and feel if there is something of value here or if it is just putting you down.
- Is there part of it that is valid?
- Is there something to listen to that is actually shaming in the situation for a reason?
- Is there something here from a past relationship or situation where you felt shamed?
- Is there something you feel shy about?
- Is there something for you to learn about shame here?

Understanding Shame

Shame is a primary emotion. The role of shame is to warn us and to protect us. Our nervous system shuts down and we actually lose cognitive ability when we are feeling ashamed. Two indicators of shame are confusion and a feeling of being stuck. Shame can freeze both mind and body. Shame is so difficult to see and to cope with because it often hides behind other emotions. Also, shame's function is to protect us by lowering our emotional intensity and capacity to act. It is important to differentiate healthy shame, which can help us pause and rethink, from toxic shame, which can produce paralysis and leave a person so frozen that he or she is incapable of action and clear thinking. Healthy shame can lead a person to take responsibility for his or her actions, to reassess, and to make changes.

In my chapter, "Embodied Life-Stories: Directing Self-Revelatory Performance to Transform Shame," in the book, *Self in Performance* (edited by Pendzick, Emmunah, & Read-Johnson, 2016), I wrote, "When we become significant to another person, as happens when we are therapist, supervisor, friend, spouse, or parent, then we can induce shame in him or her unconsciously, unintentionally, even without knowing it has happened. Failure to fully hear and understand the other's need and to communicate its validity–a look in the other direction, a frown, a disappointing facial expression–whether or not we choose to gratify that need, can sever the bridge and induce shame. Developmental needs that are not met over time can also lead to internalized shame. The child learns to feel shame that his or her needs do not matter; the rupture is from outside, from the parent who fails to validate the child's needs." I would add that it then is on the inside and the person learns unconsciously to shame themselves. Also from the chapter, "Each story in our lives is like a pebble splashing into the pond of our inner worlds and the water that ripples naturally outward. When there has been trauma, the stories that would naturally flow outward can get truncated, withheld, or lost." And, "I am creating attachment through my witnessing, which starts from the first moment: being seen in a positive way, which is counter-shaming."

Hughs (2007), in *Attachment Focused Family Therapy,* writes about why shame may be a central factor in the development of pathology and a deterrent to getting help, "First, shame places one in a fog, hidden from potentially significant others, actively avoiding the exposure to another who could provide–through intersubjective experiences of acceptance, understanding and empathy–a pathway toward both affective regulation as well as self-awareness. Second, shame prevents the development of the ability to reflect on and make sense of one's behaviors and subjective experiences" (p. 184).

In the *Eight Keys to Safe Trauma Recovery*, Rothschild (2010) notes that "shame, quite simply, tells us that something is amiss" (p. 87), and that "Rather than discharge, as an example in yelling or crying, shame dissipates, when it is understood or acknowledged by a supportive other. More than any other feeling, I find that shame needs contact to diminish" (p. 92). Rothschild describes a process for deciding when to address shame, understanding the value of shame, apportioning shame fairly, and sharing shame (pp. 98–100).

Imagination Activated via Drama Therapy and Expressive Arts Therapy

From our workshops and from an unpublished paper, "Healing Shame in the Imaginal Realm" Bret Lyon, PhD, and I, present that when a person gets stuck in shame, the most powerful way to get unstuck may be to activate his or her imagination. In the imaginal realm, logic and time are fluid and flexible. What actually happened can be explored and changed. What was stuck can be reexamined and shifted. Shaming situations from the past can be revisited, excavated through writing and expressive exercises, and thereby shifted. There are ways to give back the shame to where it belongs–through drawing, writing, and imagining past shaming experiences and through saying now what you wish you had said then. Structured writing and expressive processes can symbolically give back the shame. This is where to find resilience. This work can be done with extra care when the session is over the Internet because the person can quietly slip into the shame vortex. I develop exercises to help them have something to hold on to during and after the session.

Emunah in her book, *Acting for Real* (1994), writes about "Drama Therapy as the international and systematic use of drama and theater processes to achieve psychological growth and change" (p. 3). Drama therapy can include play, role play, psychodrama, dramatic ritual, and psychotherapy. We are helping the client to develop an observing self, an inner director that can reflect on our life (p. 32). "A dramatic enactment can include both reality and fantansy" (p. 27). Leveton (2001), from *A Clinician's Guide to Psychodrama,* wrote about the therapist becoming the client's double, and talking for the client as an emotional double or as a counselor double, or as an exaggerated double. Blatner (1988) expounded that psychodrama offers a place for replaying scenes of the past, expressing feelings now that have not been expressed, and for opening new possibilities for the future. "Individuals are invited to engage more authentically in activities that increase their sense of being alive" (p. 85).

Conclusion-Working with Counter-Shaming Metaphors

There is much to be explored in this new world of online therapy. As I was writing this chapter, I received an email and was invited to possibly set up some online groups for an eating disorder program. That would be an interesting population to work with online because when I work with them in-person, many tended to dissociate. There is much to be discovered. There is much to be explored. There is much to be created. I am excited about being able to reach people who do not live near me and who do work online.

I excited about developing ways in which to work through shyness and awkwardness and shame that many clients present, using a combination of drama therapy, expressive arts, and attachment work/psychotherapy. Homework I often suggest after online sessions dealing with shame includes to draw or write in your journal,to play music that is soothing or exciting, to dance, to meditate, to get it all out to writing and writing, and then to close the book! Now begin your life!

REFERENCES

Blatner, A. (1988). *Foundations of psychodrama: History, theory, and practice.* New York: Springer Publishing.

Emunah, R. (1994). *Acting for real: Drama therapy process, technique, and performance.* New York: Brunner/Mazel.

Fosha, D. (1992). Brief Integrative Therapy Comes of Age. Retrived May 5, 2017 from https://www.aedpinstitute.org

Hughes, D. A. (2007). *Attachment: Focused family therapy.* New York: W. W. Norton & Company.

Kaufman, G. (1974). *On shame, identity and the dynamic of change.* Paper presented at the Annual Meeting of the American Psychological Association, New Orleans, LA. Retrieved from http://files.eric.ed.gov/fulltext/ED097605.pdf

Kaufman, G. (1992). Shame: The power of caring (3rd ed.). Rochester, NY: Schenkman Books.

Leveton, E. (2001). *A clinician's guide to psychodrama* (3rd ed.). New York: Springer Publishing Comapny, Inc.

Nathanson, D. L. (1992). *Shame and pride: Affect, sex, and the birth of the self.* New York: W. W. Norton & Company.

Pendzik, S., Emunah, R., & Read Johnson, D. (Eds.). *The self in performance: Autobiographicl, self-revelatory, and autoethnographic forms of therapeutic theater.* New York: Palgrave MacMillan.

Biography

Sheila Rubin, LMFT, RDT/BCT is a marriage and family therapist, a registered drama therapist, and a board-certified trainer. She integrates somatic, expressive, and attachment modalities in her work with couples, families, and children who suffer from shame and trauma. Her private practice is in San Francisco and in Berkeley. She is an alumnus and adjunct faculty of the California for Institute Integral Studies' Psychology and Drama Therapy Program. She is also an adjunct faculty at John F. Kennedy University in the Somatic Psychology Department. Rubin has trained with the attachment theorists Diana Fosha and Sue Johnson, and the Hakomi somatic pioneer Ron Kurtz. Rubin and her husband Bret Lyon have created and co-lead

"Healing Shame Workshops" for therapists in Berkeleyand throughout the United States and Canada. Rubin developed and conducts "Embodied Life-Stories" drama therapy workshops in Berkeley since 1996. She has also directed over twenty-five Self-Revelatory Performances, as well as five of her own. She has written about her work in several publications and authored the chapter "Women, Food and Feelings" in *The Creative Therapies Treating Eating Disorders,* edited by Brooke, addressing her work incorporating drama therapy modalities into a hospital-based eating disorders program she developed. She wrote the chapter, "Myth, Mask and Movement: Ritual Theater in a Community Setting," in *Ritual Theater,* edited by Schrader. She also authored a chapter on "Self-Revelatory Performance" in *Interactive and Improvisational Drama: Varieties of Applied Theatre and Performance,* edited by Blatner; and *Using the Creative Therapies in Treating Depression,* edited by Brooke and Myers (2015). Rubin also authored *Embodied Life-Stories: Directing Self-Revelatory Performance to Transform Shame, in Self in Performance,* edited by Emunah, Johnson, and Pendzic, to be published in 2015. She can be reached at www.TheHealingStory.com or www.HealingShame.com

Part 3

MIXED EXPRESSIVE THERAPIES

Chapter 12

ASSESSING THE CREATIVE EXPRESSIVE ABILITIES OF PEOPLE LIVING WITH DEMENTIA

Dalia Gottlieb-Tanaka, Hilary Lee, and Peter Graf

Birth of an Assessment Tool

Observing, monitoring, and measuring are useful skills that have been streamlined with the addition of computer technology. When they are applied to the abilities of the underserved and vulnerable population of seniors living with dementia, they become extremely valuable. The idea for developing a tool with this potential was seeded in 1999, but the first version of the tool was not ready to be published until 2008. The story of this development links the intriguing worlds of academia and practice for the benefit of people who live with dementia.

Personal Interest in Developing an Observation Tool

In 1999, I was asked to spend time with an older woman named Ruth, who had moved from California to be near her daughter in West Vancouver, British Columbia. Ruth resided in a care facility. Except for her busy family, Ruth did not know anyone in the area. She needed company—someone to engage in conversation and to keep her mind alert. I visited her twice a week for two hours at a time; we talked about whatever topic came to mind. In fact, I was totally unprepared for the task awaiting me. With no experience interacting with a person living with memory impairment, I was not sure where to start. I looked for books that suggested activities, especially ones constructed for seniors living with dementia. I was surprised to find out that no such guides existed. Not so long ago, people with this condition were called demented patients who belonged in mental institutions. Yet, what the medical establishment and the public at large perceived as dementia did not reflect what I experienced when working with this population. Was Ruth an exception to the rule, or were other residents like her?

I searched local libraries, a local college, and the library at the University of British Columbia. I looked for two key words: creativity and dementia or creativity and Alzheimer's. No results came up in the search for relevant references. I suspect I may have been the first one to link the two keywords. There was plenty of information about dementia and, separately, about creativity, but the two together were not addressed and indicated a gap in the current literature. This was the start of my quest that led to a doctoral degree and to a postdoctoral fellowship.

Special Population: Seniors Living with Dementia

Dementia is a global term that covers about seventy-two brain diseases, of which Alzheimer's is one. "Dementia refers to the development of multiple cognitive or intellectual deficits that involve memory impairment of new or previously learned information. . . ." This definition appears in Agronin's (2004, p. 2) *Practical Guide in Psychiatry,* and is also the diagnostic classification of dementia. Ruth was the first person living with dementia I worked with; we explored creative expression activities that gave her pleasure and that added interest in her daily routine in a long-term care facility.

I began to plan my sessions with Ruth. They were all based on trial and error while I immersed myself in reading medical information on dementia, which I did not completely understand, since I came from a background in architecture. As time passed, I got to know Ruth better, observed what she was still able to do, and watched her diminishing physical and cognitive capacities. However, her condition was unpredictable and kept changing from day to day. I found that I had to be flexible and ready to go with the flow and take cues from Ruth as to what needed to be done to keep her engaged and communicative.

I was looking for a way to describe Ruth's creative expressions so that I could share them with her family and keep them for my own records. For that purpose, I tried to keep a diary, but came to the conclusion that what I needed was an observation system I could complete quickly, and with a brief glance, monitor the changes that took place over time in Ruth's creative responses. This was the beginning of work on my Creative Expression Activities Program, which I pursued with professionals, practitioners, and with seniors living with dementia in a series of settings at care facilities, at workshops, and at conferences across North America. The program won awards and gained recognition in the relatively sparse field of dementia care, specifically in the use of the creative arts as a means of communication to improve the quality of life of people with memory impairment.

My desire to develop the next step: an assessment tool for creative expression abilities for seniors living with dementia, had to wait. I had begun graduate studies and was not given the opportunity to work on my ideas at that time. The reasons given was that my ideas were too practical and graduate students in my field should focus on theoretical approaches to dementia care and not on particular solutions. Creative expression activities for seniors living with dementia were in their infancy. No one talked about reminiscence therapy, dance therapy, horticulture therapy, or drama therapy. Those therapies did not occupy mainstream teachings in academic schools nor were they employed in care facilities–at least, not with a clear purpose to engage seniors living with dementia in meaningful activities based on a person-centered approach to dementia care, which became my goal.

I graduated in 2006, and, a year later, began to think about my observation tool in earnest.

Looking for other professionals and practitioners who faced some of these problems, I founded the Society for the Arts in Dementia Care and set up conferences to exchange experiences. Lee came halfway around the world, from Australia, to attend a couple of the conferences sponsored by the society. With an occupational therapy background, she recognized the benefits of the expressive arts in dementia care and was happy to join me in developing an assessment tool. Based on our experience interacting with seniors living with dementia, we knew there was no such observation tool we could use. And this was how our collaboration began.

The Creative Approach: The Important of Creative Expression Activities for People with Dementia

Programs designed to enhance the quality of life include the creative expression programs, which harness and build on seniors' remaining abilities by engaging them in creative thinking and in spiritual contemplation in order to reaffirm their dignity and self-worth (Lee, 2007). These programs may focus on painting, listening to and creating music, dancing, singing, reminiscing, storytelling, life review, and on activities of daily life such as cooking, dressing, planning and gardening. Their specific aim is to foster psychological health and well-being–quality of life–by encouraging and developing seniors' ability to express themselves in ways that are meaningful and possibly novel to them by stimulating curiosity and self-evaluation.

Examples of Creative Expression Programs

Concretely, reminiscence programs kindle the recall of life experiences, promote interpersonal functioning, and improve emotional well-being (Kasl-Godley & Gatz, 2000). McAdam (2001) developed the *McAdam Aged Care Art Recreation Therapy (MAC.ART)* in Australia, basing it on person-centered approaches as well ason her belief that it is possible to revitalize the human capital of any aged care facility, dementia specific unit, or community setting by implementing art projects (MAC.ART, 2008).

The Breakfast Club, developed at a Jewish Home and Hospital for the Aged in the Bronx, New York (Boczko, 1994), was designed to maintain conversational and social skills, to promote recollection of early life memories, and to foster organizational, decision-making, and problem-solving skills. Other programs, such as the Creative Expression Activities Program developed in Canada (Gottlieb-Tanaka, 2006) and the self-esteem boosting Spark of Life Club Program developed in Australia (Verity, 2008, 2011) nourish the social, emotional, cultural, and spiritual needs of seniors with dementia.

Opening Minds through Art (OMA), an intergenerational art program for people with dementia, was developed by Dr. Elizabeth Lokon in 2007, and was grounded in person-centered ethics. It is based on the dual premise that people with dementia are capable of expressing themselves creatively and the growing body of empirical evidence that creative expression improves their physical and psychological well-being. Engaging in creative activities can serve to relieve boredom, depression, and anxiety, and to increase interest in life.

Ashida (2000) found that music therapy alleviates depressive symptoms in people with dementia. Additionally, Brotons and Koger (2000) found that music therapy increases language functioning in these clients. Aldridge (1993) reported that music reduces the need for tranquilizing medication. Ridder (2005), in an overview chapter on therapeutic initiatives designed for people with dementia, reviewed ninety-two studies carried out between 1980 and 2004, and based on the results, suggested that music has the ability to contribute to neurological rehabilitation. O'Toole and Lepp (2000) discovered that drama therapy helps with the integration of thoughts, feelings, and actions. Lepp, Ringsber, Holm, and Sellersjö (2003) determined that a combined program of dance, rhythm, song, storytelling, and conversation, designed especially for seniors with dementia, increased socialization. Palo-Bengtsson and Ekman (1997) revealed that dancing promoted closer relationships with caregivers, and contributed to positive feelings and better communication. Social dancing also has been found to promote a sense of identity, self-worth, and self-esteem (Trombley & Radomski, 2002).

Threats to Creative Expression Programs

In Canada, as in most regions of the industrialized world, the aging of the population will peak between 2025 and 2045, when the baby boom generation reaches 75+ years of age, and it is expected that one of every four persons over the age of 80 will have some form of cognitive impairment (Alzheimer Society of Canada, 2010). According to some estimates, 500,000 people in Canada are living with dementia today with a projection of 1,100,000 by the year 2030. About 200,000 healthy Canadians are required to provide care for today's dementia population, and the cost of care alone is $5 billion per year. The overall cost of dementia to the Canadian health care system was about $15 billion in 2008, with a projection of $75 billion by the year 2028 (Alzheimer Society of Canada, 2010). As the numbers of people living with dementia increase dramatically along with the cost of their care, we fear that the focus of care may turn to physical needs and be limited to providing basic medical services. Even today, the importance of psychosocial approaches to care that are designed to maintain or to enhance well-being and quality of life are underappreciated and often are first to be cut back when resources grow scarce.

Rationale for Developing the Creative Expression Activities Assessment (CEAA) Tool

Engaging in creative activities can contribute to or even define the quality of life at every stage in human development (Runco, Ebersole, & Mraz, 1990; Runco & Richards, 1997). New instruments have been needed for assessing and for documenting the diverse benefits of creative activities and related programs. Such programs were effective in maintaining and in enhancing the expressive abilities and quality of life of seniors with dementia. We are convinced that one major reason–perhaps the most important reason–why this basic but profound lesson is not more widely recognized, or why the value of creative expression and related programs continues to be underappreciated, stems from the lack of an easy-to-use instrument for collecting comprehensive, compelling, and solid quantitative evidence concerning the programs' numerous and diverse positive effects.

Early on, we established that no other comprehensive tools existed to assess the creative abilities of people living with dementia. We created the CEAA tool to enable the collection of this type of data, and to date, the CEAA is the only comprehensive tool of its kind.

More specifically, we created it as a tool that might be useful as well as convenient for answering important questions, such as the following:

- Are some creative activity programs more effective than others for maintaining or for enhancing the expressive abilities and quality of life of seniors with dementia?
- Which intensity of program delivery (e.g., 3 times per week vs. once every 2 weeks) is most effective in maintaining or fostering expressive abilities?
- Are the benefits of such programs similar or different for seniors with different levels of dementia?

We believe that the CEAA tool will permit health care service providers to fine tune their programming and invest their limited resources in the best interests and for the long-term benefit of the seniors in their care.

Using Technology

Developing the CEAA Tool

Based on our understanding of the relevant literature, our extensive first-hand experience with developing and delivering creative activity programs to seniors with dementia, and with the qualitative assessment of the many benefits of such programs, we drafted a first version of the instrument. Its name—Creative Expressive Activities Assessment—reflects our interest in "small-c creativity" (Cohen, 2000) where the word to create stands as a synonym for to make, to produce, to generate, and to express. The name also reflects our conviction that a person's creative abilities are crucial determinants of quality of life even in dementia.

Hilary and I both had backgrounds in qualitative research. We understood that to make the tool more credible and to achieve widespread acceptance, we would need to join forces with a quantitative researcher. We approached Dr. Peter Graf, a professor of psychology at the University of British Columbia, and the team was born. Peter would later lead the study testing the reliability and validity of the data collection phase of the tool. The data collected was later analyzed by Dr. Ruth Childs and by her graduate students, Tian Tang, Jinli Yang, and Saira Mall at the University of Toronto. Two more milestones were reached. In 2011, Dr. Julie Gross McAdam generously contributed film clips based on creative arts sessions with her clients, and in 2012, the CEAA tool was published in Lokon, Kinney, Sauer, and Kunkel's (2012) article, Wolf Project.. These results both suggest that the tool can be used in different settings and in different countries.

Embracing Digital Entry

As we started to conduct reliability and validity testing on the CEAA tool, we marked down the observed data in the traditional way by using paper and pencil. Soon, we realized that our hired observers were mostly young university students. We also noticed that those observers used computers as an integral part of their way of life. IPhones and IPads were common and were used wherever possible. In addition, care facilities often asked whether the observation forms could be downloaded directly on computers with the already entered data to save the tedious job of transferring manually recorded data onto excel forms so as to reduce time and human errors. Care facilities also wanted to be able to disseminate collected information to their staff with a click of a mouse, to caregivers who came in contact with their residents, families, administration, and medical staff. The technological advances in the care industry actually pushed us to continue to develop the tool so that it could also be used in a digital format.

Another reason for moving data collection from paper and pencil (although it still can be used) to digital format, were the needs of academia and practice to demonstrate new ideas and new understandings when submitting grant applications in a highly competitive world. We knew that if our CEAA tool was to survive in the future, we needed to provide another option for data collection. I am confident that this is not the end of the road in the development of the CEAA tool and with the predicated growing population of seniors with dementia, the tool may go through several more updates.

Developing and Testing the Tool

With the aim of developing a comprehensive assessment instrument, our first draft included over 45 items and covered 8 different ability domains. Over a period of nearly six months, this version of the instrument was used in western Australia by 8 different observers who made assessments of 88 seniors with dementia who were participants in two different creative activity programs.

Based on insights, experiences, and data from this phase, we drafted a new version of the instrument as well as a first version of the user guide. In the second phase, the new draft was used in Vancouver, Canada, by four different observers who made additional assessments of seniors with dementia who were participants in 17 different creative activity programs. Of these assessments, a total of 140 came from two individuals who observed the same seniors in the same session, and these data were used for a preliminary item analysis and for an inter-rater reliability analysis.

We combined the results of these analyses with the feedback we received from two focus groups (one with 6 participants in Canada, and the other with 10 participants in Australia) and with activity program directors who are likely users of the instrument. Based on these results, we drafted a third version of the instrument and of the user guide and used them once again to make 98 additional assessments (each of two observers made 49 assessments) in Vancouver. The data from this phase were used for the analyses reported in the next section.

Psychometric Properties of the CEAA

The current version of the CEAA consists of 25 core items, plus 2 optional items, to be used only in connection with activity programs that involve some form of writing. Most of our assessments were made in the course of programs that did not include a writing component, and thus, our data concerns only the 25-item CEAA tool. We began our work with an instrument that covered 8 different ability domains, each with approximately the same number of items, and ended up with an instrument that covers only 7 different domains (memory, attention, language, psychosocial skills, reasoning/problem solving, emotions, and culture), with the number of items varying widely among the domains (example: 1 item for attention, 8 items for language). We arrived at the final version of the instrument by removing each item on which nearly all of the participants achieved a perfect score (i.e., if the item showed a ceiling effect), as well as each item on which nearly all obtained the lowest possible score (i.e., if the item showed a floor effect). We also removed items with inter-rater reliability scores that were very low (i.e., Cohen's kappa less than .10) (J. Cohen, 1960), despite our best efforts to create clear instructions for making observations. In a final stage, we removed any items whose removal was suggested by improvements in Cronbach's alpha (Cronbach, 1951).

A statistical analysis of the data from the final 25-item CEAA showed it to have good internal consistency, with a Cronbach's alpha score=.86, thereby indicating that all of the items are sensitive to the same general underlying construct (i.e., the thing being measured). Additional research is required to clarify the precise nature of this construct, including its relationship to more familiar constructs, such as creativity and fluid intelligence, that is, the part of intelligence which involves using, as opposed to acquiring, information.

In additional analyses, we focused on the agreement between the scores produced by our two observers-raters, each of whom observed 49 different participants-sessions. Across the individual items, the Cohen's kappa scores–

a statistic which measures agreement between two raters—ranged from a low of .20 to a high of .75 (Cohen, 1960). An analysis of the total scores, defined as the sum of all of the item scores across the 25-item CEAA, produced a Cramer's V score of .825 and a contingency coefficient of .975. Both of these statistics (Cramér, 1999) also draw attention to, or indexed the association or relationship between, two sets of scores; their closeness to 1 indicates the high degree of agreement between the total CEAA scores produced by our two raters. More importantly, these findings indicate that in the hands of a properly trained individual, the CEAA can be used to make reliable and trustworthy observations on the creative-expressive abilities of seniors with dementia.

Validating the CEAA Tool

The objective of the validity study was to assess whether or not the tool is measuring the abilities it intended to measure: the creative expressive abilities of people with dementia. The CEAA tool was examined on its face, content, predictive, and convergent/concurrent validity. Two other assessment tools were used to examine the correlation with each other: the Measurable Assessment in Recreation for Resident-Centered Care (MARRC; Boothman, 2005), and the Oshkosh Social Behaviour Checklist (OSBC; McFadden, Lunsman, & Andel, 2007). Our team selected items from these two assessment tools that were relevant to creative-expressive abilities only. The assessments were used by students who were trained by Gottlieb-Tanaka and Graf. The increased knowledge about the validity of the CEAA made it more valuable as a tool for research, as well as for decision making about the kind of activity programs best suited when placing clients.

The validation took place at Cedar Village Nursing Home in Cincinnati. As part of the evaluation, 63 people were observed during the spring 2012 semester, yielding a total of 122 observations. Residents with more advanced dementia (Ruby and Pearl) were not observed (Lokon, Kinney, Sauer, & Kunkel, 2012). The use of the CEAA tool allowed the evaluators to see measurable differences between traditional activities and the enhanced arts activities that offered more opportunities to engage in and demonstrate increased creative-expressive abilities. The analysis of the data collected found that for all of the seven domains of the CEAA tool, creative expressions occurred more often during Wolf Project activities compared to traditional activities.

Benefits of Using the CEAA Tool

We have discussed how important Creative Expression Activities are to seniors with dementia. The benefits of the assessment tool extend to the other interested parties who can use it along with the User Guide.

Creative expression facilitators can observe clients' creative abilities in a systematic way and monitor any changes in those abilities over time. The documentation is easy to complete and read at a glance. It provides reliable results for reporting in meetings with colleagues, administration, and families. It can be used to get to know new clients and to follow their abilities. Facilitators can use the CEAA to monitor sessions and to assess their effectiveness by analyzing clients' responses. It serves as a guide in planning activities to suit each client.

Administrators of a care facility can use the CEAA tool to monitor how residents respond to various programs. The tool provides specific reports on residents' creative abilities to complement medical reports. The tool can be used in planning budgets for effective recreation activities and for guidance in hiring facilitators.

The CEAA tool is based on solid qualitative and quantitative research so that researchers can measure creative abilities in a quantitative and qualitative way. The CEAA tool produces consistent results among raters with 80% agreement most of the time. The tool is internally consistent in demonstrating whether the items measure the same things or different things at higher than 0.9 or 90%. In our experience, comparing ratings by two trained observers revealed similar scores in real time versus video observation, and the inter-rater agreement measured around 0.8 or 80/5. In contrast, observations of nonstructured activities as residents go about their daily routines and do not engage in creative expression activities, revealed very low scores.

A User Guide to the CEAA tool has been developed. It is available for first-time users and experienced users of the instrument. Instructions that come with the guide are easy to follow. The tool provides a reliable way to monitor people with dementia across a range of domains, including memory and attention. Users report the accompanying manual has proved to be a useful training resource. More information is available at the Dementia Activities website (Dementia-Activities.com, 2008).

Limitations and Recommendations for Future Research

In the summer of 2014, Dr. Ruth Childs and her students, Tian Tang, Jinli Yang, and Saira Mall, were asked to assist in investigating the validity of the use of our CEAA tool. As a project within a course on Test Theory, they thoroughly reviewed materials provided by the author, including a study performed by researchers at the Miami University (Ohio) in consultation with myself and with Dr. Peter Graf. Based on these materials, they developed a validity argument for the CEAA and conducted additional analyses of the data from the Miami University study to check the assumptions in the validity argument. In their report, they described the validity argument, followed by the supporting analyses. In developing the validity argument, they built on and extended the findings of the Miami University researchers, Lokon, Kinney, Sauer, and Kunkel (2012). In a report by Childs and by her students (unpublished, revised on February 26, 2015), they mentioned a number of recommendations for future research that would further strengthen the validity argument. An article on the report is forthcoming.

As I was working on this chapter, new information continued to emerge from Childs and from her students which stated among other things: "Investigate whether changes in the client's performance in creativity activity programs over time correspond with a change of the client's dementia level. It might also be possible to investigate whether these relationships are consistent across creative activity programs. If so, this might provide support for using the CEAA to compare the effectiveness of programs in eliciting creative expression" (Revised February 26, 2015, p. 8).

This recommendation actually supported an earlier desire of our team to find a link between the level of dementia and the benefits of being engaged in creative expression programs. However, we quickly realized that there were some limitations we could not overcome at the time of our data collection. Some medical records of residents who participated in our studies revealed a lack of clear diagnosis of dementia and of its level. Could it be to spare the patient/client from being linked to an unwanted stigma which is so misunderstood and feared?

We are aware that having the CEAA tool produced in the English language only limits its use to English-speaking facilitators and observers. We are planning to translate the CEAA tool into Hebrew next. As feedback started to come back from users of the tool, we realized that lack of training, whether self-taught by using the CEAA tool guide, or facilitated by the authors of the tool, led to unintended usage of the tool. The developing team made an effort to simplify the academic jargon (yet built on solid research) by making the tool friendly and easy to be used. In addition to language limitation and the need for proper training on the tool, we are aware that dementia is a medical condition which could be unpredictable in its symptoms and in its course of progression. Therefore, we suggest conducting several observations over time for a more comprehensive understanding of the kind and level of creative expression abilities of a person living with dementia. The CEAA tool covers only the responses that are linked to creative abilities. It does not cover physical or functional abilities of daily life such as driving or grocery shopping. It is meant to complement other geriatric assessments that measure mental status such as the Folstein Mini-Mental State

Examination known as MMSE as published in the *Journal of Psychiatric Research, 12*(3): 189-198, 1975 & 1998.

Definitions

Dementia–Medical Definition

Dementia is a global term that covers about seventy-two brain diseases, of which Alzheimer's is one. "Dementia refers to the development of multiple cognitive or intellectual deficits that involve memory impairment of new or previously learned information. . . ." This definition appears in Agronin's (2004, p. 2) *Practical Guide in Psychiatry–Dementia. Diagnostic and Statistical Manual of Mental Disorders* (4th ed.), *Text Revisions* (DSM-IV-TR).

Traditional Way of Collecting Data

A common way that is still used as an observation technique is by mounting an $8^1/_2$ x 11-inch page on a clipboard with a predesigned table for marking what is being observed. The scores are usually marked down with a pencil. The data on the paper forms can then be analyzed and scores are summarized manually. For a large sample of participants, data that was marked down on paper may be transferred to an Excel form on the computer and then analyzed using quantitative methods.

Wolf Project–Evaluation of the Arts in Aging at Cedar Village July 2012

The purpose of this research was to evaluate the Creative Arts in Aging Program at Cedar Village. New funding from the Wolf family that began in January of 2012, allowed Cedar Village to expand and to build upon its existing creative arts programming. In the spring semester of 2012 (January–May), the funding provided residents with opportunities to participate in art activities conducted by Joan Hock (artist) and additional music therapy sessions conducted by Jude Jones (music therapist). This document reported the first round of evaluations of art/music activities; the evaluation was conducted by Scripps Gerontology Center at Miami University during this first semester of the expanded arts programming.[12]

---

12. Source: Lokon, E., Kinney, J., Sauer, P., MGS, & Kunkel, S. (2012). The Wolf Project. Retrieved March 12, 2015, from http://www.dementia-activities.com/PDF/WOLF_Report_July2012.pdf

Small-c Creativity

"Building on Howard Gardener's concepts, two aspects of creativity are important to appreciate. One is to look at creativity with a capital C, which is the typical way we look at it, the type of creativity that can influence the course of a community or culture. But equally important is creativity with a little c, the creative acts that can change the course for individuals or for their families, and bring something new into existence in terms of how they deal with their jobs, a hobby, a new career, interpersonal relationships, family life, and community and volunteer work. These are ripe opportunities for creativity with a little c.[13]

Inter-rater Reliability Analysis

In statistics, inter-rater reliability, inter-rater agreement, or concordance is the degree of agreement among raters. It gives a score of how much homogeneity, or consensus, there is in the ratings given by judges.[14]

Additional Definition on Inter-rater Reliability

We use inter-rater reliability to ensure that people making subjective assessments are all in tune with one another. Generally measured by Spearman's Rho (continuous/ordinal variables) or by Cohen's Kappa (nominal variables that cannot be ordered), the inter-rater reliability helps create a degree of objectivity.[15]

We also recommend watching *Issues in Psychological Classifications: Reliability, Validity & Labeling* and *Issues in Psychological Assessment: Reliability, Validity, and Bias.*

Creative Expression Activities Programs

The Creative Expression Activities Program was developed by Dr. Dalia Gottlieb-Tanaka. It is based on a variety of planned and spontaneous activities addressed to healthy seniors and to clients with mild to moderate to

13. Cohen, G. (2000). *Creativity and Aging.* As published in: *GIA Reader, 11,* 2 (Fall 2000). Retrieved March 12, 2015, from http://www.giarts.org/article/creativity-and-aging

14. Inter-rater reliability–Wikipedia, the free encyclopedia. Retrieved March 12, 2015, from en.wikipedia.org/wiki/Inter-rater_reliability

15. Retrieved March 12, 2015, from http://study.com/academy/lesson/inter-rater-reliability-in-psychology-definition-formula-quiz.html

severe dementia. It is also based on solid academic research and on years of practical experience. The program includes topics such as health and family matters, fears, anxieties, achievements, life and death issues, food, arts, making music and music appreciation, pets, and seasonal celebrations and holidays which materialize into creative expressions. The program emphasizes the use of clients' present abilities that may encourage them to tap into their past and present life histories with hopes for the future by expressing their feelings creatively through drawings, writing poems, storytelling, music, dance, and reminiscing. Gottlieb-Tanaka takes cues from her program participants and adjusts the topics to fit the needs of her clients. The key issue to facilitation is to be flexible, to be kind, and to respond with compassion. All of the participants have the right to express themselves and to be valued.

Psychometric Properties

Quantifiable attributes (e.g., validity or reliability) that relate to the statistical strength or weakness of a test or measurement.[16]

Good Internal Consistency

Internal consistency is typically measured using Cronbach's Alpha (?). Cronbach's Alpha ranges from 0 to 1, with higher values indicating greater internal consistency (and ultimately reliability). Common guidelines for evaluating Cronbach's Alpha are:

- .00 to .69=Poor
- .70 to .79=Fair
- .80 to .89=Good
- .90 to .99=Excellent/Strong

If you get a value of 1.0, then you have "complete agreement."[17]

Traditional Activities vs. Enhanced Arts Activities

As mentioned in the Wolf Project (2012, p. 2): "Residents were also observed during traditional structured activities such as bingo, Shabbat, coffee & news.

---

16. *Medical Dictionary for the Health Professions and Nursing* © Farlex 2012. Retrieved March 12, 2015, from http://medical-dictionary.thefreedictionary.com/psychometric+properties
17. Retrieved March 12, 2015, from http://www.statsmakemecry.com/smmctheblog/confusing-stats-terms-explained-internal-consistency.html

Arts & crafts and sing-along activities that *were not conducted by the art and music therapists* were grouped as part of the traditional ongoing activities at Cedar Village."[18]

REFERENCES

Aldridge, D. (1993). The music of the body: Music therapy in medical settings. *The Journal of Mind-Body Health, 9*(1), 17–35.

Ashida, S. (2000). The effect of reminiscence music therapy sessions on changes in depressive symptoms in elderly persons with dementia. *Journal of Music Therapy, 37*(3), 170–182. doi: http://dx.doi.org/10.1093/jmt/37.3.170

Boczko, F. (1994). The Breakfast Club: A multi-modal language stimulation program for nursing home residents with Alzheimer's disease. *American Journal of Alzheimer's Disease, 9*(1), 35–38.

Boothman, S. (2005). *The measurable assessment in recreation for resident-centered care (MARRC).* Paper presented at the Eleventh Canadian Congress on Leisure Research, Nanaimo, BC.

Brotons, M., & Koger, S. (2000). The impact of music therapy on language functioning in dementia. *Journal of Music Therapy, 37*(3), 183–195. doi: http://dx.doi.org/10.1093/jmt/37.3.183

Cohen, D. G. (2000). *The creative age: Awakening human potential in the second half of life.* New York: Avon Books.

Cohen, J. (1960). A coefficient for agreement for nominal scales. *Education and Psychological Measurement, 20*(1), 37–47.

Cramér, H. (1999). *Mathematical methods of statistics.* Princeton, NJ: Princeton University Press.

Cronbach, L. J. (1951). Coefficient alpha and the internal structure of tests. *Psychometrika, 16*(3), 297–334.

Dementia-Activities.com. (2008). Welcome to the dementia activities website! Retrieved August 5, 2014 from http://www.dementia-activities.com/index.html

Gottlieb-Tanaka, D. (2006). *Creative expression, menentia and the therapeutic environment.* Unpublished dissertation (PhD). Vancouver, BC: University of British Columbia.

Kasl-Godley, J., & Gatz, M. (2000). Psychosocial interventions for individuals with dementia: An integration of theory, therapy, and a clinical understanding of dementia. *Clinical Psychology Review, 20*(6), 755–782. doi: http://dx.doi.org/10.1016/S0272-7358(99)00062-8

Lee, H. (2007). *The impact of the spark of life program on the personal and emtional well-being of people with dementia, carers and families perceptions.* Unpublished dissertation (MSc). Perth, WA: Curtin University of Technology.

---

18. Lokon, E., Kinney, J., Sauer, P., MGS, & Kunkel, S. (2012). The Wolf Project. Retrieved March 12, 2015, from http://www.dementia-activities.com/PDF/WOLF_Report_July2012.pd

Lepp, M., Ringsberg, K. C., Holm, A. K., & Sellersjö, G. (2003). Dementia–involving patients and their caregivers in a drama programme: The caregivers' experiences. *Journal of Clinical Nursing, 12*(6), 873–881. doi: http://dx.doe.org/10.1046/j.1365-2702.2003.00801.x

Lokon, E., Kinney, J., Sauer, P., & Kunkel, S. (2012). *Wolf project: Evaluation of the arts in aging at Cedar Village.* Oxford, OH: Miami University, Scripps Gerontology Center. Also available on http://www.dementia-activities.com/PDF/WOLF_Report_July2012.pdf

Mac.Art. (2008). Mac.art: McAdam aged care art recreation therapy. Retrieved Jly 29, 2014 from http://www.macart.com.au/sitemap.htm

McFadden, S. H., Lunsman, M., & Andel, R. (2007). *Comparative analysis and interrater reliability of the Oshkosh Social Behaviors Checklist (OSBC) for persons with dementia.* Poster session. Paper presented at the Gerontological Society of America, San Francisco, CA.

O'Toole, J., & Lepp, M. (2000). *Drama for life. Stories of adult learning and empowerment.* Brisbane, QLD: PlayLab Press.

Palo-Bengtsson, L., & Ekman, S. (1997). Social dancing in the care of persons with dementia in a nursing home setting: A phenomenological study. *Scholarly Inquiry in Nursing Practice, 11*(2), 101–118.

Ridder, H. M. (2005). An overview of therapeutic initiatives when working with people suffering from dementia. In D. Aldridge (Ed.), *Music therapy and neurological rehabilitation: Performing health* (pp. 61–81). London: Jessica Kingsley Publishers.

Runco, M. A., Ebersole, P., & Mraz, W. (1990). Creativity and self-actualization. *Journal of Social Behavior and Personality, 6*(5), 161–167.

Runco, M. A., & Richards, R. (1997). *Eminent creativity, everyday creativity and health.* London: Ablex Publishing Corporation.

Acknowledgments

Special thanks to Hilary Lee, MSc and Peter Graf, PhD. Both were instrumental in developing the CEAA tool. Hilary Lee, with a background in occupational therapy, implements person-centered and holistic approaches in her projects. She is the Director of the Society for the Arts in Dementia Care in Australia and has published her work in age care and peer reviewed journals. Hilary works with Dementia Care Australia and is the President of *Spark of Life*. For more details in Hilary's work, see www.dementiacareaustralia.com. Email address: hilary@dementiacareaustralia.com

Peter Graf is a professor in the University of British Columbia's Department of Psychology, where he is the director of the Memory & Cognition Laboratory, and an investigator with the Brain Research Centre. His expertise is on human memory and related abilities. Peter has published extensively and presented his work at national and international conferences.

Biographies

Dalia Gottlieb-Tanaka, PhD, graduated in 1976, from the Bezalel Academy of Arts & Design in Jerusalem, and received a Master's of Architecture degree in 1980, from the University of British Columbia. She is the founder of the Society for the Arts in Dementia Care. The Creative Expression Activities Program she developed for seniors with dementia, won awards from the American Society on Aging and from the MetLife Foundation. She continues to do research and to deliver presentations and workshops internationally. Gottlieb-Tanaka supports interdisciplinary collaboration with other professionals who share an interest in the use of visual and performing arts in health services provided to seniors with dementia.

The Society for the Arts in Dementia Care: www.cecd-society.org
The Society Facebookwww.facebook.com/TheSocietyForTheArtsInDementiaCare
For more information on the arts in dementia care: www.dementia-activities.com

Hilary Lee, MSc, has a background in occupational therapy. She completed a Master's in Science degree with a focus on dementia research in 2007. With over twenty years of practical experience in dementia care, Lee has been implementing a person-centered and holistic approach with projects, such as the early identification and prevention of depression in dementia, and in designing innovative and creative programs to enable people with dementia to express themselves in new ways. She established a chapter of the Society for the Arts in Dementia Care in Australia after connecting with the Society in Canada and is its chair. Lee has published her work in age care and peer-reviewed journals and is sought after as a presenter both nationally and internationally. She is now working with Dementia Care Australia as the president of *Spark of Life*. For more details about the *Spark of Life* philosophy, please log on towww.dementiacareaustralia.com. Email address: hilary@dementiacareaustralia.com

Peter Graf, PhD, is a professor in the University of British Columbia's Department of Psychology, where he is the director of the Memory & Cognition Laboratory, and an investigator with the Brain Research Centre. His expertise is on human memory and on related abilities, on how these abilities function in normal intact adults, how they change across the adult lifespan, and how they are affected by trauma or diseases such as Alzheimer's. He has published extensively and presented his work at national and international conferences

Chapter 13

FOCUSING-ORIENTED ARTS THERAPY–INTERNET PROTOCOL (FOAT-IP) FOR DEPRESSION IN SOUTH ASIAN[19] WOMEN

RASHMI CHIDANAND

"Go see a doctor and get medicine." My health had rapidly started to deteriorate, ranging from digestive problems and stomach pains escalating to spinal back pain and vertigo. Despite being born and raised in the United States, the South Asian cultural stigmas around mental health were prevalent all around me. Psychotherapy or going to see a therapist did not even cross my mind as an option to manage my somatization of stress, anxiety, and depression as a result of my life stressors. The South Asian mentality to fix somatic health symptoms was to get medicine from a physician. It was only through my own journey of FOAT that I discovered a private way to process life stressors and to alleviate somatic symptoms. Inspired by personal experience while being mindful of the cultural need for privacy and upholding family honor in society, I wanted to help reduce the gap with the introduction of a *nonverbal* alternative technique to traditional "talk therapy." As a bridge between "no therapy" to "therapy," I explored FOAT-IP as a segue well-being tool to initiate the healing process in South Asian women. (Chidanand, 2014)

As a clinician, trying to bring therapeutic services to even the most resistant or hard-to-reach populations is an ongoing challenge. As with some other ethnic groups, South Asians may not be as receptive to traditional talk therapy due to stigmatas around psychotherapy held by this population. Even though a majority of the working-aged South Asian adults are medical

---

19. South Asians (those comprising of Indian, Pakistani, Nepali, Sri Lankan, Bangladeshi, Bhutanese, and Maldivian heritage).
*Note: The entire protocol with FOAT-IP Manual is outlined in Chidanand (2014) and is available at http://gradworks.umi.com/36/36 /3636779.html

professionals, the community as a whole minimizes the use of any mental health services (Ahmed, Mohan, & Bhugra, 2007; Prathikanti, 1997). The cultural and religious framework of traditional South Asian values is founded in family structures and in community life. According to Das and Kemp (1997, as cited in Prathikanti, 1997) and to Jayakar (1994, as cited in Prathikanti, 1997), psychotherapy is underutilized due to cultural stigmatas on bringing shame to the entire family and to one's ethnic group. The South Asian concept of family generally refers to the large and dynamic entity that is composed of several households dispersed all over the world, yet that manages to function as a single unit. Exposing personal conflicts outside a family not only undermines family honor, but also compromises the South Asian community's image of being the model minority in the United States. Consequently, mental illness is considered a sign of instability or weakness, and thus, hidden from the public eye (Prathikanti, 1997; Yoshioka, Gilbert, El-Bassel, & Baig-Amin, 2003). Because South Asians are hesitant to talk openly to anyone, such as a therapist, outside of their family circles, adjunct approaches that draw on aspects of Gendlin's (1996) Focusing-oriented Therapy (FOT) and the expressive arts (i.e., art, movement, and poetry) can help facilitate meaning-making in a nonverbal manner that also respects their need for privacy. Therefore, with the collaboration and guidance of Dr. Laury Rappaport, I adapted Focusing-oriented Arts Therapy (FOAT; Rappaport, 2008, 2009, 2010, 2014) into Focusing-Oriented Arts Therapy-Internet Protocol (FOAT-IP); Chidanand, 2014) as a supplemental technique to help South Asian women, a population at risk for Intimate Partner Violence (IPV).

This is important because 2 in 5 South Asian women experience interpersonal violence within the context of their marital relationship (Raj, Liu, McCleary-Sills, & Silverman, 2005). This statistic is disproportionately higher than other ethnic groups, including Asian and Pacific Islanders. Yet, as a subset of Asians or Asian Americans, South Asian women are one of the less studied populations; practically the only examination of this group consists of a limited amount of research on South Asian IPV (Hurwitz, Gupta, Liu, Silverman, & Raj, 2006). In summary, South Asian women residing in the United States who are survivors of IPV, may not be receptive to conventional verbal therapy due to familial, cultural, and societally imposed stigmatas surrounding psychotherapy. Hence, I developed FOAT-IP as an adjunct method to clinical work to help manage post-traumatic stress disorder (PTSD) precursors such as stress, anxiety, and depression in South Asian IPV survivors.

This chapter includes a brief overview of FOAT-IP as a well-being tool for South Asian women. Specifically, it discusses (1) the overview of Gendlin's FOT and Rappaport's FOAT that was adapted to the Internet (i.e., FOAT-IP); (2) the promising potential of FOAT-IP as an adjunct technique for existing interventions to bring therapeutic support through the Internet for highly reluctant populations (e.g., South Asian women) that would otherwise not seek mental health services; and (3) research participant's FOAT-IP artwork and writing examples to illustrate the potential effectiveness of this online tool.

THEORETICAL FRAMEWORK

Focusing-oriented Therapy (FOT)

Focusing-oriented Therapy is the application of Gendlin's original Focusing method (1981) with psychotherapy (Gendlin, 1978, Madison, 2014a, 2014b; Purton, 2004). Gendlin's FOT evolved from his research with Rogers and is categorized as client-centered psychotherapy (Gendlin, 1996). Roger's client- or person-centered psychotherapy (PCP) is based on self-theory, where a client has failed to develop a healthy sense of self. *Self-theory* strives for *congruence* between the self and the entire realm of an individual's experience. PCP is a form of humanistic therapy "that enable[s] the client to access feelings, strengthen reliance on inner resources, develop self-esteem, and become less dependent on the approval of others" (Ingram, 2006, p. 327). PCP also incorporates an existential therapeutic approach "in which the therapist self-discloses, offers honest feedback, and presents a model of healthy interpersonal functioning" (p. 327).

PCP therapists adopt and convey a particular attitude toward a client before displaying any skills. Specifically, they experience and express congruence, unconditional positive self-regard, and accurate empathy for the client (Flannagan & Flannagan, 2007). The congruent therapist is authentic, open, and honest, and is able to express both positive and negative feelings present in the therapeutic relationship with a client. *Unconditional positive regard* for a client is evident by the therapist openly accepting and valuing the entire being of a client. In this safe and trustful container, clients explore what they really want and who they really are, which leads to clients accepting themselves. In conjunction with congruence and unconditional positive regard, *accurate empathy* is a powerful component in therapy that promotes insight for the therapist to see and to feel a client's world from the client's point of view. Contemporary PCP therapists are more active and directive than traditional PCP therapists. For example, Rappaport's (2008, 2009) integration of the expressive arts with Gendlin's (1978, 1996) FOT represents the variation of the nondirective stance of PCP. In essence, PCP therapists come across to clients as, "I am listening and doing my best to understand your life experiences and how you are experiencing them in life and in yourself."

Based on research about what contributes to effective psychotherapy, FOT helps clients to become aware of one's *felt sense*–the direct preverbal bodily experience residing within an individual. Fundamental to the approach is the Focusing Attitude–mindful awareness of the felt sense with an attitude of friendly curiosity. The felt sense is an embodied experience, accessing a bodily sensation that has meaning. During the Focusing process, one finds a *handle* or a symbol that may arise in the form of an image, gesture, word, phrase, or sound. FOT also integrates compassionate listening and the safety of the relationship with the Focusing process.

Focusing-oriented Arts Therapy (FOAT)

FOAT® is an umbrella term for *Focusing-oriented Expressive Arts* and includes both clinical and nonclinical applications. There are four main approaches: FOAT Basic Step; Clearing a Space with Arts (CAS-Arts); Theme-Directed FOAT; and FOAT-Psychotherapy (Rappaport, 2009, 2014). FOAT Basic Step consists of bringing the Focusing Attitude of "being friendly" to the bodily felt sense, seeing if there is a symbol or a handle that matches the felt sense–such as a word, phrase, image, gesture, or sound–and then externalizing the handle through expressive arts (Rappaport, 2009, p. 27). For example, a word or a phrase may be expressed through writing; an image through art; a gesture into movement or dance; and sound into music or sound expression.

Rappaport (2009) defined the approaches as follows: In CAS-Arts, the client uses the imagination and the arts to symbolically place stressors and issues in the way of feeling "All Fine" and also to express the "All Fine Place" (an inherent place of well-being; p. 37). Rappaport developed CAS-Arts after Gendlin's (1978, 1996) method for Clearing a Space in which the Focuser accesses the felt sense and imagines placing the issues in the way of feeling fine outside of the body, and also then gets a felt place that is separate from those stressors (a place of well-being). The arts help to place the issues outside of the body, as well as to provide a concretization of the issues and "All Fine Place." CAS-Arts is "beneficial for centering, stress reduction, clarifying and dis-identifying with issues, and helping clients to have an experiential knowing of their intrinsic wholeness" (Rappaport, 2009, p. 92).

FOAT-Psychotherapy is "primarily applied to individuals and couples where the orientation is toward authenticity, congruence, empathy, depth-oriented insight, communication skills, and change" (Rappaport, 2009, p. 92). In FOAT Psychotherapy, the therapist follows the client's experiential unfolding moment-to-moment and then responds with listening, Focusing, and expressive arts in a carefully attuned manner. A *Theme-Directed* FOAT approach is most often used in groups, and can also be used with individuals and with couples. A theme, such as fear, trust, or strengths, is selected that matches the client or group needs. Although FOAT is "primarily a *Person-Centered Approach,* it is applicable to all orientations, including, psychodynamic, cognitive, behavioral, etc." (Rappaport, 2009, p. 92).

Development and Overview of FOAT-IP

Initially, my research was intended to be an eight-week-long workshop that met for about two hours in a group setting. However, during recruitment, the anticipated challenge in obtaining participants was grossly underestimated. The clock was ticking and as weeks and months passed by, I was forced to reevaluate and to revisit the research design. In that contemplation, it occurred to me that I am residing in Silicon Valley, heavily saturated with South Asians; yet, I am not even getting one participant. What am I missing? What is the fragrance that will attract my participants to the sweet nectar of FOAT-IP? Marketing strategies of appealing to their highly affluent and achievement-oriented mindset by presenting it as a free workshop to help with work-home balance, burnout prevention, and/or self-growth all failed. Reducing the duration to four weeks and offering a $500 gratitude gift card through a raffle drawing, also resulted in no participants. Then, it dawned on me. Silicon Valley meant tech-savvy individuals, where a majority of the South Asians were software engineers, computer scientists, and webpage builders.

With the collaboration and guidance of Dr. Laury Rappaport, *FOAT-IP* is my adaptation of FOAT to a web-based protocol for the purpose of reaching a population that is highly reluctant to utilize mental health services. The FOAT-IP for this research includes a Theme-Directed FOAT approach on well-being/empowerment that also includes FOAT Basic Step and CAS-Arts. FOAT-IP integrates FOT and expressive arts to facilitate emotional and spiritual healing (Rappaport, 2009, 2014). FOAT-IP offers a direct way of working through central emotions without any self-disclosure, and consequently may perhaps be more accessible to South Asian clients who are not acculturated to traditional talk therapy (Maker, Mittal, & Restog, 2005). South Asian women communicate unhappiness by behaving in a subdued manner (Prathikanti, 1997). Because explicit expression of anger is considered a shameful act of impatience and lack of self-control, an outlet for expressing any negative emotions may be found through the expressive arts. Because South Asians are hesitant to talk openly to anyone outside of their family circles, such as a therapist, adjunct approaches such as Gendlin's FOT and Rappaport's FOAT that integrate Focusing with the expressive arts (i.e., art, movement, and poetry) may help facilitate meaning-making in a non-verbal manner that also respects their need for privacy.

Moreover, research on this population is significantly deficient, which includes research on the effects of alternative psychotherapeutic interventions to augment conventional talk therapy. Therefore, FOAT-IP was explored as a potentially promising well-being technique to manage stress to reduce anxiety and depression symptomology in South Asian IPV women survivors.

CLINICAL APPLICATION

FOAT-Internet Protocol (FOAT-IP)

FOAT-IP is framed in a wellness and prevention model by managing post-traumatic stress disorder (PTSD) precursor symptoms of stress, anxiety, and depression through FOAT activities focusing on stress management, self-awareness, compassion, and spiritual empowerment. A pre-and posttest quantitative design was utilized in this four-week pilot research for a Web-based intervention. Participants (N=16) were South Asian women who completed four quantitative measures (Perceived Stress Scale, State Trait Anxiety Inventory, Beck Depression Inventory, and Positive State of Mind) at the beginning and end of the study. FOAT-IP was piloted in the United States, based out of the San Francisco Bay Area but included participants from California, Texas, and New York. Participants accessed and engaged in FOAT-IP activities right from the convenience of their home through the internet.

The FOAT-IP activities were all directly from Rappaport's FOAT book (2009) from which were compiled into a FOAT-IP Manual (Chidanand, 2014, p. 114). One diversity hurdle that was encountered during the recruiting stage was the word therapy in FOAT. To clarify to the participants that this was not online therapy but rather a self-care skillset or well-being tool, FOAT-IP was referred to as *Focusing Expressive Arts Technique* (FEAT). This reframing assisted in easing any concerns or uneasiness around inadvertently part-taking in therapy.

Culturally, the participants were familiar with meditation and with the arts being primarily Indians and of the Hindu faith, which has a strong emphasis on such mindful and creative practices. However, to make sure the participants were familiar and comfortable with both, there was an Orientation Week prior to Week 1, which focused on helping the participants foster the Focusing Attitude, access the felt sense, and become familiar with the expressive modalities (e.g., the visual arts of drawing or painting).

The FOAT-IP activities were all delivered through the Internet. Specifically, the FOAT activities were audio formats (.mp3) that the participants listened to that directly streamed off the webpage. At their own pace, participants engaged in their creative activity; they either took a photo, video, or wrote on a word document, and upon completion, uploaded directly to the webpage. Following the creative activity, the participants were invited to journal about the experience as a way to briefly dialogue and to process the FOAT activity. The goal of the journaling component was to take the *nonverbal* experience and to provide an opportunity to transform it into a *verbal* experience, which deepens the process of insight and inner healing in the privacy of one's own home (see the Immigrant Housewife's journal entries in this chapter).

Outline of FOAT-IP Weekly Activities

Orientation Week
- Check in
- Exercise 0.0 FEAT Grounding Exercise and Mindful Breathing
- Exercise 0.1 Focusing Attitude and Felt Sense (Rappaport, 2009, p. 31)
- Optional: CHOOSE 1:
  - Exercise 0.2 Exploring the Language of Artmaking (Rappaport, 2009, p. 81) or
  - Exercise 0.3 Name Drawings (Rappaport, 2009, p. 149)
- Journal

Week 1 Stress Reduction for Mind, Body, and Spirit: Clearing Space
- Exercise 1.0 FEAT Self Check-in (Rappaport, 2009, p. 97)
- CHOOSE 1:
  - Exercise 1.1 Clearing a Space with Art I (Concrete Imagery) or
  - Exercise 1.2. Art II (Directive Imagery) (Rappaport, 2009, p. 121)
- Exercise 1.3: Well-being Self-care (FOAT Self-care Exercise © Laury Rappaport, 2012)
- Journal

Week 2 Stress Management for Mind, Body, and Spirit
- Exercise 2.0 Peaceful Place (Rappaport, 2009, p. 141)
- Exercise 2.1 Accessing Inner Wisdom (Rappaport, 2009, p. 141)
- Journal

Week 3 Accessing Acceptance, Compassion, and Inner Strength
- Exercise 3.0 Acceptance and Compassion (Rappaport, 2009, p. 95)
- Exercise 3.1 Strengths (Rappaport, 2009, p. 174)
- CHOOSE 1:
  - Exercise 3.2 Walking Meditation (Rappaport, 2009, p. 232) or
  - Exercise 3.3 Exploring Movement to Music
- Journal

Week 4 Spirituality
- Exercise 4.0 Where I Am Now/Where I'd Like to Be Spiritually (Rappaport, 2009, p. 231)
- Exercise 4.1 Pebble Meditation (Rappaport, 2009, p. 208)
- Exercise 4.2 What I Want to Carry With Me? (Rappaport, 2009, p. 175)
- Journal

Examples of FOAT Activities and Artworks from Participants

The examples of the FOAT-IP artworks are from two of the participants. One participant was an American-born, South Asian computer animator working for Disney Animation Studios with no reported health issues. As a result, working in abstract medium is most therapeutic after being employed all day in concrete details at Disney. The other participant was an immigrant, South Asian housewife with reported health issues, and having no prior art background. She found solace working in concrete images and in trying out different mediums (e.g., painting and watercolors) and creative modalities (e.g., movement and writing).

Clearing A Space (CAS) with Art

EXERCISE. ART II: Clearing a Space with Directive Imagery:
(*Rappaport, 2009, p. 120*)

Goal: This exercise is useful for centering and forstress reduction. This exercise includes a guided Focusing of listening inwardly (more like guided imagery or meditation).

First, find a comfortable position in your chairs or on the floor, and take a few deep breaths, inviting your body to relax. . . . If you feel like it, you may close your eyes . . . or keep them open . . . whichever is more comfortable to you.

---

continued

Clearing A Space (CAS) with Art—*Continued*

When you're ready, ask, "How am I from the inside right now?" . . . Turn your attention like a searchlight inside to your body, just noticing whatever you find there, without judgment. . . . Now imagine yourself in some peaceful place. . . . It may be a place you know already or it may be one you create in your imagination. Imagine you have a beautiful kite to which you can attach all of the things between you and feeling "All Fine." Or, you may imagine tying each issue or concern you have to a balloon, and imagine that the string lets the balloon float at just the right distance from you. Or, check to see if you'd like the balloon to just float off into the sky. If the kite and balloon images do not resonate with you, imagine someone from your life (friend, therapist, family member, teacher, or spiritual figure) who can hold each issue or concern for you. Or, imagine putting each concern or issue in a different-colored suitcase and putting it on baggage claim carousel to set at some distance from yourself. You can go claim it anytime you are ready to. With each issue or concern, check in with yourself and ask, "Except for all that, I'm "All Fine," right?" . . . If more comes up, continue to tie it to a balloon or to set in a suitcase for the baggage carousel. Keep a comfortable distance from you and your kite, balloon, or suitcase.

Keeping everything at a distance, now, I'd like to invite you to bring your attention to this "All Fine Place" . . . See if there is an image that matches or acts like a "handle" for the "All Fine Place." . . . Check it against your body to make sure it is right. If not, invite a new image that matches or acts like a "handle" for the "All Fine Place" to come. . . . If what comes is a word or phrase, that's fine. . . . Be accepting of that. I invite you to mark this "All Fine Place" in a meaningful way for you, so that you can return to this cleared space of feeling All Fine during times of stress and ungroundedness. When you are ready, use the art materials, music, gesture, movement, and/or words to create something expressing your felt sense of the "All Fine Place."

During the first week of FOAT-IP, both participants engaged in CAS-Art and resonated with distancing their stressors with the balloon-imagery. Figure 1 shows how the computer animator had stressors concerning family expectations, duties, and other familial responsibilities she was in the midst of grappling with. The CAS-Art helped her experience relief from the heavy weight of her familial, Indian obligations, versus her desire to be bicultural by balancing her Indian and American sides of her value and belief system. In Figure 2, the Immigrant Housewife is experiencing the freedom of letting go of all the worries in her body and moving freely in life. As a recent immi-

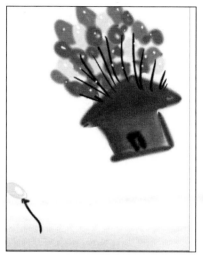

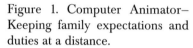

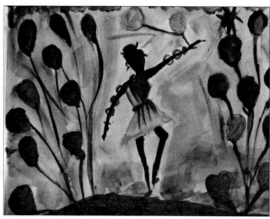

Figure 1. Computer Animator–
Keeping family expectations and
duties at a distance.

Figure 2. Immigrant Housewife–Letting go of all
the worries within the body.

grant, she has been struggling with balancing her life in America with her
husband through an arranged marriage, while also maintaining ties to her
homeland. Both participants are experiencing lightness from the heavy
weight of being women holding strong South Asian familial, cultural, and
societal beliefs and value systems.

Halfway through the FOAT-IP workshop, participants were asked to
explore movement as a modality. Figure 3 is the visual representation of the
computer animator's positive experience from engaging in the Walking
Pebble Meditation (Exercise 3.2). Notice the vibrant colors, the sense of
movement, and the use of abstract imagery she utilized to capture the positive energy moving through her after participating in the FOAT-IP activity.

Here is the Immigrant Housewife's journal entry in response to her experience with Movement with Music (Exercise 3.3), which captured the process
and effectiveness of FOAT activities.

*Every week I always mention and talk about my favorite exercise of the week. This
week I really enjoyed this exercise. Listening to the music helped me relax and the
movement helped me calm my nerves. When I turned on the Pandora Radio and
the Bollywood music started to play, I slowly started to move without my knowledge. I started to carefully analyze and to enjoy every beat of the drums and instruments' sounds.*

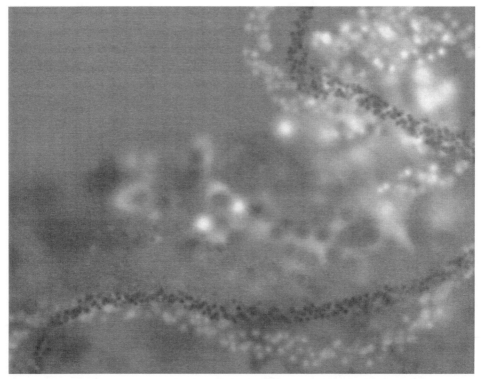

Figure 3. Computer Animator–After engaging in the Walking Pebble-Meditation (Exercise 3.2), there is movement and positive energy in the creative piece.

For a few moments, I forgot everything and I was engrossed into the music and dance. Dancing made me happy and feel good about myself. When I was dancing, I started noticing the anger, irritation, and agitation starting to slowly go away. Then, I told all my negative thoughts and negativity to go away with my dance moves. In the process, I was bringing in positivity to my mind and body. After dancing for a while I noticed changes in my mind and body. The tightness was gone and I was feeling great. This exercise was great for self-acceptance. For that moment I felt calm and forgot all the worries and tension. I started to appreciate instruments, music and choreography. This exercise really helped me to explore my inner talents and made me aware that music, and dance makes me happy more than any other activity. I preferred Exercise 3.3 compared to meditation and walking exercise because it's difficult to control my wandering thoughts in that exercise. Whereas music and dance distracts me completely from everyday worries, [and instead] I will be more focused on rhythm, beats, choreography, and music.

Participants' Artworks–Where I Am Now/ Where I Would Like to Be Spiritually?

Through this FOAT-IP activity, participants visually captured the before (i.e., where I am now) and after (i.e., where I would like to be spiritually) states of their mind, body, and spirit. Specifically, the participants were asked about their spirituality–"where I am now spiritually?" (before) and "where I would like to be spiritually?" (after) and created two drawings accordingly. Figure 4 captures the computer animator's spirituality (i.e., yellow) being hidden, covered up by dark shadows (i.e., black cloudiness). The Computer Animator's current stance on spirituality is unknown, amorphous, and possibly still being discovered given she is in her mid-20s. Her sense of self is still being defined and formulated. Figure 5 clearly captures her positive outlook on the bright clarity she would achieve by embracing spirituality or vy connecting more with her spiritual self.

The Immigrant Housewife's artworks reflect more of the traditional Hindu perspective on spirituality. Her spirituality is rooted in the religious Hindu practice of going to the temple and worshiping an idol of a Hindu god like

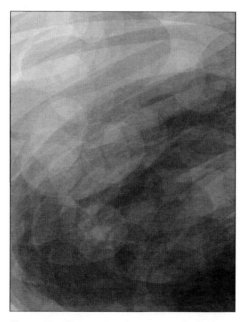 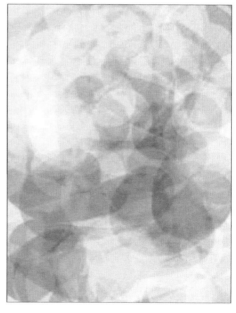

Figure 4. Computer Animator–Currently, spirituality is covered with Dark Shadows.

Figure 5. Computer Animator–Ultimately, would like Spirituality to be without the shadows and in the presence of Light (yellow circles).

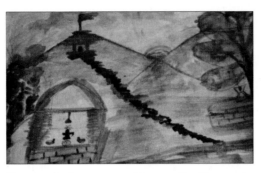

Figure 6. Immigrant Housewife–Currently, going to the temple is the spiritual practice.

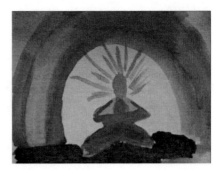

Figure 7. Immigrant Housewife–Ultimately, would like to experience self-actualization (enlightenment).

the Shivalinga in her Figure 6 drawing. As a Hindu devotee, she would like her spirituality to evolve to the level of attaining self-actualization (enlightenment), where she is one with herself (see Fig. 7). The Immigrant Housewife summarized the felt sense of the entire FOAT-IP experience in her final journal entry: "What I want to carry with me?"

Journal Entries on "What I Want to Carry with Me"

I decided to participate in this workshop because I wanted to change myself. I wanted to bring focus back into my life; basically to bring back my real identity which was lost in the process. Instead of working on it, I had accepted my chaotic life. It was overwhelming and way out of control. It caused a huge amount of stress because even though I wanted to change, it was like, "where do I start?"

The exercises really helped me to accept my flaws and to take a small step every day [to help me change] instead of doing everything at once, which is practically impossible. "Clearing a Space" exercise really helped me to let go of all my blockages, worries, and issues. Looking inside for [a] "source of strength" really helped me have a positive attitude toward problems while acceptance helped me to accept myself. I have many flaws but "I will try to work on it eventually" is a new motto of mine. . . . Practicing self-care was a huge step for me. Working to keep my focus on my body and soul is very important.

I joined a yoga class again because I realized during the workshop that self-care really helps to stay fit and calm. I started going on walks and I love it because it gives me personal space to think and plan for the rest of the day. Creativity exercises really helped me to relax and also gave me joy in using different colors and art materials. The process also revealed to me some hidden creative talents that I did not know I possessed before. Spirituality and meditation really helped to instill calmness and hope for the future.

From this workshop I learned many things like taking small steps to reach a goal, practicing self-care, compassion, and especially self-acceptance (because sometimes I can be too self-critical, which can be bad for the body and soul). So acceptance work was a great exercise. I also learned to handle my stress by visualizing a happy place along with happy moments in my life. By incorporating spirituality and meditation, it helped to ease my unknown fears by giving me hope and confidence.

The workshop was a great experience and great journey toward positivity in life and I wished that the workshop [had] *continued for a few more weeks.*

As can be seen in the Immigrant Housewife's journal entries, the FOAT-IP activities cultivated her awareness, especially around the importance of taking care of the body as well as the spirit (soul) for overall health and happiness. With this new awareness, she was motivated to change her old habits and to develop new ones by integrating yoga classes, daily walks, creative arts, and meditation into her new lifestyle. In essence, her journal entries captured the experience of many of the FOAT-IP participants.

Findings of FOAT-IP

The findings of my quantitative research (pilot study) demonstrated that 47% of the participants' improvement may be attributed to the FOAT-IP intervention on the depression measure. The findings on stress, anxiety, and positive states of mind measures were found inconclusive, which may have been due to the study's small sample size, appropriate of the measures or the length of the protocol. However, the high percentage of the reduced depression appears to be quite significant since the intervention was short, and depression is a dynamic variable that has other probable contributing factors (e.g., income, health, self-worth, career, and family). It is noteworthy that the results were statistically significant despite the complexity of factors contributing to symptoms of depression and the limitations in sample size and study duration. These results strongly suggest FOAT-IP's potential value as an effective therapeutic technique for this potentially highly resistant and stigmatized population.

Briefly mentioned earlier, meaning-making is important to positive health (Park & Ai, 2006; Silberman, 2005; Thombre, Sherman, & Simonton, 2010). As a result of my study, I speculated that engaging in the FOAT-IP activities facilitated meaning-making for the participants to the extent that their state of mind significantly improved on the depression scale. Depression is a dynamic variable that has numerous causes; however, it may also be one of the most challenging to treat in South Asians due to the cultural stigmas, denial, and secrecy (Ahmad, Riaz, Barata, & Stewart, 2004; MySahana, 2011a, 2011b, 2011c; PAMF, 2012a, 2012b, 2012c). At the end of my study, I speculated that FOAT-IP seems to have crossed cultural barriers and allowed an improvement in feeling depressed by creating meaning from one's felt sense to create a more positive mindset.

In addition, my research may have reflected culturally familiar practices, which may have helped facilitate engagement with felt sense handles in FOAT-IP. The demographics of the participants suggest that the majority of the participants engaged in meditation (N=6), yoga (N=5), art (N=8), dance (N=8), writing (N=7), singing (N=5), and/or musical instruments (N=3) as part of their existing self-care practices. Given that a majority of the South Asian participants also identified themselves as Hindu, and that meditation, yoga, and the arts are all part of the practice of Hinduism, FOAT-IP seemingly created a natural bridge for these women to utilize practices with which they are already familiar to facilitate improvements in their mental health.

CONCLUSION

The unspoken need for any intervention, let alone a well-being tool like FOAT-IP, is the openness for new experiences and for allowing change to evolve from the felt sense level through bodily awareness. Atkinson and Gim's (1989) study, "Asian-American Cultural Identity and Attitudes Toward Mental Health Services" suggested a possible acculturation factor influencing the decision making of Asian Americans seeking mental health assistance. In other words, the more acculturated the Asian American was in adapting to Western thinking, the more likely the he or she was open to psychotherapy. Similarly, I speculate that South Asians who are younger, more educated, and more modern (i.e., Western) in worldview perspectives are more likely inclined to new experiences to facilitate change, especially self-change.

Delimitations and Limitations

As with any research, a number of limitations and delimitations existed for my research such as the researcher bias limitations, the small sample size delimitation and limitations, and the measures limitations. For the purpose of this chapter, I will highlight the most noteworthy limitations: the methodological delimitations and limitations, the South Asian perspective limitation, and the attrition limitation.

Methodological Delimitation and Limitations

I opted to implement FOAT-IP through the Internet to facilitate participation within what appears to be a highly reluctant population, which served as a primary delimitation in this study. Even though there are growing studies on web-based interventions, especially working with mental disorders, there are some limitations as well as advantages to Internet-delivered interventions. First, studies have found Internet interventions effective for mild-to-moderate mental issues, while efficacy with more severe mental disorders (e.g., bipolar and schizophrenia) still needs to be explored (Anderson, Carlbring, Ljotsson, & Hedman, 2013). Second, there is the challenge to establish a consistent model for Internet implementation as technology evolves, and as the Internet is more commonly being accessed through smartphones than a computer. Future studies would have to investigate various models that would take into consideration the different environments of implementation (e.g., computer, smartphone, and tablet). Yet, the likelihood of adherence to treatment and to relapse prevention may be improved with such open accessibility to users. Web-based interventions augment conventional psychotherapy, which may accelerate therapeutic healing between clinical sessions. Future studies may conduct a comparison study to research the efficacy between conventional therapy and conventional study augmented by online intervention. Even though the majority of literature for Internet-delivered interventions was for CBT, FOAT-IP's initial results suggested that FOAT-IP intervention was feasible and has the potential to be efficacious as a Web-based intervention to augment treatment modalities for depression in South Asian women, who are at risk for IPV.

The implementation of the study online is a methodological limitation when it comes to uniformity; in other words, ensuring that the participants opted to do the FOAT-IP activities in one sitting versus over a week, did not influence the outcomes. In this study, the researcher noted that all of the participants consistently did the FOAT-IP activities in one sitting at approximately the same time each week. However, future studies should note this as a possible methodological limitation, which is harder to control with larger, heterogeneous sample sizes.

South Asian Perspective Limitation

Recruitment of South Asian women was one of the most challenging phases and the South Asian community's attitude is the greatest limitation that impacted recruitment in this study. I was aware that culturally there would be a barrier potentially due to stigmatas and to upholding family values. However, the extent of the reluctance was unexpected. For example, I attended a large South Asian fundraising walkathon event in the San Francisco Bay Area. The walkathon was aimed to set the standard as the largest social and service platform of its kind. It recognized, supported, and nurtured the spirit of giving by empowering individuals of diverse backgrounds to unite and to strengthen their communities. I had also read that it had one the largest gatherings of all of the various South Asian organizations in the Bay Area.

Lack of participation by the South Asian population was grossly underestimated by the researcher. There is no statistical information available for this population to explain the possible reasons for this except through the following anecdotal data. As I approached the vendor booths holding flyers in hand, the South Asian volunteers at the booths were skeptical, hesitant, and uncooperative. Despite explaining the purpose of the research workshop, the flyers were repeatedly placed under the table pending approval by the organization's manager (offsite).

I also encountered the "business mindset" of the South Asian community; "business mindset" in this community means that there is an expectation of a quid pro quo or reciprocation for any services rendered. For example, I approached the spiritual organization that one family has been an active member of since 1990. However, they were not members of the San Jose chapter. The booth representatives handed the researcher the schedules of classes, workshops, and events at the spiritual center, encouraged her to first invest time in attending and in building relationships with the members, and said, "Then we can see how we can help you with your research workshop." This spiritual organization is supposed to be founded on helping the community and humanity in a gracious, generous manner. Yet, here were representatives from her own spiritual organization asking her to invest time and money she did not have, and to attend classes and workshops before they would volunteer any assistance in recruiting. This experience suggests a possible set of limitations that would need to be addressed, which mentioned is in the Future Studies section of this chapter.

I consulted about different recruiting attempts with her family, and was surprised by her parents and sisters' responses: "What were you thinking wanting to recruit our people? Desis [South Asians] don't help each other like that. You know that. In fact, have your friends help you recruit. They are more responsive to non-Desis than their own kind. That's just how they are." The supervisor at my internship site also had concurred with what my parents had shared. The Indian supervisor mentioned how the South Asians who seek counseling, insist on working only with non-South Asian therapists. I speculate that the reason is to not feel guilt or shame associated with seeking psychotherapy. Further speculating, the chances of the non-South Asian therapists running into other South Asians in the area, and potentially "out-ing" them to their community, may be slightly less risky compared to seek-ing therapy with a South Asian.

At the next recruiting event, I took my Caucasian male friend with me. He managed to distribute nearly 80% of the flyers within two hours by sim-ply saying, "Help South Asian women," while I took longer with more dia-logue effort. Another future study would be to examine this preference for non-South Asian therapists by conducting a survey for the preference be-tween a non-South Asian therapist versus a South Asian therapist.

As part of the recruiting efforts, the flyer underwent different modifica-tions. Originally, the study was designed to be marketed in the San Francisco Bay Area only as a women's group (i.e., no online format). The researcher created the first flyer using words "Stress . . . Anxiety . . . Depressed," hav-ing heard South Asians (especially in the Silicon Valley) express such senti-ments on numerous occasions. However, through the distribution process, it was found that South Asians quickly took offense to the word stress, which is perceived as a benign and common experience in the workplace by Amer-icans. To illustrate, when one of my Caucasian female friends approached her South Asian co-worker and asked, "Would you be willing to help my friend with her dissertation research?" The co-worker took one glance down at the flyer and took offense, "*You* think I'm stressed?" The friend remarked, confused by the defensiveness, "Who isn't? We all work for big hi-tech com-panies with high-demanding jobs." This type of response from South Asian women was commonly encountered during the recruitment phase. As men-tioned in the literature, the South Asian population is extremely reluctant to seek traditional talk therapy, which is partially due to the cultural stigmata surrounding psychotherapy and its demeaning association with being dys-functional and abnormal (Maker, Mittal, & Rastogi, 2005; Prathikanti, 1997; Yoshioka et al., 2003).

In my research, the first flyer was eventually modified into a more achievement-oriented empowerment workshop and used catch phrases such as "work and home balance" and "burnout prevention." I extended this workshop to volunteers at domestic violence shelters in the Bay Area as a way to work through secondary traumatization and burn-out prevention. Fly-ers were also marketed online through social media platforms such as Face-book. In addition, the assistance of students belonging to South Asian orga-nizations at local universities such as Stanford University and other col-leges/universities in the Bay Area were recruited in marketing the flyers through their mailing lists. The South Asian students were quite open to pro-moting the flyers; however, despite these diverse modes of marketing and distributing flyers, recruiting efforts still yielded zero participants. Transforming the FOAT-IP into a Web-based intervention made it accessible to more people while creating the convenience for participation from the privacy of their homes. In addition, when the study was modified from an 8-week empowerment group Bay Area workshop into an 8-week Web-based workshop, the recruiting efforts started to yield some participants (N=40). However, by the time the workshop started, the potential participants withdrew, and I had to reduce the study to 4 weeks and to reduce the number of participants (N=25).

To expedite the recruiting process for the shorter study, I had enlisted my family and friends to reach out to their South Asian friends all over the United States. In summary, for the purpose of yielding significant results to demonstrate the effects of FOAT-IP on this population, the study originally was designed to be an 8-week study. However, as a result of recruiting challenges and limited time to complete the study, the design was reduced to 4 weeks to facilitate participation, which ultimately yielded participants. The study's duration was a delimitation because I speculate that a larger impact of FOAT-IP may have resulted with a longer study, thereby potentially resulting in statistically significant numbers. Future studies may benefit from a longitudinal study to demonstrate the effectiveness of FOAT-IP over a longer duration than 4 weeks. Future studies may also benefit in exploring this recruitment limitation by investigating how to motivate South Asians to participate in workshops and research.

I also observed the participants' lowest priority was emotional self-care practices by how the participants, especially in the control group, had difficulty finding thirty minutes out of an entire week to complete the posttests. Some participants agreed to participate but a week later ended up dropping out because they were "too busy." I speculate that the items that the South Asian woman prioritizes ahead of her own health and well-being on her "to-do" list may come into balance if she made taking care of her mental and spiritual self a priority. However, the culture and societal message of "family comes first" seems to force self-care practices at the bottom of their unbalanced lifestyles (Hurwitz, Gupta, Liu, Silverman, & Ra, 2006; Prathikanti, 1997; Yoshioka et al., 2003). The responsibility of family obligations outweighs any beliefs to fulfill individual desires of a family member (Venkataramani-Kothari, 2007).

Expounding on this above concept of putting family ahead of self, especially in the context of IPV, a question surfaced: Are South Asian women viewing marriages as a *black hole*? In this context, I am defining a black hole as a concept of whatever goes in, does not come out. Similarly, I speculate the South Asian IPV women may feel stuck in unhealthy relationships because of cultural stigmatas and fears of guilt and shame in dishonoring their families. As a result, they may view outside help, such as couples' therapy, as hopeless because there is no motivation for compromise and change in a black-hole marriage. Both parties may believe that divorce is unlikely, especially for immigrant South Asian women who are dependent on their husbands for livelihood and for support. I further speculate the power dynamic may be skewed to the extent that South Asian women endure marital problems and sometimes abuse because they cannot go outside for help. Even if help was sought, the marriages would remain unchanged behind closed doors. Perhaps it is this fear that is preventing these women from seeking help and from feeling unstuck in these unhealthy marriages.

I speculate that unless South Asian women feel empowered and as independent equals to their spouses, the problems and abuse will continue to get sucked into the black hole. Until South Asian women give their husbands a reason for change, such as the possibility of leaving him, compromise and change will not occur. However, I speculate that South Asian IPV survivors would need to realize that such abusive relationships will not change and that the only way to take care of themselves is through empowerment and through eventually leaving the husband to start a new life. Future studies with South Asian IPV survivors would need to explore this concept through a qualitative study after building strong rapport with the participants.

Attrition Limitation

Another limitation consideration is minimizing, if not eliminating, attrition when studying this population. Recruiting South Asians was extremely challenging, let alone reducing attrition in this population. A total of 25 participants (experimental group=12, control group=13) had been recruited, but only a total of 16 participants completed the study. The control group incurred attrition because of participants unexpectedly taking a trip to India and unable to complete the posttests until their return to the United States. Other participants in the control group reported simply being "too busy" and "forgetting" despite the multiple email reminders. These reasons could also be further evidence of the South Asians' resistance and reluctance to participate in research. Four of the participants, randomly assigned into the experimental group, signed the consent forms to participate but chose not to participate for the entire duration of the study. Two of the four, who were students who would have found the $500 raffle gift card incentive appealing, also chose not to participate. The other participants were quite representative of the South Asian community, consisting of affluent, well-educated working professionals.

How to motivate an affluent population to participate and to remain an active participant throughout the entire study? One possibility is to individually pay each participant a weekly amount that accrues with each week's submission to encourage weekly compliance. However, it would have to be in a manner to prevent introducing research bias and validity issues into the research design and implementation. South Asians are achievement-oriented and money-minded; if research participation can be presented in a manner that answers, "What can I gain or get out of this?" then perhaps research participation would increase and/or attrition be reduced when conducting studies with this population. Another option is building an alliance with South Asian organizations by being an active member for a couple of years, and utilizing this relationship to run the research study as a workshop within the organization.

Future Studies

Future studies should explore a more heterogeneous sample of South Asians, as well as validating these preliminary findings with a larger sample. Without this, the findings of such a study may not be generalizable to the broader South Asian population residing in the United States. In addition, future studies might benefit from explicitly examining whether there is any measurable South Asian tendency toward emotional suppression and the possible relationship of such behavior to states of mind and/or somatization. This is an important consideration because the literature indicates that this group seems to suffer disproportionately from psychosomatic health issues, which may indicate that South Asians tend to translate their psychological stressors into physical bodily symptoms (Hurwitz, Gupta, Liu, Silverman, & Ra, 2006; Raj et al., 2005; Reavey et al., 2006). Additionally, future studies might also include a somatic symptoms inventory to assess for somaticized issues. Other future studies might explore the presentation of stress, anxiety, and depression in South Asians and compare symptomology with the diagnostic criterion of the DSM-5 to determine whether these conditions show cultural variation within a South Asian population. It would also be worthwhile for future studies to investigate whether there are demonstrable South Asian tendencies toward perfectionism and procrastination that may influence states of mind, depression, anxiety, and stress.

With regard to recruitment and minimization of attrition, future studies involving South Asians should consider the need to build strong relationships with local organizations for an extended period of time–perhaps a year or more–before expecting any collaboration in recruiting and/or participation in research. Future studies may also want to consider a comparison study between a Web-based intervention and a non-Web-based group intervention, examining the effectiveness of each in mitigating attrition and in motivating participation within this highly reluctant and private population. Moreover, future studies would have to address questions such as how to encourage emotional self-health over family and self-materialistic professional gains.

In my research, several cultural inquiries surfaced that future studies should investigate further. Even though meditation, yoga, and Eastern philosophies are becoming more popular in mainstream culture in Western countries, people in India are moving away from traditions and toward a materialistic mindset. One way that traditionalism may manifest, is in a reluctance to participate. By being set in their cultural ways, South Asians most likely are not ready to take risks such as volunteering for a stranger's research study. This is a result of the cultural wiring under which younger generations were raised, in which they blindly do as their parents did. This is also an important consideration when assessing the likelihood of South Asians' willingness to help strangers or openness to change in the context of self-actualization.

The unspoken need for any intervention, let alone a well-being tool like FOAT-IP, is the openness for new experiences and allowing change to evolve from the felt sense level through bodily awareness. Atkinson and Gim's (1989) study, "Asian-American Cultural Identity and Attitudes Toward Mental Health Services" suggested a possible acculturation factor influencing the decision making of Asian American seeking mental health assistance. In other words, the more acculturated the Asian American was in adapting to Western thinking, the more likely he or she was open to psychotherapy. Similarly, I speculate that South Asians who are younger, more educated, and modern (i.e., Western) in worldview perspectives are more likely inclined to new experiences to facilitate change, especially self-change. Therefore, future studies exploring South Asian upbringing, worldviews, and openness to change would be informative for future research designs, recruitment approaches, and attrition reduction.

REFERENCES

Ahmad, F., Riaz, S., Barata, P., & Stewart, D. (2004). Patriarchal beliefs and perception of abuse among South Asian immigrant women. *Violence Against Women, 10*(1), 262–282. doi:10.1177/1077801203256000

Ahmed, K., Mohan, R., & Bhugra, D. (2007). Self-harm in South Asian women: A literature review approach to assessment and formulation. *American Journal of Psychotherapy, 61*(1), 71–81.

Anderson, G., Carlbring, P., Ljotsson, B., & Hedman, E. (2013). Guided Internet-based CBT for common mental disorders. *Journal of Contemporary Psychotherapy, 43,* 223–233. doi:10.1007/s10879-013-9237-9

Atkinson, D., & Gim, R. (1989). Asian-American cultural identity and attitudes toward mental health services. *Journal of Counseling Psychology, 36*(2), 209–212. doi:0022-0167/89

Chidanand, R. (2014). *Quantitative Study Exploring the Effects of Focusing-Oriented Arts Therapy–Internet Protocol (FOAT-IP) on Stress, Anxiety, Depression, and Positive States of Mind in South Asian Women.* Retrieved from: http://search.proquest.com/docview/1616602141

Gendlin, E. (1978). *Focusing.* New York: Bantam Books.

Gendlin, E. (1996). *Focusing-oriented psychotherapy: A manual for the experiential method.* New York: Guilford Press.

Flannagan, J., & Flannagan, R. (2007). *Counseling and psychotherapy theories in context and practice.* Hoboken: John Wiley and Sons.

Hurwitz, E., Gupta, J., Liu, R., Silverman, J., & Raj, A. (2006). Intimate partner violence: Associated with poor health outcomes in the U.S. South Asian women. *Journal of Immigrant and Minority Health, 8*(3), 251–262. doi:10.1007/s10903-006-9330-1

Ingram, B. L. (2006). *Clinical case formulations: Matching the integrative treatment plan to the client.* Hoboken, NJ: John Wiley and Sons.

Maker, A., Mittal, M., & Rastogi, M. (2005). South Asians in the United States: Developing a systemic and empirically based mental health assessment model. In M. Rastogi & E. Wieling (Eds.), *Voices of color: First-person accounts of ethnic minority therapists* (pp. 233–254). London: Sage.

Madison, G. (Ed.), (2014a). *Theory and practice of focusing-oriented psychotherapy–Beyond the talking cure.* Vol. I. London: Jessica Kingsley Publishers.

Madison, G. (Ed.). (2014b). *Emerging practice in focusing-oriented psychotherapy–Innovative theory and applications.* Vol. II. London: Jessica Kingsley.

MySahana. (2011a). *How South Asian stereotypes and discrimination create mental health stigma.* Retrieved from http://www.mysahana.org/2011/08/how-south-asian-stereotypes-and-discrimination-create-mental-health-stigma/

MySahana. (2011b). *Biggest risk factor for heart disease: Depression.* Retrieved from http://www.mysahana.org/2011/11/biggest-risk-factor-for-heart-disease-depression/

MySahana. (2011c). *South Asian emotion: The link between stress and depression.* Retrieved from http://www.mysahana.org/2011/08/south-asian-emotion-the-link-between-stress-and-depression/

MySahana. (2011d). *Stress.* Retrieved from http://www.mysahana.org/2010/11/stress/

MySahana. (2011e). *Emotion suppression: Effects on mental and physical health.* Retrieved from http://www.mysahana.org/2011/05/emotion-suppression-effects-on-mental-and-physical-health/

MySahana. (2012a). *Six common reasons for lack of motivation.* Retrieved from http://www.mysahana.org/2012/04/six-common-reasons-for-lack-of-motivation/

MySahana. (2012b). *Signs of perfectionism.* Retrieved from http://www.mysahana .org/2012/04/signs-of-perfectionism/

PAMF. (2012a). *Depression and anxiety.* Retrieved from http://www.pamf.org /southasian/risk/concerns/depression.html

PAMF. (2012b). *Health concerns.* Retrieved from http://www.pamf.org/southasian /risk/concerns/

PAMF. (2012c). *South Asian women's mental health.* Retrieved from http://www.pamf .org/southasian/healthy/women/mentalhealth/

Park, C., & Ai, A. (2006). Meaning making and growth: New directions for research on survivors of trauma. *Journal of Loss and Trauma, 11*(1), 389–407. doi:10.1080 /15325020600685295

Prathikanti, S. (1997). *East Indian American families. In E. Lee (Ed.), Working with Asian Americans: A guide for clinicians* (pp. 79–100). New York: Guilford Press.

Purton, C. (2004). *Person-centered therapy: The focusing oriented approach.* New York: Palgrave Macmillan.

Raj, A., Liu, R., McCleary-Sills, J., & Silverman, J. (2005). South Asian victims of intimate partner violence more likely than non-victims to report sexual health concerns. *Journal of Immigrant Health, 7*(2), 85–91. doi:10.1007/s10903-005-2641-9

Rappaport, L. (2008). Focusing-oriented Art Therapy. *The Folio, 21*(1), 139–155.

Rappaport, L. (2009). *Focusing-oriented Art Therapy: Accessing the body's wisdom and creative intelligence.* London: Jessica Kingsley.

Rappaport, L. (2010). Focusing-oriented Art Therapy: Working with trauma. *Person-centered and experiential psychotherapies, 9*(2), 128–142. doi:1477-9757/10/02128 -15

Rappaport, L. (2014). Focusing-oriented expressive arts therapy: Cultivating mindfulness and compassion, and accessing inner wisdom. In L. Rappaport (Ed.), *Mindfulness and the arts therapies: Theory and practice* (pp. 193–207). London: Jessica Kingsley.

Rappaport, L. (2014). Focusing-oriented expressive arts and mindfulness with children and adolescents with trauma. In C. Malchiodi (Ed.), *Creative interventions for traumatized children* (2nd ed.). New York: Guilford Press.

Silberman, I. (2005). Religion as a meaning system: Implications for the new millennium. *Journal of Social Issues, 61,* 641–664.

Thombre, A., Sherman, A., & Simonton, S. (2010). Posttraumatic growth among cancer patients in India. *Journal of Behavioral Medicine, 33,* 15–23. doi:10.1007/s10865-009-9229-0.

Venkataramani-Kothari, A. (2007). Understanding South Asian immigrant women's experience of violence. In S. Dasgupta (Ed.), *Body evidence: Intimate violence against South Asian women in America* (pp. 11–23). Piscataway, NJ: Rutgers University Press.

Yoshioka, M. R., Gilbert, L., El-Bassel, N., & Baig-Amin, M. (2003). Social support and isclosure of abuse: Comparing South Asian, African American, and Hispanic battered women. *Journal of Family Violence, 18*(3), 171–180.

Biography

Rashmi Chidanand earned her PhD in Clinical Psychology with a specialization in Expressive Arts Therapy from the Institute of Transpersonal Psychology. She is certified in Focusing-Oriented Therapy from The International Focusing Institute in New Chidanand's background includes research at Stanford University, teaching at ITP, University of East-West Medicine, California Institute of Integral Studies, and at John F. Kennedy University in their Continuing Education program. Dr. Chidanand's clinical experience includes working at the Community Health Awareness Council and at the Mountain View-Whisman School District as a mental health specialist for special education. She currently has a private practice—*TheraVie Wellness*—that focuses on life empowerment for children and for adults. As part of her self-care practices, Dr. Chidanand engages actively in yoga, creative writing, Indian classical dancing, and other mindfulness practices that she also utilizes in her clinical work. Derived from her dissertation on FOAT®-IP, Chidanand's vision is to make quality mental health care services accessible to the South Asian population, while continuing to find ways to serve the community and to work with diverse populations.

Chapter 14

A CASE STUDY USING CYBERCOUNSELING AND DIGITAL ART THERAPY WITH A CLIENT DIAGNOSED WITH HIGH-FUNCTIONING LEARNING DISABILITY

PRIYADARSHINI SENROY

Introduction

With recent technological advancement and growing popularity in the use of the Internet, various forms of technology are being used to deliver mental health services online. According to Barak, Hen, Boniel-Nissim, and Shapira (2008a), cybercounseling is one such delivery model that has seen tremendous growth in the past ten years. Like cybercouseling, the field of art therapy has also been growing and developing, and it is constantly integrating and complimenting new techniques, mediums and tools to meet the needs of clients. Technology is one such tool that has received increased attention recently as being a modality of offering digital art therapy. The author will be drawing on her experience as a cybercounselor, as a creative arts therapist, and as a disability educator to share counseling sessions undertaken with the protagonist of the case study. The case study will use parts of session vignettes, and share highlights of success and challenges encountered during the cybercounseling sessions. The author will also draw from new developments in the field and practitioners within the field of cybercounseling and creative arts therapy while referencing as well to informing her own understanding of best practices while using this medium. Some of the literature reviewed for this case study will include theory and practice including journal articles, case studies, and reports by experts and by researchers in the area of cybercounseling, digital art therapy, and disability.

Definition

Before delving into the history of when and how cybercounseling came into being, let us try and define it. There are many terminologies that have been used over the years to include the many ways in which telecommunications has been used in mental health and well-being settings. Research by Barak, Hen, Boniel-Nissim, and Shapira (2008b) have suggested that interchangeable terminologies–"cyber counseling," "online counseling," "web-based counseling," and "online support"–can be used, depending on the way in which the service is delivered. The deliverables will differ with respect to participants, delivery location, communication medium, and interaction process. A concise explanation of these forms (Shiller, 2009a) explains that counseling participants can be individuals, couples, or groups. The location for counseling delivery can be face-to face or at a distance with the assistance of technology. The communication medium for counseling can be what is read from text, what is heard from audio, or what is seen and heard in-person or from video. The interaction process for counseling can be synchronous or asynchronous. Synchronous interaction occurs with little or no gap in time between the responses of the counselor and the client. Asynchronous interaction occurs with a gap in time between the responses of the counselor and the client.

History

So when did cyber ounseling start? A presentation on online counseling (Wittes, Speyer, & Mani 2010a) informs us that one of the earliest distance communication technologies were written correspondence. The modality is well-documented; in fact, Freud was an advocate of letter-based counseling. Following a chronological timeline, in the sixties, a computerized "therapist" named Eliza, who emulated a Rogerian psychotherapist, became the most famous computer program in clinical psychology. Continuing the journey, Santhiveeran (2004) dated the use of computers in psychotherapy to 1972, with the advent of bulletin boards and online support groups. The earliest known organized service to provide mental health advice online was Ask Uncle Ezra, a free service offered to students of Cornell University in Ithaca, New York and has been operational since 1986. Following the successes of such initiatives, the International Society of Mental Health Online was established in the late-1990s. Since then, several psychological associations including the American, the Australian, the British, and the Canadian, have set up guidelines regarding ethical online counseling. These professional counseling associations have demonstrated the importance that technologies are having in their fields and for their clients by devoting entire journal issues to technology-related topics as stated by Peterson, Stovall, Elkins, Parker-Bell & Barbara (2005). Cybercounseling is also subjected to all practice and ethical considerations stipulated by these professional organization and in the law, rules, and regulations governing licensed practice as determined by different states and areas, where the practice takes place. Cybercounseling is a field that has seen tremendous growth in the past twenty years (Barak, Hen, Boniel-Nissim, & Shapira, 2008). In the present day, cybercounseling is offered as courses in universities around the world and Employment Assistance Programs recognize these modalities enough to offer them as complimentary services to the traditional face-to-face counseling. Wittes, Speyer, and Mani 2010(b) shares that an Employment Assistance Program company has been offering e-counseling in Canada since 2000. It is a professional, confidential, counseling service available directly through their website. The service allows the client to connect with a counselor from any computer with Internet access. This short-term service is an effective means of addressing personal issues by means of letters to and from the assigned e-counselor. Clients can post messages at any time of the day or night, from anywhere in the world.

Effectiveness

How is cybercounseling effective as a modality of offering distance therapeutic or counseling to clients? In their works (Murphy & Mitchell, n.d.) identified numerous benefits of conducting therapy online. Their research tells us that Internet-based counseling can provide important services to clients who might not otherwise be willing or be able to meet with professional counselors in their offices. This is emphasized by who specially refers to the geographically isolated, or to those isolated by their various physical or emotional conditions, including the elderly and physically challenged. Online services can also be incredibly cost-effective as they can minimize travel costs and office related expenses. Online counseling is intended to provide services that are most suitable for clients who have either previously engaged in formal counseling services and/or are seeking short-term support for issues that are unrelated to major crises, severe mental health issues,; and suicidal, homicidal, or violent behavior (past and present) as not all issues are suitable for cybercounseling.

To validate that cybercounseling is effective, there is a growing body of evidence based literature in this field, that is supported by the following: Collie, Mitchell, & Murphy, n.d.; Derrig-Palumbo & Zeine, 2005; Hsiung, 2002; Kraus, Zack, & Sticker, 2004; Murphy & Mitchell, n.d.; Mitchell &

Murphy, 2004; Murphy, MacFadden, & Mitchell, 2008; and Tyler & Sabella, 2003. One of the studies conducted by (Murphy & Mitchell, n.d.) highlighted several of the benefits of online counseling via email. Like these authors, they have found that the recordkeeping of counseling via cybercounseling and the space for the clients to go over them and keep them for future references, are what makes it a unique experience. As Barak (1998) noted, the delayed-correspondence technique enables thinking, planning, and editing of any message. A study by authors Murphy, Mitchell, and Hallett (n.d.) shares that cybercounseling is a field that has seen tremendous growth in more than a decade. This research confirms the results of reviewed research and makes plain that online counseling can provide client satisfaction and counseling outcomes, as good as those in face-to-face counseling. The findings from research studies by authors (Barak et al., 2008) have also studied the outcomes and the therapeutic relationship or working alliance that has had an impact on satisfaction as reported by clients. A study conducted by an Employment Assistance Provider (Shepell, 2015) that provides cybercounseling services, presented statistics on the success of this modality within their client base. They collected data from a sample of 407 chats taken from December 5, 2011, to January 31, 2012, and the findings indicate that 94% of First Chat users reported feeling comfortable using chat as a clinical counseling service. 90% reported that the counsellor understood their problems and concerns, and 81% agreed that their provider helped then consider the options and solutions to resolve their problems. The overall level of client satisfaction was 87% who also indicated that they would recommend First Chat to others.

When it comes to talking about the efficacy of using text-based communication, research suggests that the written word is more than capable of communicating emotion, especially if the clinician is well-versed in the use of creative text-based communication. Suler (2000) reported that some clients may be more comfortable and expressive when they believe a human therapist in not present. Clients also self-disclose, self-reflect, and feel less fearful of being judged in this setting, as noted in the research (Yaphe & Speyer, 2010). This also helps to build the significance of a supportive, healthy, and therapeutic working environment between the client and the counsellor, which is equally important online as it is in a face-to-face session. This finding can also be found in the research by Reynolds, Stiles, and Grohol (2006) who suggested that a therapeutic alliance can be constructed online and can be equal to that in face-to-face counseling. What might differ, is the medium and experience of how this relationship may develop. Anthony (2011) found that the rapport between counselor and client in cyberspace is developed not by relating to another person's physical presence and spoken work, but through the client's mental constructs via the written word. Efficacy of therapeutic alliance is also found in the work of Horvath and Luborsky (1993) who stated that there are various techniques that have been developed to establish the therapeutic alliance as it was to address the lack of tone of voice and nonverbal in text-based work. Emotional bracketing, descriptive immediacy, descriptive imagery, and time presence, collectively known as the presence techniques, have been created to address this issue by providing ways for counsellors (and clients) to communicate essential nonverbal and tone-of-voice information that is not be contained in the words used to describe a problem, to ask a question, or to explain a therapeutic task (Murphy & Mitchell, n.d.). Some of these presence techniques will be demonstrated in the case study further in the chapter.

Digital Art Therapy and Disability

Internet communication has seen a plethora of new developments which continue to change the terrain of not only online communication, but also the possibilities for providing methods and materials for artistic communication within the context of art therapy, states Machioldi (2015). In her earlier work, Malchiodi (2000) explained further, that for art therapy, the progress made in computer technology and in digital imagery may have even a greater impact as these advances have created opportunities to make digital media such as photography, videography, computer -based painting, and photo programs an integral part of art psychotherapy. For nearly two decades, digital media has offered clients new ways to express themselves creatively. Digital media as another complementary art medium that has unique therapeutic qualities, has also been corroborated by other authors (McNiff, 1999; Orr, 2006, 2010). Digital media and digital art therapy can be shared in a variety of platforms like video games and digital art programs, and also in social media. The last one, according to Chapman (2010), has been emerging as an important and unique vehicle for people with developmental disabilities to control the expression of their own ideas and concerns and, as a result, promote self-advocacy and "smash" stereotypes. The protagonist of the case study in this chapter has been diagnosed with having a disability and throughout the study, various social media and networking sites like blog posts, Facebook, Instagram, Second Life, and Skype have been explored as tools of communication and self-expression. For youths with learning disabilities, communicating via text or visual imagery, for example, Instagram, Pinterest, or Snapchat, does not does not need attention to facial cues, to gestures, or to nonverbal expressions.

The Client

Sonali (name changed for confidentiality) is in her mid-20s. She was considered for a promotion at her current employment. In her interview, Sonali had mentioned that she always had problems keeping and maintaining employment, managing relationships, and has dealt with social anxiety most of her growing and adult life. The supervisor suggested that she perhaps get a psychological assessment done. Sonali was diagnosed as having high-functioning global learning disability along with social anxiety disorder. After her diagnosis, Sonali was also encouraged to seek counseling to help resolve feelings and to define issues that could help make sense of what she may be experiencing as being a newly diagnosed person. Counseling was also suggested as it was evident that the diagnosis and disclosure had a big impact on her self-esteem and on her self-image. Sonali was referred to see me initially for face-to-face counseling.

In the first meeting, I noticed that Sonali was finding it challenging to get comfortable with the face-to-face setting. She was not making any eye contact, and she was not able to communicate or problem solve within the given amount of time. I could see in her body language that she was anxious during most of the session. Upon probing, she said that she was uncomfortable with the one-on-one situation. She also mentioned that she was not a talking person but more of a writing person. When it came to booking the next session, she said that she would email me her availability.

After a few weeks, she emailed, saying that she could not come as she was traveling home to India and she would like to keep in touch as she had given a lot of thought and really wanted to continue the exchanges, so cyber-counseling was suggested. Many clients use this service when they are vacationing or on extended travel as it provides them with the flexibility and the accessibility unlike face-to-face counseling which can be conducted in-person only. For Sonali, this seemed to be convenient as there was a continuation of service and it also helped her to navigate her anxiety and her social skills, without causing any discomfort. Some individuals with developmental disabilities found that they may interact more successfully with computers and with their associated programs than with traditional media (Beck, 2011). Limited social skills that are attributable to their diagnoses, may impede dynamic face-to-face interactions. Technology makes the attainment of these skills more linear and less time dependent.

Sonali also expressed an interest in experiencing how counseling could be conducted online. She did not have any problem understanding or grasping the technical details and her learning disability did not play any role in accessing the service. Sonali represents a growing number of emerging adults who are among the most avid users of digital communication technologies, including texting, instant messaging (IM), and video chat (Duggan & Brenner, 2013; Lenhart, Madden, Smith, Purcell, Zickuhr, & Rainie, 2011). Further, today's older youths are often described as "digital natives" because they have grown up using these technologies, utilizing text-based tools to develop existing friendships during adolescence, a sensitive period for socio-emotional development (Baird, 2010; Prensky, 2001; Steinberg, 2005). A mutual decision was made that writing might also help to give her that space to work on her thoughts and not to make her anxious by only using spoken words to express and to communicate. Like Sonali, it has been reported that cybercounseling may also be beneficial for those who are socially phobic (Lange, Ven, & Schrieken, 2003) and those who are afraid to seek face-to-face therapy due to anxiety (Fenichel, Suler, Barak, Zelvin, Jones, & Munro, 2002). By writing out her thoughts and feelings, Sonali would be able to focus on her concerns and issues and not on how she talks or expresses herself.

With progressing sessions, Sonali mentioned that she loved journaling and was thinking of blogging. This seemed to tie in perfectly with cyber-counseling as it involves the process of writing and externalizing clients' thoughts. Writing, according to White and Epston (1990), allows clients to develop some distance from their problems and to see themselves and their relationships as distinct from the problem itself. Research has shown that the act of putting thoughts and feelings into written words is healing in itself (Pennebaker & Chung, 2007). Writing allows the author to witness the experience from a safe distance, making it possible to form a new perspective (Pennebaker & Chung, 2007). It is interesting to mention that this research is in line with the media richness theory, proposed by Daft and Lengel (1986), which states that some media allow for the exchange of richer information due to the number of cues and channels available for communication

Sonali was apprehensive about the cybercounseling modality at first, as she was concerned about her privacy and confidentiality. She had heard many negative comments about this modality. Keeping in line with the guidelines of the Canadian Counseling and Psychotherapy Association (CCPA) (2015), Sonali was also informed about boundary issues, jurisdictions, duty to report, counselor credentials, and so forth. In their section on possible pitfalls when offering e-counseling services, CCPA informs that while there are many ethical and practical issues related to counseling strangers, there are certain key issues to keep in mind when deciding whether or not to venture into the world of e-counseling. Like many authors, Murphy and Mitchell (n.d.) have also explored the advantages, challenges, and ethical issues when considering the delivery of cybercounseling services in-depth. No matter what the pros and cons are, it is evident that regardless of the technology used, counsellors should retain their responsibility for the maintenance of the ethical principles of privacy and confidentiality, for decisions made during the counseling sessions (Shiller, 2009b).

Sonali had a mixed response to the first session. She had to also deal with technical issues which arose, requiring troubleshooting and emails expressing her frustrations from time to time. Sonali had to navigate practical issues like finding time to reply and ensuring that she had a quiet, secure space. Additionally, she had to guide through some of the techniques used and examples had to be given to reduce her anxiety level. She was also informed about the ways in which the communication could occur. Communication could take place in both synchronous (live chat) and asynchronous (with a time delay) format as mentioned in the introduction. Sonali chose the asynchronous format as she shared that she was able to express herself more effectively if she did not feel rushed. Asynchronous communication, for example, offers youths with cognitive disabilities, more control over the pace of conversation than face-to-face or real-time mediated communication.

Asynchronous conversations permitted both me and the client the time to compose a thought or question that precisely reflects the concern or issue (Tate & Zabinski, 2004). It also allows the convenience of replying when the client is ready and able to reply (Suler, 2000). Speyer and Zack (2010) have found that the client can always (even years hence) re-read, rehearse, and reinforce the solutions and resolutions it contains. When the client has words to hold onto, hope is established. With many clients, this is literally true. They carry printouts in their pockets, purses, and briefcases. In this way, online counseling becomes an open-ended, ongoing session with healing words accessible at any time. This was true for Sonali who really appreciated the time delay and who took advantage of it. In one of the conversations she writes: "My last correspondence with you was a week ago now[eager hands—can't wait to type]. I have printed off every written word we shared and I can't tell you how many times I have gone back to those letters to reread the words [feel like teddy bear–warm, fuzzy, cared for]. The whole experience has been so much more than I expected it to be [folded hands]. Thank you for giving me the time to think &reply" [smiling with wide eyes]. By this time, Sonali had become familiar with the various techniques that guides cyber-counseling expressions. Two techniques suggested by Murphy and Mitchell (n.d.) are emotional bracketing and descriptive immediacy. Emotional bracketing employs the use of square brackets wherein we write about inner nonobservable thoughts and feelings. For example, folded hands allows the client to hear the intended vocal tone in the words. Descriptive immediacy provides the client with information about the counsellor's observable, nonverbal behavior toward the client, for example, smiling with wide eyes. I became aware of Sonali's creative side when she started to insert photographs along with words.

I decided to meet Sonali where her interest was and asked her if she would be interested in incorporating other creative art modalities like multimedia, phototherapy, and digital art making in some form or the other in our sessions moving forward. I explained to her that this would be different than using the traditional form of art therapies. Art therapy for clients with intellectual disability has been evolving over the last quarter century. According to White, Bull, and Beavis (2008), when therapists started using it with this client group, they tended to focus on the therapeutic value of making art but it is now used as a direct therapy to understand emotions, relationships, and the client's interpretation of their experiences. Combining art therapy and digital media is one such form that Orr (2006, 2010) describes in that it has inherent therapeutic benefits for some clients. In fact, the art of using photography was researched and written about as an art therapy medium as early as 1974. She also cautions that when choosing media to use with a client, it is always important to determine client interests, personal associations, and experience with any medium before working with that medium as it can also be detrimental to other clients.

I found this to be true in Sonali's case, as over the course of staying in India, Sonali used different multimedia tools including using photography, to reflect her moods and thoughts. She seemed to have found a nonverbal cathartic medium and the next couple of session, was comprised of images only and no words. Additionally, Sonali said that she found that the images spoke more than words than she had thought. I then introduced her to numerous digital arts-making websites which she used to create images and to share her days as a way of photojournaling. She started to post them on Facebook, on Youtube, and on Instagram, as well as in her blogs as she recorded her journey through India . The websites and the programs worked well as in this case as they were virtually available for her use at her own convenience. She posted them in her blog and also began to use the artwork in her messages. She found that while written journaling was good for her, incorporating images into them was definitely more therapeutic. In one of our conversations about her parents, Sonali wrote to say, "I'm so frustrated [angry with myself]. My parents don't understand. But, hmm, now that I think about what you said again, I think I'm actually angrier with them than with myself. [Whoa. Weird. I feel pretty good just now, sharing this. IS THIS AN "AHA" MOMENT PRIYA THAT YOU HAVE TALKED ABOUT?????]." Then she put up a series of images which she said reflected how she felt before, during, and post her conversations with her parents. The therapeutic effect that the digital images and photographs had on Sonali is the by-product of a technique used by Weiser (2015) a pioneer on phototherapy. She mentions that using clients' personal snapshots and family photos to connect with feelings, thoughts, and memories during their counseling sessions, are ways that words alone cannot do. For Sonali, these images when used within the cybercounseling context, opened a whole new way of communicating, relating, and understanding of herself.

Sonali was nearing the halfway mark of her vacation and during this time she made a request. She wanted to Skype and to talk to me as she wanted to see me in person and to hear my voice, which was missing from her interactions. This visual and audio request falls in line with what Suler (2000b) suggests that feeling the therapist's presence may be powerful when multiple sensory cues are available, which can enhance the impact of the therapist's interventions, the sense of intimacy, and the commitment to therapy. I found this interesting and brought this to her attention by asking how this was different than face-to-face and she mentioned that "you are here but there—I am less nervous. During the first Skype session, I noticed and acknowledged that she was relaxed in her surroundings, in her tone, and also in her body language. In a CCPA blog, Martin agrees that "videoconferencing (via Skype, for example) offers something "closer" to face-to-face counselling where counselors and clients can enjoy the benefits of hearing verbal intonation, observing some body language and seeing each other's eyes" (cited in CCPA, 2015). While Skyping, she mentioned that she had attended a dance workshop and learned a technique which she wanted to share with me. She did some actions and wanted me to follow her. I mentioned that perhaps this is like mirroring. I could relate to this as I have a background of drama and movement therapy and have often used it with clients. In her book, *The Creative Arts Manual,* Brooke (2006), states that in dance movement therapy terms, congruence would be expressed through using the technique of mirroring or shaping and nonverbally reflecting complimentary quality of the client. This used with empathy and with unconditional acceptance, can have an immense healing effect. Using the construct of kinesthetic empathy within in the context of cybercounseling, was an interesting transition of doing mirroring with her on Skype. Considered one of dance movement therapy s major contributions to psychotherapy, Berger explains this construct of synthesizes as an approach of the dynamics of the therapeutic relationship that includes nonverbal communication, bodily movement, dancing, and verbal expression (cited in Fried, Katz, Kleinman, & Naess, 1989). Sonali did another movement and said that it represented her feelings of freedom and when I mirrored it back to her, she said, "Priya, you understand how I feel." It felt as if we were able to share expressions and able to connect on different levels.

It was nearing the end of Sonali's vacation and she was planning her return. She felt that she could not wait to come for her face-to-face sessions. She shared that the initial sessions had been uncomfortable and that the process at that time was causing her anxiety. As she traveled and discovered different ways of expressing herself online, along with her newfound interest in using the digital art media, she became more confident in her communication, both verbal and nonverbal skills, and in her social skills and in her interpersonal skills. As our online interactions came to an end for the time being, once her initial concerns had been dealt with, she summed up her experience with this "My experience with cybercounseling has been very empowering. First of all I found writing to be easier than talking. I was able to put my thoughts in order without thinking–am I saying the right thing. . . . The best part of it is that I could go back any time and read again and reflect on other things and know how my thoughts on some matters have evolved. I also found the whole process very easy . . . no pressure, no stress . . . Ahhhhhh." And the photos and websites and pictures were just amazing every time I look at them, every time I upload a movement piece, Priya, I can't believe that this is me and let's not even talk about those friends I have met on Facebook. And the feedback I get including all the likes and shares would not have been possible just with words alone!!!! #AWESOME, Priya!!!!!

Conclusion

When Sonali returned, she came for her face-to-face session and the person I saw that day sitting across from me was someone who I had not met before. Firm handshake, eye contact, confident posture, and the ability to communicate openly, was noticed and acknowledged. She was able to identify these changes in herself and was observed by her employers. Sonali was upgraded to another position in her current employment. Evaluating the case, there was a mutual agreement that her transformation was a combination of her visit to India, discovering cyberounselling and off course digital art therapy. She had become an avid photo blogger, using videos, and art along with uploading her movement pieces on Youtube, to give voice to her expressions with a high number of followers. This had a great impact on her social anxiety. She has been befriended and liked by her Facebook acquaintances and by her friends. She also ventured to socially connect with others in the virtual world of Second Life, which is a free 3D virtual world where users can socialize, connect, and create, using free voice and text chat, a platform which she was thinking of using in the counseling context in the future.

Cybercounseling along with using digital art therapy, proved to be successful for Sonali in more than one way. There were challenges along the way when she had to wait for websites to express how she felt instead of just drawing and showing it to me. She also shared that sometimes the artwork did not feel real, as she could not touch it like traditional paper. Throughout the case study, literature reviews, works by pioneers in the field of digital art therapy and of course, the lived experience of Sonali, has shown that for people with developmental disabilities, regardless of their cognitive abilities, a wide range of digital-based art techniques, and programs in conjunction with cybercounseling is now possible and hopefully will continue to expand as technology advances. It is also a necessary topic to research further as technology is the way of the future. Although the literature and research papers reviewed indicate that the field of art therapy may be ready to embrace the medium of cybercounseling once there is sufficient proof of effectiveness and benefits, this can only be achieved through further research.

REFERENCES

Anthony, K. (n.d). The nature of the therapeutic relationship within online counselling. *Online Therapy Institute, 12, para. 1.* Retrieved from http://www .onlinetherapyinstitute.com/wpcontent/uploads/2011/02/thesis2000Anthony .pdf

Baird, A. A. (2010). The terrible twelves. In P. D. Zelazo, M. Chandler, & E. Crone (Eds.), *Developmental social cognitive neuroscience* (pp. 191–207). New York: Psychology Press.

Barak, A. (1999). Psychological applications on the internet: A discipline on the threshold of a new millennium. *Applied & Preventive Psychology, 8,* 231–245.

Barak, A., Hen, L., Boniel-Nissim, M., & Shapira, N. (2008). A comprehensive review and a meta-analysis of the effectiveness of Internet-based psychotherapeutic interventions. *Journal of Technology in Human Services, 26*(2),109–160.

Beck, E. (2011). Stitched together: Working with dually diagnosed developmentally disabled adults. *FUSION, 3*(1), 26–27.

Berger, M. R. (1956). Bodily expression of experience and emotion. In J. Fried, S. Katz, S. Kleinman, & J. Naess (Eds.), (1989). *A collection of early writings: Toward a body of knowledge, 1.* Columbia, MD. American Dance Therapy Association.

Brooke, S. L. (2006). *Creative arts therapies manual: A guide to the history, theoretical Approaches, assessment, and work with special.* Springfield, IL: Charles C Thomas, Publisher.

Canadian Counselling and Psychotherapy Association. (2015). *Did you know?– Possible pitfalls when offering E-counselling services.* Retrieved from http://www.ccpa -accp.ca/en/ecounselling/

Chapman, G. (2010). *Internet an equalizer for people with disabilities.* Retrieved from http://www.physorg.com/news202909285.html

Collie, K., Mitchell, D. L., & Murphy, L. J. (n.d). *Skills for on-line counseling: Maximum impact at minimum bandwidth.* Retrieved from http://therapyonline.ca/files/Skills %20for%20On-Line%20Counseling.pdf

Daft, R. L., & Lengel, R. H. (1986). Organizational information requirements, media richness and structural design. *Management Science, 32,* 554–571.

Derrig-Palumbo, K., & Zeine, F. (2005). *Online therapy: A therapist's guide to expanding your practice.* New York: Norton.

Duggan, M., & Brenner, J. (2013). The demographics of social media users–2012. *Pew Internet & American Life Project.* Retrieved from http://pewinternet.org /Reports /2013/Socialmedia-users.aspx

Fenichel, M., Suler, J., Barak, A., Zelvin, E., Jones, G., Munro, K. et al. (2002). Myths and realities of online clinical work. *CyberPsychology & Behavior, 5*(5), 481–497

Fried, S., Katz, S., Kleinman, S., & Naess, J. (Eds.). (1989). *The art and science of dance/movement therapy: Life is dance* (2nd ed.). New York: Routlege.

Heyman, C., & Speyer, C. (2010). The writing cure: Therapeutic effectiveness via the Internet. *TILT Magazine: Therapeutic Innovations in Light of Technology, 1*(1), 9–11.

Horvath, A. O., & Luborsky, L. (1993).The role of the therapeutic alliance in psychotherapy. *Journal of Consulting and Clinical Psychology, 61*(4), 561–573.

Hsiung, R. C. (Ed.). (2002). *Etherapy: Case studies, guiding principles, and the clinical potential of the Internet.* New York: Norton.

Kraus, R., Zack, J., & Sticker, G. (Eds.). (2004). *Online counseling: A handbook for mental health professionals.* San Diego: Elsevier Academic Press.

Lange, A., van de Ven JP., & Schrieken, B. (2003). Interapy: treatment of post-traumatic stress via the Internet. *Cognitive Behaviour Therapy, 32*(3), 110–124.

Lenhart, A., Madden, M., Smith, A., Purcell, K., Zickuhr, K., & Rainie, L. (2011). Teens, kindness and cruelty on social network sites. *Pew Internet and American Life Project.* Retrieved from http://pewinternet.org/Reports/2011/Teens-and - social-media.aspx

Malchiodi, C. (2000). *Art therapy & computer technology: A virtual studio of possibilities.* London and Philadelphia: Jessica Kingsley Publishers.

Malchioldi, C. (2015). *Digital art therapy.* Retrieved from http://www.cathymalchiodi .com/art-therapy-resources/digital-art-therapy-2/

McNiff, S. (1999). The virtual art therapy studio. *Art Therapy: Journal of the American Art Therapy Association, 16*(4), 197–200.

Mitchell, D., & Murphy, L. (n.d.). *Confronting the challenges of therapy online: A pilot project.* Retrieved from http://www.therapyonline.ca/files/Confronting_the_challenges .pdf

Mitchell, D. L., & Murphy, L. (n.d). *E-mail rules! Organizations and individuals creating ethical excellence in telemental-health.* Retrieved from http://www.therapyonline.ca /_old_site _sept_2010/Publications/E-mail%20Rules.pdf

Murphy, L. J., & Mitchell, D. L. (n.d.). *Overcoming the absence of tone and non-verbal elements of communication in text-based cybercounselling.* Retrieved from http://www .therapyonline.ca/files/Overcoming%20the%20absence.pdf

Murphy, L. J., & Mitchell, D. L. (n.d.). *When writing helps to heal: E-mail as therapy.* Retrieved from http://www.therapyonline.ca/files /When%20Writing%20Helps %20To%20Heal.pdf

Murphy, L. J, & Mitchell, D. L. (n.d.). *Overcoming the absence of tone and non-verbal elements of communication in text-based cybercounselling* (pp. 216–218). Retrieved from http://www .therapyonline.ca/files/Overcoming%20the%20absence.pdf

Murphy, L. J., MacFadden, R. J, & Mitchell, D. L. (2008). Cybercounseling online: The development of a university-based training program for e-mail counselling. *Journal of Technology in Human Services, 26,* 447–469.

Murphy, L., Mitchell, D., & Hallett, R. (n.d). *Client satisfaction and outcome comparisons of online and face-to-face counselling.* Retrieved from http://therapyonline.ca /cybercounselling/_protected/resources/Readings/Client_Characteristics_in _Cyber _and_In-Person_Counselling.pdf

Orr, P. (2006). Technology training for future art therapists: Is there a need? *Art Therapy: Journal of the American Art Therapy Association, 23*(4), 191–196.

Orr. P. (2010). Social remixing: Art therapy media in the digital age. In C. Moon (Ed.), *Materials and media in art therapy* (pp. 89–100). New York: Routledge.

Pennebaker, J. W., & Chung, C. K. (2007). Expressive writing, emotional upheavals, and health. In H. Friedman & R. Silver (Eds.), *Handbook of health psychology* (pp. 263–84). New York: Oxford UP.

Peterson, B., Stovall, K., Elkins, D., & Parker-Bell, B. (2005). Art therapists and computer technology. *Journal of the American Art Therapy Association, 22*(3), 139–149.

Prensky, M. (2001). Digital natives and digital immigrants. *MCB University Press, 9*(5), 1–6.

Reynolds, D., Stiles, W. B., & Grohol, J. M. (2006). An investigation of session impact and alliance in Internet based psychotherapy: Preliminary findings. *Counselling and Psychotherapy Research, 6*(3), 164–168.

Santhiveeran, J. (2004). E-therapy: Scope, concerns, ethical standards and feasibility. *Journal of Family Social Work, 8*(3), 37–54.

Sheppell.fgi. (2015). *Attracting new EAP users through online text-based chat services.* Retrieved from Through%20Online%20Text-Based%20Chat%20Services_SFGI .pdf

Shiller, I. (2009a). Online counselling: A review of the literature. *East Metro Youth Services.* Retrieved from http://www.emys.on.ca/pdfs_fordownload/online counselling_literaturereview.pdf

Shiller, I. (2009b). Online counselling: A review of the literature. *East Metro Youth Services.* Retrieved from http://www.emys.on.ca/pdfs_fordownload/onlinecounselling_literaturereview.pdf

Speyer, C., & Zack, J. (2010). Online Counseling: Beyond the Pros and Cons. Retrieved May 6, 2017 from https://www.easna.org/wp-content/uploads/2010 /08/WS2B-E-CounselingBeyondthatProsandCons-Handout.pdf

Steinberg, L. (2005). Cognitive and affective development in adolescence. *Trends in Cognitive Sciences, 9,* 69–74.

Suler, J. (2000). *Psychotherapy in cyberspace: A 5-dimensional model of online and comput-er-mediated psychotherapy.* Retrieved from http://gsb.haifa.ac.il/~sheizaf /cyberpsych/05-Suler.pdf

Tate, D. F., & Zabinski, M. F. (2004). Computer and Internet applications for psychological treatment: Update for clinicians. *Journal of Clinical Psychology: In Session, 60*(2), 209–220.

Tyler, J. M., & Sabella, R. A. (2003). *Using technology to improve counseling practice: A primer for the 21st Century.* Alexandria, VA: America.

Weiser, J. (2015). *PhotoTherapy, therapeutic photography, & related techniques.* Retrieved from http://phototherapy-centre.com/

White, I., Bull, S., & Beavis, M. (2008). Isobel's images–one woman's experience of art therapy. *British Journal of Learning Disabilities, 37,* 103–109.

White, M., & Epston, D. (1990). *Narrative means to therapeutic ends.* New York: W.W. Norton and Company.

Wittes, P., Speyer, C., & Mani, M. (2010a). *HealingWords: Short-term E-counselling in an EAP Setting* [PowerPoint slide 2]. Retrieved from https://www.easna.org/wp -content/uploads/2010/08/HealingWords.Short-termE-counsellinginanEAP Setting.pdf

Wittes, P., Speyer, C., & Mani, M. (2010a). *HealingWords: Short-term E-counselling in an EAP Setting* [PowerPoint slide 6]. Retrieved from https://www.easna.org/wp -content/uploads/2010/08/HealingWords.Short-termE-counsellinginanEAP Setting.pdf

Yaphe, J., & Speyer, C. (2010). Text-based online counseling: Email. In *Online counseling: A Handbook for Mental Health Professionals* (2nd ed., Chapt. 8).

Biography

Priyadarshini Senroy , MA, CCC is a counselor who uses creative arts therapy and cybercounseling in her practice. She has been working as a certified Canadian counsellor with at-risk youths and their families for over ten years including clients with disabilities. Adapting to the changing needs of her client group and their needs, Senroy offers cybercounseling mixed with creative multimedia using popular social media sites and applications. Before immigrating to Canada, she worked as a drama and movement therapist in India and in England with clients from different diverse cultural group and she is also a published author, blogger, facilitator, and educator.

Chapter 15

LIQUID VIBRATIONS–
MUSICAL HYDROTHERAPY

Joel Cahen

Introduction

Liquid Vibrations was formed as a continuation of the underwater sound art concert series by Joel Cahen called Wet Sounds, which began touring pools in the United Kingdom in 2008. Adèle Drake, founder and former CEO of Drake Music in the UK, had made the connection between the properties of underwater sound perception and the potential benefits this could have on children with special and complex needs and together with Cahen they began setting up the organization in 2009.

Having set up as a charity in 2013, Liquid Vibrations has been providing training in Musical Hydrotherapy to staff at special needs schools. The combination of the benefits of hydrotherapy combined with music therapy and underwater listening, has been researched in collaboration with Roehampton University and Kent University. The lack of verbalization that most of the participants exhibit, creates difficulties in fully assessing the effect the sessions on their well-being, hence the team has conducted careful observations in each of the sessions provided since 2010, by filming the activity with two or more cameras; interviewing the peers, the headmaster, and the children themselves where possible; and sending out feedback forms to the parents.

The questions that guided the research were: Do the listening sessions affect a positive change in the participants' movement and awareness? Is there a discernible progression throughout the sessions? Do the sessions contribute to the development of meaningful communication and interaction with their surroundings?

This chapter will look at an analysis of the listening experience, a necessary consideration of all practice based on music and on sound and is the conceptual background of Musical Hydrotherapy practice. It will then describe the aims and motivations behind Musical Hydrotherapy and how Liquid Vibrations achieves them. The chapter ends with a case study by Hannah Newman of Kent University. UK.

Background

Liquid Vibrations is a charity organization that engages children and young people with special and complex needs in listening through the medium of water facilitated by aquatic body therapy in hydrotherapy pools. Underwater speakers are placed inside the pool and sound is heard through them when any part of the head is placed in the water. Additionally, vibrations can be felt in the body when it is in certain proximity to the speaker.

The properties of sound in water greatly affect the work. Sound travels 4.5 times faster in water than in air (Etter, 2013). This changes the perception of directionality. The difference of the arrival time of the sound between the two ears is too short for the brain to identify the direction of the sound or any reverberation and therefore sense of space. Underwater, sound is perceived by bone conduction by the skeletal system as well as by the eardrum (Parvin & Nedwell, 1995). Mostly affected are the spine and skull. The vibrations travel from the water to the bone and stimulate the inner ear directly, and so the listener actually perceives the sounds as if they are heard from inside their head. The result is a perception of sound that is incredibly detailed and immediate. The sound is perceived as detached from its spatial origin due to the lack of spatial signature usually recognizable by reverberation of the space. This gives the impression of a very personal and intimate experience. Despite being in a public space, the listener can feel as inhabiting a very private space, a womb-like environment.

The Listening Experience

Listening and attentiveness is important in creating meaningful communication (Purdy, 1996). Additionally, listening is an important part of meaningful musical interaction. Therefore, the practice of deep listening could open up new vistas of communication in that it increases attentiveness to one's surroundings and can increase tolerance to unfamiliar circumstances and improve musicality in the individual. Liquid Vibrations has devised sessions at hydrotherapy pools with an emphasis on listening and enabling an optimal position for listening. The beneficiaries of our service are children aged under 16 with special and complex needs and profound and multiple learning disabilities (PMLD) who have severe communication difficulties. Some cannot vocalize or have restrictions in movement and gestures; some are sight or hearing impaired.

The idea with which we approached the project, is the assumption that although everyone responds to sound differently, the factors that affect the listening experience, are shared by everyone. As most musical experiences whether being created or perceived involve listening, various factors would apply to the experience of musical interaction and creation. These are briefly explained as follows.

The Listener

Physical Capabilities

Can the Listener Hear? Most hearing occurs through activation of the eardrum; however, some hearing occurs through bone conduction, especially underwater. In cases where the cochlea and neural pathways from the inner ear to the receptors in the brain are damaged, hearing is lost entirely. In the water one can feel sound waves if they are played using underwater speakers.

Do the Listeners Have Any Conditions that Prevent Them from Listening? These could be neural disorders that affect their tolerance of sounds or their attention span or they may be under medication.

Are They Restricted from Inhabiting the Listening Space? This can occur in an auditorium without wheelchair access or in case of listening in water then this medium is restricted for some listeners who may not be able to be in water due to skin sensitivities or physical condition.

Comfort and Listening Position. Physical comfort affects the degree of attention; thereby discomfort can affect listening negatively.

Mood. The listener's mood is affected by experiences directly preceding the listening experience. The mood can affect the listener's interpretation and receptivity to the present experience. This is a general statement, but in the case of children with special and complex needs, the mood is volatile and can affect their ability to participate in the session and in their consequent degree of attention.

Cultural Background

Do the Listeners Have a Preconception of What Constitutes a Sound that Demands Listening? To listen is already to focus one's attention, to exert a particular effort (Barthes, 1985), some listeners may not regard some sounds as worthy of a focus of their attention, thereby ignoring them or regarding them as noise.[20]

Do the Listeners Have a Sense of Aesthetic Appreciation? Exposure to art forms through practice and guidance can develop a sense of aesthetic appreciation that enriches an experience. The listening sessions offer a platform for the aesthetic appreciation of sound.

The Environment in Which the Sound Is Perceived

Physical Affects. Perception of sound is influenced by the spatial dimensions of the space the sound is played in, as these determine which frequencies are accentuated and reverberations, and the materials in the space (reflective, resonant, porous, etc.).

Cultural Affects. The cultural context, or the institutional context that define the listening environment, informs the listener's expectation and contextualizes the sound heard, thereby affecting its perceived meaning.

Company. The presence of other people can be a distraction, which affects the listening process and interaction. As music is a time-based media, continuity helps give meaning to the sounds perceived; if that continuity is affected by other people in the space, then their presence would affect the listening experience and the meaning given to the sounds.

The Sound

The Compositional Elements of the Sound. Semiotic, aesthetic, cultural, and its progression and rhythm.

The Psychoacoustic and Bioacoustic Properties. Frequency, dynamic, rhythmic, and binaural properties.

The Method of Production. The type of speakers, high or low fidelity, and the sound's relations to an action or gesture and the performance aspect all affect how the sound reacts in the space and in the meaning of its production.

Interaction

The element that binds these three factors together is interaction. The interaction of the listener with these elements and between the elements

---

20. This breadth of the scope of what is called noise and what is called Music has been determining the transformation of musical structures in the last 100 years. This liminal point is largely affected by the degree of exposure to a variety of different music of different structures and, with reference to art music, an aesthetic appreciation of sound perception.

themselves, actively feeds back onto the experience itself and makes the listening experience an active process. As discussed by Clarke (2005), Gibson's (1966) ecological approach sees organisms immersed in a continual process of perceptual learning. This is progressive differentiation as perceivers become increasingly sensitive to distinction in the stimulus information. Perception is essentially an exploratory engagement, a "tuning in" and adapting to the environment, optimizing its resonance with the environment and developing awareness to the information that characterizes it. The aims of a therapeutic practice take into consideration the expectations of the treatment. In the case of music and listening practice, by considering and utilizing these factors, the expectations are more closely aligned with the experience of the participant.

The Aims of the Practice

As Liquid Vibrations began looking into adapting underwater sound to use in an educational and artistic context with children with complex needs in the hydrotherapy pools, we developed the following aims:

Confidence and Awareness. Developing a sense of individuality and sense of self in the listener despite being in a public space. To create a basis for linking proprioceptive and internal awareness with auditory perceptions, promoting external awareness.

This could facilitate communication as well as musical expression in movement or in sound. The creation of a mental connection between relaxation and contemplative listening in combination with a sense of individuality, can suggest a sense of mental control over one's environment and communication. The sense of intimacy occurs as a result of special properties of listening to underwater sound and to the sense of privacy it evokes.

To Promote Well-being. This is achieved by the provision of a relaxing experience that gives a lasting positive feeling, encourages vocalization and increases movement for those with limited mobility. As the sound is only audible inside the water the listener has to intend to listen, the sound does not impose itself on the listener as it does in most life situations. This motivation develops intention and displays the curiosity of the participant.

To Promote Awareness of the Art of Music in Particular. To increase the aesthetic appreciation of sound content in order to create immersion through observational separation. This could be beneficial in two ways:

1. An exercise in concentrated listening that does not demand any response as expected in many musical activities in the children's lives (e.g., singalong, play-along, and dance-along). Deep listening allows

for introspection whether as a result of a daydream or as a result of assessment of the sounds heard and activation of the imagination. Sound is separated from the communal context that is often presented in schools.

2. This could expand and empower the participant's musicality and tolerance of various environments as they have other tools by which to assess sounds, rather than just as signifiers of action to which they submit.

How Do We Achieve These Aims?

Sound

To this effect, Liquid Vibrations present a variety of music, classified as Tonal/Familia, Abstract Music, and Narrative Sounds. The movement between these three types of sound follows the sequence in which they are written here.

1. *Tonal/Familiar.* This refers to music that has a harmonious and melodic tonal progression and/or steady rhythm.[21] It serves to attract the participants into the new sensation and to increase their interaction with each other.

2. *Abstract Music.* Music that is characterized by its use of unconventional sounds, flexible structure, wide frequency spectrum, and its focus on sonic texture. The low frequencies are physically felt as vibrations on the body and extend the sonic sensation beyond the aural; this is particularly effective with participants with impaired hearing. The varied uses of the frequency spectrum is intended to invoke an interest in sound resulting from attention to textural sonic aesthetics rather than particular melodies, song- or rhythm-based sound structures, which compose a large majority of the recorded sound content to which the participants are often exposed.

   "The wide-open sonic world of electroacoustic music encourages imaginative and imagined extrinsic connections because of the variety and ambiguity of its materials" (Smalley, 1992, pp. 514-554). In the same way that visual puzzles and optical illusions make conscious the borders between stimulus and image recognition and thus confuse the brain to find an explanation, so does abstract and unfamiliar music encourage the listener to pay attention to the textures and to the

---

21. Generally speaking, the intention behind the term *familiar music* points to familiar and harmonic chord sequences and rhythmic structures of Western music.

sonorous qualities of the sound in order to create meaning using imagination.

3. *Narrative Sounds.* Narrative sounds are regarded as sonic signifiers, sound objects that, much like a photograph, represent the original but that are only reproductions. Part of assimilation into a society that is saturated in reproductions would include exposure to reproductions, in sound, image, and object. Narrative sounds shift the listening reference from the internal world, which the sonic textures are intended to immerse the listener in, to the external world, evoking the imagination to the familiar external environment that is nameable and identifiable. Examples of narrative sounds are the sound of whales, bird songs, a dog barking, voice, traffic, or rain. Underwater, they can be heard in isolation. Because narrative sounds are usually heard in an experiential context, their isolation and disassociation from the actual event, as reproductions, bring to attention sonic qualities, which might otherwise be masked by the event. This could also expand the sound palate of the listener and their aesthetic idea of sound and find expression in their musicality.

Relaxation

Liquid Vibrations conduct basic aquatic body therapy training sessions for the staff and for peers in each of the participating schools. Watsu is an aquatic body therapy through movement in water where the practitioner guides the participant using minimal contact and the weightless buoyancy in water to achieve a state of total muscle relaxation (Dull, 2004). This also facilitates the ideal position for underwater listening with the back of the head immersed in water, rearranging the posture for deep relaxation. The benefits include increased mobility and flexibility, muscle relaxation, fuller deeper breathing, reduction in anxiety and stress levels, decreased pain, improved sleep and digestion, and a general sense of well-being (Dull, 2004).

Listening Sessions

The listening sessions usually last 20 minutes to 30 minutes. Some of the participants in the sessions have had their peers support them one-on-one to facilitate underwater listening by supporting their body in the water according to the training they received. Other participants, mainly those within the Autistic Spectrum Disorder, have attended the pool unaided and explore the space above and below the water independently.

Developing Intention and Action. Unaided, the participants initiate listening themselves as part of their playful use of the pool. Moreover, the underwater listening is by choice and is a musical, and abstract artistic experience.

The Pool as a Playful Social Space. Hydrotherapy pool sessions sometimes become playful and encourage curiosity and social interaction between the participants and are a positive environment. The pool is a social space, which transforms into a private and intimate space as soon as the participant places their head in the water.

Case Study–Spring Term 2015

The following is an adaption of the report written by Hannah New-man.[22]

Nine sessions occurred in a special needs school in Canterbury, UK. The participants were three females under the age of 16, all diagnosed with Profound and Multiple Learning Difficulties. They experienced the sessions in the school's own hydrotherapy pool in which music created for the piece was played through underwater speakers. The piece of music was 10 minutes long and consisted of different sounds and moments of silence. The participants also experienced Watsu and Aquatic Bodywork in the pool, which was carried out by either the specialist involved in the project, Steve Karle, or by the participant's teaching assistant (TA). All of the sessions were filmed.

In addition to this, "dry" sessions occurred. This was where the same music was played in a quiet classroom, with the participant being accompanied by a member of the staff. These sessions occurred at three points across the research period and were filmed.

The methods of analysis chosen and developed were based on the previous research that had been carried out with Liquid Vibrations. One method, was the established Sounds of Intent (SoI) which is a method for the evaluation of musical development. This is a framework developed which analyzes the musical development of individuals with special needs, from children who have PMLD, to those on the autistic spectrum (with or without savant skills) (Sounds of Intent). The framework was developed from extensive observational data of children, psychological research into "typical" music development, and underpinned by the zygonic theory "which seeks to explain how music makes sense to us all" (Dull, 2004). The framework consists of three domains: reactive, proactive, and interactive, which each have six levels of development. This is a tool for assessing musical development (Vogiatzoglou, Ockelford, Welch, & Himonides, 2011; Welch, Ockelford, Carter, Zimmermann, & Himonides, 2009, Welch, & Ockelford, 2010).

---

22. Researcher and current PhD student. (An executive summary of the research can be found on the Liquid Vibrations website. The full report is available on request.)

In addition to this, an observation document was developed for the purpose of this research which noted specific behaviors that looked for any changes or responses to the research. Questionnaires were also developed for the TAs who worked with the participants, to document the behavior of the participant, and any changes. Questionnaires were also given to parents and staff to document behavior changes. At the same time as the "dry" sessions, interviews were also carried out with the TAs and teacher in which similar questions to the observation form that was supplied on a weekly basis were asked, as well as typical behavioral cues for each individual and an overall perspective on the experience. This was carried out in the second and third dry session. An interview was also conducted toward the end of the project with the Head Teacher of the school. Unfortunately, there were difficulties in attendance with the participants, as due to the complex natures of the conditions of each participant, medical issues often meant that they were unable to go into the pool or were not in school.

Results

Child One

In the first few sessions no physical reaction was noted. In later sessions she had clear reactions suddenly changing her physical behavior when the music started, or holding her weight and swaying her body from side to side. In later sessions, the physical reaction was reduced to smiling. There were no vocalizations that could be specifically linked to the music, as she vocalized throughout sessions.

With SoI, her grading started at R1 and developed to R2 after her third interaction with the session. In the "dry" sessions she displayed happy sounds throughout, even able to complete one of them after her TA thought she would not be able to because she was in a bad mood. From the TA forms it can be concluded that there were no negative alterations to her mood or behavior. The sessions increased her relaxation and half of them caused her to make her happy sounds. The interviews supported this with her class teacher commenting that she seemingly danced, which he had never witnessed her doing before. Only one parent/staff form was returned and this did not provide much information, as it coincided with a week when she was unable to go into the pool.

Child Two

Physical reactions were noted in the first few weeks via smiling. She developed this to dance in later weeks. Toward the end, her physical reactions were less frequent. There were no vocalizations that could be specifically linked to the music, as she vocalized throughout the sessions. Her SoI grading was ranked at R2 in all of the sessions, bar the last one in which it was reduced to R1. She was only able to attend the final "dry" session so not a lot can be concluded from it, although she did put her fingers in her ears, which she had not done during the pool sessions. The TA form indicated that there were no negative effects on her mood or on her behavior, with most of the sessions having at least a slight positive effect. The majority of the sessions caused a change in her physical presentation or in her vocalizations. The TA felt that her interaction with the participant was increased during the sessions. The interview complemented the forms, although she did state that she had not noticed a change in mood or in behavior, other than an increase in happiness which had been generally happening. She noted that the participant enjoyed the sessions very much. No parent/staff form was received.

Child Three

No verbalizations were made at any point during the research. There were some physical changes when she heard the music for the first time in some of the cases. In the final week, she worked with us, there was a very strong reaction to the music where she lifted her head toward the speaker, started moving her hands rapidly, and the eyes became active. Her SoI grading was ranked consistently at R2. She attended the first and second "dry" session. In the first she showed no response and in the second she seemed to enjoy the music: smiling as it went on. No TA forms or parent/staff forms were returned. An interview with her TA indicated that it was a positive experience for her, and that there had been change in, for example, her relaxation. We were able to interview this participant using eye pointing. She responded positively to all of the questions asked, except to one question about the Watsu, to which she responded that it surprised her.

Summary of Study

All of the participants showed at least once clear example of a reaction to the music. Another thing that can be concluded from the observation documents and supported by the forms and interviews, is that all of the children enjoyed the sessions. There were many instances of happiness and enjoyment which occurred in both the pool sessions and in the "dry" sessions. The fact that these occurred in the "dry" sessions, indicates that the children are responding positively to the music that was created, aside from the hydrotherapy pool and Watsu. There was also an indication across-the-board of the experience being very relaxing and calming, which is another positive outcome of the project.

The SoI ratings were inconclusive: one participant improved, one decreased, and the final stayed the same. This is, however, expected due to the complex nature of the conditions that can cause fluctuations in behavior. In addition, there was an indication of change and development with all of the participants, albeit relatively small. With individuals with PMLD the targets that are set for them can be very small and require a longer period of time to achieve. It is unlikely that a 9-week experience (approximately 10 minutes per week) would have a profound affect. However, the fact that there was some change indicates this could be a positive tool to use.

This research has had a positive impact on the school. They have purchased their own floats, similar to the ones that were used with Watsu, and the staff are very positive and enthusiastic about continuing and developing the training of Watsu that they experienced. There are also discussions about purchasing underwater speakers.

This research project provides sufficient evidence to warrant further investigation into the role of underwater sound and Watsu on children with PMLD. This was an overview analysis of the work. The results that we can see from this, warrant further investigation into this material to more closely analyze the effects (if any) that the music may be having over the period of time.

One strand to this research, which was not fully explored, was the effect that this experience had on the group students with autism (ASD). Some of them showed clear changes in experience outside of the pool and then inside the pool, for instance: one child would wear headphones and did not like noise; however, once in the pool, he would spend most of the time underwater near a speaker, actively seeking the noise and vibrations. Close analysis could occur of the footage that was taken to see if there were any significant differences but from the surface analysis that occurred, these children could benefit from such an experience.

Conclusion

As of 2016 ,Liquid Vibrations has conducted training sessions in several schools for children with special and complex needs in England and in Athens while continuing research. These were kindly funded by the Milton Keynes Foundation, Awards for All, Sound Connections, University of Kent,

SEMPRE, the Henry Smith Foundation, Arts Council of England, and the Onassis Foundation. The researchers from the University of Roehampton, the University of Kent, and The Institute of Education, have produced reports for each of these sessions which are available on the Liquid Vibrations website.

Additionally, Liquid Vibrations has begun conducting music workshops for people with disabilities to compose for underwater listening, encouraging creative dialogues and exchange. The artistic experience and the listening activity under leisurely conditions are seen to promote curiosity, relaxation and, at times, a positive change in movement or in vocal expression. The lasting effects beyond the session can only be assessed after a more prolonged period of observation involving their families and continuing hard and soft data analysis.

One of the greatest functions of art is, arguably, the space it clears up in the beholder's mind for reflection, imagination, and repose. Similarly, sound, and its use in art and in music, has functions that lie beyond the social interaction that surrounds its presentation. These functions are supported by phenomenological considerations as to its mode of presentation, whether for listening or for playing; these considerations shape the experiential effects that the work has on its creators and on its listeners. By customizing and crafting the experience to cater for physical limitations and spatial parameters, while endeavuring to expose listeners to the wide mutations of sonic frameworks, Liquid Vibrations brings an aesthetic artistic experience to a public to which it may not be otherwise exposed.

REFERENCES

Clarke, E. F. (2005). *Ways of listening.* New York: Oxford University Press.

Dull, H (2004). *Watsu: Freeing the body in water* (3rd ed). Trafford Publishing.

Etter, Paul C. (2013). *Underwater acoustic modelling and simulation* (4th ed.). Boca Raton: CRC Press.

Gibson, J. J. (1966). *The senses considered as perceptual systems.* Boston: Houghton Mifflin.

Kim, J., Wigram, T. & Gold, C. (2008). The effects of improvisational music therapy on joint attention behaviors in autistic children: A randomized controlled study. *Journal of Autism and Developmental Disabilities, 38,* 1758–1766.

Kim, J., Wigram, T., & Gold, C. (2009). Emotional, motivational and interpersonal responsiveness of children with autism in improvisational music therapy, *Autism, 13*(4), 389–409.

Parvin, S, J., & Nedwell, J. R. (1995). Underwater sound perception and the development of an underwater noise weighting scale. *Underwater Technology, 21*(1), 12–19(8). doi:10.3723 /175605495783328836.

Purdy, M. (1996). What is listening? In M. Purdy & D. Borisoff (Eds.), *Listening in everyday life: A personal and professional approach* (pp. 1–20). Seabrook, MD: University Press of America.

Smalley, D. (1992), The listening imagination: Listening in the electroacoustic era, In J. Paynter, T. Howell, R. Orton, & P. Seymour (Eds.), *Companion to contemporary musical thought* (pp. 514–554). London: Routledge.

Sounds of Intent. (n.d.). *About SoI.* Retrieved April 10, 2015 from http://soundsofintent.org/about-soi

Vogiatzoglou, A., Ockelford, A., Welch, G., & Himonides, E. (2011). Sounds of intent: Interactive software to assess the musical development of children and young people with complex needs. *Music and Medicine, 3*(3), 189–195.

Welch, G., & Ockelford, A. (2010). Music for all. In S. Hallam & A. Creech (Eds.), *Music education in the 21st century in the United Kingdom: Achievements, analysis and aspiration* (pp. 36–52). London: Institute of Education.

Welch, G., Ockelford, A., Carter, F. C., Zimmermann, S. A., & Himonides, E. (2009). Sounds of intent: Mapping musical behaviour and development in children and young people with complex needs. *Psychology of Music, 37*(3), 348–370.

Biography

Joel Cahen is an audio and visual practitioner based in London. His artwork interrogates the effects of sound in various spaces (the physical, the cultural, and the body). Since 2008, he has been performing worldwide with Wet Sounds, an underwater concert project that sonifies both wet and dry areas of the swimming pools. He has had a long-standing weekly radio show on London's Resonance 104.4fm exploring culture jams and cacophony. Since 2012, he has created Interzone Theatre, a work exploring the possibilities of locative sound-based augmented reality as a performative platform. He is also co-founder of Scrap Club, a public Destructivist activity where the audience smash household items with sledgehammers, and co-founder and artistic director of Liquid Vibrations, a charity which provides training sessions for musical hydrotherapy for children with special needs. Cahen's work has been presented and performed in galleries and festivals in the UK and abroad such as Tate Modern, Whitechapel Art Gallery, AV Festival, International Symposium on Electronic Arts, International Symposium for Music Education, Red Bull Music Academy, All Tomorrow Parties, and Nu Musik.

Part 4

E-COUNSELING AND SUPERVISION

Chapter 16

THE GOOD AND BAD OF ONLINE THERAPY: PERSPECTIVES FROM THREE ONLINE THERAPISTS

Dorothy A. Miraglia

When you make a connection with someone online, oftentimes it feels a little limited, but also safe. And people, strangely, are more comfortable sharing information about themselves with strangers online, simply because it's someone who is outside of their normal circle of friends, much in the same way you share things with a therapist.
–Nev Schulman (Montgomery, 2013, from the TV Show, Catfish)

The Internet has become a legitimate social tool, so it is no surprise the field of online therapy is flourishing. Online therapy, or e-therapy/e-counseling, can be defined as "therapeutic services delivered by a helping professional over the internet via text, audio and/or video" (Finn & Barak, 2010, p. 268). Online therapists use a variety of technologies to communicate with patients. These technologies include email, video chat, instant messaging (Kolog, Sutinen, & Vanhalakka-Ruoho, 2014), and text messaging (Gibson & Cartwright, 2014). Researchers continue to emphasize that online therapy cannot replace traditional face-to-face therapy, even though it has proven to be effective (Kolog, Sutinen, & Vanhalakka-Ruoho, 2014).

As cited in Prabhakar (2013), online therapy can be traced back to Freud in the early 1900s, in which he used letters to communicate with his patients. As early as 1982, mental health services emerged on the Internet in the form of self-help groups. Because of the growing field of online counseling, The International Society for Mental Health Online (2015) was formed in 1997, to promote information and the understanding about online communication for the mental health community.

Online therapy communication has increased from the computer to the smartphone. Clients can participate in an online therapy session via email or via real time interaction, which consists of video chat, telephone conversation, or text messaging. Because online therapy can occur globally, clients can seek services from another country and in another language. Furthermore, online therapy sessions can occur individually or in a group setting (Prabhakar, 2013).

This chapter will explore the benefits and drawbacks of online therapy as well as ethical considerations. To help understand online therapy better, three online therapists were interviewed as part of a case study. Their responses focused on why they pursued a career in online therapy, what they find are the benefits and drawbacks of online therapy, and challenges they face as an online counselor. Furthermore, each online therapist provided an example of a client identifying how online therapy was effective to this individual. Finally, each therapist offered his or her insight into the future of online therapy. The next section focuses on the perceived benefits of online therapy.

Benefits of Online Therapy

The biggest advantage of online therapy is convenience and flexibility. Individuals who travel often can seek treatment wherever they are. Online therapy is also convenient for those living in rural areas where treatment is not available and for those who cannot physically travel to a face-to-face therapy session (Prabhakar, 2013). Online therapy allows the client to choose the mode of communication he or she would like, which includes telephone, email, live video chat, or text messaging. A person can receive therapy from the comfort of their own home and when it works best for them.

Another advantage of online therapy is anonymity. In a 2004 study by Suler, he identified the online disinhibition effect. He explained that communication through disembodied forms may encourage more emotional expression and self-reflection. Additionally, he noted that clients experience a more equal relationship with their counselor when therapy session takes place using communication technologies. This is similar to Prabhakar (2013) who explained that clients are more open and honest and explore deeper concerns in a shorter time span in online therapy sessions as opposed to face-to-face therapy.

Callahan and Inckle (2012) interviewed 9 counselors and a focus group composed of 5 adolescents, aged 12 to 17 years, who were part of a consultation groups with a children's helpline in Ireland. The researchers found that online therapy sessions with adolescents focused on a greater variety and more sensitive topics than face-to-face topics. Results also indicated that adolescents might feel less intimidated talking to a counselor online and exercise more power and control. The results of this study are similar to Hanley (2012) who found that adolescents had a positive experience with online therapy sessions. Adolescents created good quality relationships with their counselors from their initial engagement, developed a rapport, and established control within the sessions.

In another study, Durrani, Irvine, and Nolan (2012) conducted an e-counseling trial by evaluating the influence of psychological stress and depression on individuals' motivation to adhere to recommended guidelines for diet and exercise. Subjects with hypertension ranged between the ages of 44 and 74 with participants being 59% female. This group completed assessment within two weeks after a four-month e-counseling program. Results showed e-counseling is significantly associated with therapeutic improvements in lifestyle change, which included a decline in depression and in stress and in the motivation or readiness to exercise. However, participants' willingness to change their diet was not associated with a change in depression and stress levels. This suggested that this relationship might be mediated by situational factors that were outside the scope of Durrani, Irvine, and Bolan's (2012) analysis. The researchers noted this was the first study to show how e-counseling with motivational interviewing significantly improves an individual diagnosed with hypertension readiness to change their exercise and diet behavior.

As discussed, there are many advantages to online therapy. Online therapy has proven to be effective to adolescents and adults. However, online therapy does have its drawbacks.

Drawbacks of Online Therapy

Prabhakar (2013) identified online therapy challenges in relation to the provider, industry, and patient. As for the provider, he or she may misdiagnosis the patient in a text only therapy session because nonverbal cues may be compromised. In addition, social norms may be taken out of context and a time lapse may not account for an immediate intervention. Prabhakar (2013) also noted how the online therapist may not be familiar with the legal, political, or cultural subtleties of the client's environment.

The healthcare industry is facing pressure to change their rules and regulations to accommodate the forms of communication. Insurance companies currently do not cover online therapy sessions. For the provisions of online counseling, legislation needs to "include web-based counseling services, reimbursement concerns, security and encryption of patient health records, maintaining confidentiality over an increasingly unregulated medium such as the Internet, verifying provider and patient identities, and defining jurisdiction" (Prabhakar, 2013, pp. 213–214).

The patient may misinterpret an email or text only session. In a face-to-face session, the patient can immediately verify the information with the therapist (Prabhakar, 2013). Another concern is eye contact during a live video session. A client and a therapist typically look at each other's faces when talking via the computer. However, the camera is usually perched at the top of the computer screen causing their gazes to be off-kilter (Hoffman, 2011). Therefore, a patient may think the therapist is not looking them in the eye.

Anonymity is a danger with online therapy (Hoffman, 2011). Most individuals avoid treatment because they feel shame or would like privacy. Some online therapists do not require patients to fully identify themselves, but this can be a cause for concern. If a patient has an emergency, the therapist will not be able to send help, and if the patient has a breakdown the therapist is limited in helping (Hoffman, 2011). Many online therapists will not treat someone who is suicidal, an alcoholic, or those who are severely mentally ill. One therapist refused to treat an alcoholic online because he could not smell his breath (Hoffman, 2011). Also, many psychologists find online therapy is suitable for those suffering from agoraphobia, anxiety, depression, and obsessive-compulsive disorder and that Internet addiction can be treated through live video therapy sessions (Hoffman, 2011).

Some therapists do not feel comfortable treating patients online. Hertlein, Blumer, and Smith (2014) surveyed 227 marriage and family therapists to identify how often they use online communication with their clients and how comfortable they felt communicating this way. Half of the sample rarely communicated with clients via email and stated they never use this form of communication with clients. Forty-seven participants stated they often communicated with clients via email while 9 participates stated they always communicate with clients this way. Therefore, a majority of the therapists were uncomfortable treating couples and families exclusively online and even more therapists were uncomfortable treating individuals exclusively online. This may be due to impaired warmth, empathy, and sensitivity when communicating online (Rees & Stone, 2005; Hertlein, Blumer, & Smith, 2014). These ethical concerns are worthy of more attention, particularly in the literature.

Ethical Guidelines

As most therapists know, the American Psychological Association (APA) developed a Code of Ethics to guide mental health professionals with their clients. The APA may need to extend to online therapy because the language does not specifically address online therapy services (Prabhakar, 2013). For example, APA may want to change how long information is stored from an online therapy session because the information, such as a video chat session, could be stored online posing the risk of the therapist's computer being hacked.

Competency is an important issue in terms of online therapy. Any person can misrepresent oneself on the Internet as a therapist to a client who is unfamiliar with the industry standards. In turn, clients may also misrepresent themselves to "save face" (Prabhakar, 2013, p. 214). Although competency falls under the responsibility of the therapist, the client must be competent in a virtual environment. Just like face-to-face therapy, the online therapist should present his or her credentials to clients before beginning therapy so that the client can verify the information. It is also important that the online therapist continue educating himself or herself about online therapy to reduce the possibility of miscommunication and misdiagnosis (Prabhakar, 2013). Additionally, an online therapist may adhere to his or her cultural upbringing and not fully understand the culture of the client. For example, Prabhakar (2013) pointed out that in India's language, a word does not exist for depression. The researcher suggested that communication subtleties be an added skill for online therapy programs.

Confidentiality is a concern because online therapy occurs in an unregulated environment. There is a risk of security becoming breached. This becomes more of an issue when the therapist communicates from a different geographic region than the client (Prabhakar, 2013). Furthermore, what may be considered private information in one society, may be considered public information in another.

Electronic signatures are often used to verify identities via the Internet. Prabhakar (2013) suggested that when online clients and their therapist electronically sign a consent form, they should each include their full information, addresses, and pictures to prove their identity. This information will help ensure the disclosure and identify of all parties involved.

Case Study

For the purpose of this chapter, I sought out online therapists to participate in an email interview. Participants were recruited via email after conducting an online therapist web search and posting a recruitment flyer on LinkedIn via therapy pages. Three online therapists contacted the researcher. The researcher emailed each therapist a consent form, which explained the purpose of the study and outlined the benefits as well as minor risks, and an open-ended questionnaire. The therapists digitally signed the consent form and emailed it back to the researcher along with responses to the ten open-ended interview questions. The researcher reviewed each of the responses and if she needed clarification or additional information, she emailed the therapist for clarification. The three online therapists answered questions pertaining to online therapy, which included the advantages and disadvantages of online therapy; the type of clients who participate in this therapy; and what they see as the future of online therapy. Their responses are discussed in this section.

About the Participants/Therapists

Scott Boyd is a licensed professional counselor and a national certified counselor in the Commonwealth of Pennsylvania. He works as an online counselor using video chat technology through www.breakthrough.com. Additionally, he uses doxy.me to for video chat therapy. He noted that as of May 2015, doxy.me would have an iOS and Android application to provide smartphone access to his office. He pursued a career in online counseling because he recognized that many individuals who wanted or needed therapy do not seek treatment. The main reasons why people do not seek treatment include lack of time, cost of services, stigmata, and lack of access to mental health providers. Because Boyd values his time and that of others, he believes technology is a means to provide quality mental health care to busy professionals and individuals with disabilities. He also believed that online therapy is beneficial to those who worry about the stigmata of seeking services via traditional means. He further explained that individuals living in rural areas, like Pennsylvania, often suffer the most and do not have access to quality and affordable counseling.

Dr. Lisa Herman, who goes by the name, Dr. Lisa, is a licensed clinical psychologist who started a private online therapy practice two years ago (www.drlisa-etherapy.com). Email, phone, and Skype chat are the technologies she uses to communicate with her e-therapy clients. Dr. Lisa began her online practice because she realized that many face-to-face patients wanted to call and to talk to her by telephone but that was not always convenient for her because insurance companies would not cover phone therapy sessions. This influenced her decision to start her own online therapy practice similar to a private practice, but only online.

Jay Ostrowski is an e-counselor and helps develop online therapy programs. When counseling his online clients, his technology of choice is video chat. He explained that a career in online therapy initially intrigued him. He was asked to see clients overseas for a mission organization and did so for the term of those clients. Furthermore, he discussed how he moved to a different state and online counseling allowed him to continue services with his previous clients.

Advantages of Online Therapy

The advantages of online therapy were consistent among all three online therapists. Convenience was the biggest advantage along with individuals not having to worry about childcare. Ostroski cited the advantage of online therapy: "Increased confidentiality, especially in smaller towns where one is likely to see someone they know in the lobby or parking lot (This happened a lot when I had my in-person offices)."

Disadvantages of Online Therapy

The disadvantages of online therapy included technology issues, such as a slow Internet connection or lack of computer skills. Boyd and Dr. Lisa both explained that insurance companies do not cover online therapy causing the client to pay out of pocket. Dr. Lisa also explained how confidentiality is an issue because of email hacking and Skype and how online therapy is not for every patient. She emphasized how "both client and therapist need to be mindful of the lack of privacy online." It is also not for the severely mentally ill or suicidal patient." Dr. Lisa also noted a disadvantage was that online therapy misses a lot of nonverbal cues that are important to therapy. This statement is similar to Boyd's viewpoint of the disadvantages of online therapy. He explained that depending on the type of online therapy (asynchronous email or synchronous chat), it requires the counselor to clarify a great deal more due to an inability to read the tone of the client. Conversely, the counselor's communication could easily be misread or misinterpreted by the client. In video chat sessions, this disadvantage is mitigated.

Health Insurance Portability & Accountability (HIPPA) was also an issue among two of the online therapists. Dr. Lisa explained how there are little to no laws around e-therapy and that each state have their own regulations (if any). She noted on her website (http://drlisa-etherapy.com) that "clients must reside in the State of Minnesota or New York to receive E-therapy Services from Dr. Lisa." Boyd expanded on this issue explaining how licensure boards in each state do not necessarily have policies governing the practice of e-therapy. As a licensed professional counselor, his board looks to the American Counseling Association (ACA) and National Board of Certified Counselors (NBCC). They have guidelines and require all the same policies for private practitioners, such as HIPPA privacy policy, Informed Consent, Clients Rights, and responsibilities. The one policy Scott has added is a social media policy to ensure respect for the client's confidentiality. HIPPA and HITECH rules are very important and costly if an e-therapy practitioner violates these laws. It is very important that the platform he uses for video chat is encrypted and compliant with HIPPA and HITECH law. If they are, the provider of the platform will sign a Business Associate Agreement between me (the user) and their company.

Online Therapy Clients

Online therapists were asked what types of clients pursue online therapy. Clients of various ages seek online therapy, especially those in rural areas who do not have access to treatment as Boyd noted. Ostroski mentioned that he counsels clients of varies ages who are "tech savy and tech phobic." Convenience and those suffering from anxiety were common reasons clients seek online therapy. Dr. Lisa explained how she is working with a family with a 12-year-old boy who has anxiety issues. Online therapy allows them to seek treatment from the comfort of their own home. They have the option to talk with Dr. Lisa after his homework or before dinnertime. Another client of hers has medical issues and cannot travel to a clinic. Dr. Lisa emphasized how online therapy is perfect for this client and for those who cannot travel to a session weekly. Additionally, she noted how online therapy is beneficial to teenagers. She explained how the Internet is their main source of communication in today's world and, therefore, Skype is a great way to get them invested in treatment.

The three therapists provided a general example of a client who benefited from their online therapy. Boyd worked with a shy, middle-aged man who sought online therapy because of conflict in his marriage. This client was struggling with anxiety, adjustment to the idea of divorce, and deeply committed to reconciling with his wife. Their sessions focused on self-awareness, communication styles, and conflict resolution styles during conflict.

Dr. Lisa worked with a 12-year-old boy whose anxiety was greatly reduced through online therapy. He learned about what anxiety is and how to control it using techniques they practiced each week through Skype. Dr. Lisa also included his parents in sessions (typically by phone) so that they were aware and able to help their son implement what he learned.

Ostroski provided generic descriptions of the types of clients he has worked with. One client was an executive who struggled with anxiety and could not take time out of work to travel to a clinic for services. A second client was a firsttime mother who struggled with depression and who did not want to leave the house. Another client was a physician battling alcoholism who could not be seen in his small town because his own clients would recognize him.

The Future of Online Therapy

As previously discussed, online therapy is a convenient method to help clients seek treatment. The future of online therapy is heading in the direction of additional accessibility via smartphone applications, according to the online therapists. Furthermore, this means that more clients will seek online treatment when they do not feel comfortable in a face-to-face setting or when they do not have access to a therapist in terms of where they live.

Boyd emphasized how the growth of technology will increase accessibility to online therapy. He explained how Mhealth devices, such as ginger.io and wearable technologies, are providing individuals with tools to take ownership over their healthcare. These smart technologies and applications help individuals get help when they need it. He further emphasized how Big Data and healthcare analytics are here to stay, providing innovative new methods to assist providers and their clients with the care they need, when they need it.

Dr. Lisa hopes she is on the cutting edge for licensed clinical psychologists to move their practice online stating it is convenient for everyone. She elaborated by saying how e-visits for physicians and for nurses are accepted everywhere now and that mental health therapy should not be too far behind. She emphasized how we must keep up with where things are going in society and that technology has a lot to offer in mental health relationships. Dr. Lisa stated that just because online therapy is new and different does not necessarily mean it is going to be less effective than face-to-face therapy. "In many cases, we will reach an entire subset of the population who disparately need it, thus reducing ER and inpatient visits and increasing positive mental health in our communities."

Ostroski sees online therapy rising dramatically within the next two to three years. He based this on how Accountable Care Organizations are required to use telehealth services and that many government bodies are contributing together over a billion dollars in creating services. Therefore, online therapy will be part of the telehealth services.

Discussion

There are many benefits to online therapy. Those afraid to seek treatment in a face-to-face setting or do not have treatment options in their community, now have the ability to use the Internet and to seek help. With the advancement of video chat and smartphone applications, an individual can seek treatment anywhere in the world. With the advancement of online therapy, it is hopeful that more people will be treated for issues they are coping with, such as anxiety or a troubled relationship.

Each of the therapists noted the advantages and disadvantages of online therapy with the good outweighing the bad. Parents no longer have to worry about taking off from work or finding childcare if they need a therapy session. A client who moves away from his or her therapist now has the accessibility of continuing treatment via online therapy instead of finding a new therapist. Although HIPPA is a concern, it is hoped that within the next few years, each state will begin to recognize the importance of online therapy along with insurance companies providing coverage for this treatment.

Boyd discussed working in the rural state of Pennsylvania and how most people living in rural areas seek online therapy. He found this important because face-to-face services are lacking in these areas. His point of view aligned with Hertlein, Blumer, and Smith (2014) who found that therapists were more favorable using online therapy in rural settings. The researchers emphasized that training programs should incorporate information explaining which "online therapy is useful as an adjunct to traditional treatment, and in which circumstances it is useful as a stand-alone treatment (p. 65).

Dr. Lisa emphasized how teenagers benefit from online therapy because this is their main source of communication. Her opinion is consistent with Gibson and Cartwright's (2014) study that found that text counseling benefited adolescents. Participants in this study felt that their autonomy was protected and that they could bypass their parents' authority and felt assured of their privacy. Furthermore, the convenience of online therapy was a factor and that adolescents felt they could really get to know the counselor.

As Ostroski pointed out, online therapy is on the rise. Many people rely on the Internet for communication. Having the ability to instantly connect with a therapist is not only convenient, but provides a sense of security and reliability. A client seeking treatment in the comfort of his or her own home, may feel less anxious about sitting in a face-to-face setting.

Hopefully, insurance companies and legislation will change the ways in which they view online therapy and implement coverage. Keeping up with the times is important. There is a lot of focus on mental health issues so the option of having another form of therapy that is accessible, should be a priority. Online therapy allows a client to take control of their emotions and to let them choose which form of online communication is best for them.

Because this book focused on the creative therapies and technology, it is important to mention that upon researching online therapy, I did not find any information regarding a creative therapy conducted via online therapy. This is an area that future creative therapists should explore. It seems possible that an art therapist and a client can paint together via video chat as well as a music therapist and a client composing a song via email, sharing song lyrics or singing on video chat. As of right now, it seems that there is a standard level of online therapy but more needs to be implemented. Expanding different types of creative therapies to the online therapy world is not only beneficial, but also imperative with keeping up with the times and technology. The more options there are for an individual to seek therapy, the better the individual will be in the long run.

REFERENCES

Callahan, A., & Inckle, K. (2012). Cybertherapy or psychobabble? A mixed methods study of online emotional support. *British Journal of Guidance & Counseling, 40*(3), 261–278.

Durrani, S., Irvine, J., & Bolan, R. P. (2012). Psychosocial determinants of health behaviour change in an e-counseling intervention for hypertension. *International Journal of Hypertension,* 1–5.

Finn, J., & Barak, A. (2010). A descriptive study of e-counsellor attitudes, ethics, and practice. *Counselling & Psychotherapy Research, 10*(4), 268–277.

Gibson, K., & Cartwright, C. (2014). Young people's experiences of mobile phone text counselling: Balancing connection and control. *Children and Youth Services Review, 43,* 96–104.

Hanley, T. (2012). Understanding the online therapeutic alliance through the eyes of adolescent service users. *Counseling and Psychotherapy Research: Linking Research with Practice, 12*(1), 35–43.

Hertlein, K., Blumer, M., & Smith, J. (2014). Marriage and family therapists' use and comfort with online communication with clients. *Contemporary Family Therapy: An International Journal, 36*(1), 58–69.

Hoffman, J. (2011, September 23). When your therapist is only a click away. *The New York Times.* Retrieved from http://www.nytimes.com/2011/09/25/fashion /therapists-are-seeing-patients-online.html?pagewanted=all&_r=1

The International Society for Mental Health Online. (2015). *About* ISMHO. Retrieved from http://ismho.org

Kolog, E. A., Sutinen, E., & Vanhalakka-Ruoho, M. (2014). E-counselling implementation: Students' life stories and counselling technologies in perspective. International *Journal of Education and Development using Information and Communication Technology, 10*(3), 32–48.

Montgomery, J. (2013). Manti Te'o hoax: 'Catfish' star Nev Schulman weighs in. MTV News. Retrieved from http://www.mtv.com/news/1700336/manti-teo - catfish-nev-schulman/

Prabhakar, E. (2013). E-Therapy: Ethical considerations of a changing healthcare communication environment. *Pastoral Psychology, 62*(2), 211–218.

Rees, C. S., & Stone, S. (2005). Therapeutic alliance in face-to-face versus videoconferenced psychotherapy. *Professional Psychology: Research and Practice, 36*(6), 649–653.

Suler, J. (2004). The online disinhibition effect. *CyberPsychology & Behaviour, 7*(3), 321–326.

Biography

Dorothy A. Miraglia, PhD earned her BS in music and sociology from Adelphi University (2004). She attended Hofstra University (2006) earning her MA in Interdisciplinary Studies and earned a MS in Industrial and Organizational Psychology from the University of Phoenix (2011). Dr. Miraglia graduated with distinction from Capella University (2014) earning her PhD in Advanced Studies in Human Behavior. Her dissertation is titled, *The experiences of adult women ages 30-44 who log on to Facebook daily using their smartphone: A generic qualitative study.* Dr. Miraglia co-wrote a chapter in Dr. Stephanie Brooke's book, *The use of the creative therapies in treating depression.* Additionally, they co-edited the book, *Using the creative therapies to cope with grief and loss.* Their next project together is *The use of the creative therapies with bulling and aggression.* Dr. Miraglia works as an online instructor for West Coast University and for Florida State College at Jacksonville teaching humanities. She also writes blog articles for The Babb Group, which is an educational consultant company, related to online teaching.

Chapter 17

THE USE OF TECHNOLOGY TO SUPPORT THE SUPERVISION PROCESS

Theresa Fraser

Introduction

Do you remember your first supervision session as a clinician? You probably had paperwork from your university or college in hand. You were probably feeling both nervous and excited. After attending all of your theory classes, you were now going to have the opportunity to learn from someone who has been working in the field. You hope that you will like them. Additionally, you hope that they will like you and then you realize later that like has little to do with the potential learning. You hope that your supervisor will observe the skills that you have developed intuitively and relationally prior to becoming a therapist. Furthermore, you hope that your supervisor will appreciate the skills that you are developing as you do "the work." You hope they are comfortable sharing and teaching you what you don't know.

This excitement about supervision is what motivates us to initially come to supervision. Then as the supervisory relationship develops, you experience the value of having an "elder" challenge you, affirm your work, listen to your struggles, and share their wisdom of doing the work with you. There are times you may resent supervision or your supervisor. Also, there are times you may resent having to spend time reviewing sessions that you may wish you could forget because they impacted you in a place you did not expect would be impacted. There will be other times where you are eager to go back and to share what happened in specific client sessions after your last supervision session. You may have exciting news about how an intervention worked or you may have frustrated news about how it did not. However, all of it matters, and all of it is part of the supervisory process.

This chapter will talk about supervision but will also address how supervision can happen in the twenty-first century using tools that were never available before, and tools that will change and adapt as time continues. We, as clinicians, also have to change and adapt and be flexible both in our service provision and in regards to our professional growth as clinicians. We can use these tools to help our work, but they should never drive our work. Tools are only effective if they serve the purpose that we need them too. Landreth says that play therapy tools are "toys and materials should be selected, not collected" (Landreth, 2002, p. 133). Technology tools need to be looked at in the same manner.

Supervision of a clinician's effectiveness versus an agencies service provision only gained importance after the 1920s. When it began to be acknowledged as an important part of the training and the certification process where the applicant had to engage in a supervisory relationship to have their work with vulnerable individuals overseen (Kadushin & Harkness, 2014). The purpose of this was to

- ensure that administrative tasks were accurately completed in order to secure and to maintain funding.
- make certain that the clinicians learned the skills they needed in order to meet client needs.
- see that the supervisor supported the supervisee in their professional development so that he or she could do the job.

It was understood therefore that the supervisor generally maintained these three functions: "administrative educational and supportive" (Kadushin & Harkness, 2014, p. 4). Bernard and Goodyear (2004) defined supervision as

> an intervention provided by a more senior member of a profession to a more junior member or members of that same profession. This relationship is evaluative, extends over time, and has the simultaneous purposes of enhancing the professional functioning of the more junior person(s), monitoring the quality of professional services offered to the clients, she, he, or they see, and serving as a gatekeeper for those who are to enter the particular profession. (p. 8)

Milne (2009) defined clinical supervision as "the formal provision, by approved supervisors, of a relationship-based education and training that is work-focused and which manages, supports, develops and evaluates the work of colleagues" (p. 15).

Supervision was not only important to paid workers, but also became part of human service internship programs at both the college and university levels. "ClientField placements provide students with the opportunity to integrate their classroom learning with knowledge and skills in a range of human service programs as well as offering specific models of practice for the future" (as cited in Cleak & Smith, 2012, p. 243). These work-related learning experiences can be identified as work-integrated learning, placements, practicums, and co-ops. Married with these true to life experiences was, and is always, supervision, this occurring often weekly in a formal sense and more often as needs arise. "In conjunction with practice, supervision seems to be a key component of professional development beyond initial helping skills training" (Hill, Stahl, & Roffman, 2007, p. 369).

In the past, supervision has been highly dependent on the verbal interaction between supervisee and supervisor. However, participants in group and/or individual supervision may have difficulty articulating what it is they want out of supervision and/or from the clinical The supervisor (Drewes & Mullen, 2008). The supervisee may bring clinical updates on service provision, seek feedback on draft reports or court documents, perhaps pose questions that relate to the interventions (planned or used), or even discuss the therapeutic relationship shared with the client (Fraser, 2014).

The seasoned supervisor enters into a supervisory relationship understanding what their own strengths/challenges and supervisory goals are: ". . . self-assessment, in addition to supervisor assessment, is important in recognizing an individual's strengths and identifying areas for growth" (Swank & Lambie, 2016, p. 92). The supervisor should also be clear on the needs of the supervisee (often as a result of introductory interviews or screening tools). The supervisor should assess the supervisee new to the field, or if they are experienced clinicians who may have specific expertise in their discipline. Both the skill level of the supervisee and abilities of the supervisor will determine the interventions or activities required to support the supervisee. "This relationship is characterized by acceptance of the supervisee by the supervisor, empathy, support, a nonjudgmental stance toward the supervisee, the supervisor's belief in the supervisee, and flexibility" (Donald, Culbreth, & Carter, 2015, p. 66).

An important consideration is the dual roles that the supervisor may hold in the supervisory relationship. For example, is the supervisee clear about what they are looking for from the supervisory relationship? Do they intuitively or reflectively know what they need specific direction and support in? Is the supervisor an internal supervisor who also shared responsibility for the successful operation of the whole program? Or is the supervisor an external supervisor whose primary goal is to help the supervisee develop as a clinician? These variables inform the cadence, occurrence, and purpose of the supervisory relationship and the role that the supervisor needs to assume.

> The role of the supervisor is not to function as an omnipotent authoritarian; rather, the supervisor must act reciprocally and deliberately as teacher-learner-facilitator working in tandem with the person whom is seeking supervision. Above all, the wellbeing of those who are and will be served is central in supervisory relationships and power within those relationships must be used toward and for the betterment of how and what one does as a human service profession. (Pool, 2010, p. 69)

Supervisors and supervisees alike may have varied perceptions of the supervisory relationship. This may be based on prior supervisory relationships, workload as compared to available resources, and feelings of confidence or vulnerability in the service provision arena (Fraser, 2016). "My approach to supervision, has been partly shaped by my experience of what it felt like not to have what, with hindsight, I can see that I needed" (Shore, 2011, p. 89).

Most regulated professions clearly define the number of supervision hours required as well as who can provide these hours, how they are provided, and where they are provided. Supervisors are usually seasoned clinicians who may or may not have specific training in supervision but have extensive experience working with like populations or with specific therapeutic approaches. Judy Ryde in Shohe (2011) observed that "my supervisees have said that it is important to them to have a supervisor for this work who knows what it is to work with this client group" (p. 130).

Special Population–(Children, Teens, Adults)

Supervisor agreements or contracts need to include informed consent including confidentiality discussions and payment arrangements, as well as agreements around processes if there are conflicting beliefs between supervisor and supervisee around client intervention. Malpractice insurance information should be shared as well as clarity around what code of ethics each clinician adheres to. This is particularly important information to review if supervisee and supervisee hold different memberships in regulated colleges for their profession.

The occurrence of supervision may be impacted by immediate client needs. Thus, when there is a great deal going on in a community, educational, medical, or residential program, it is not uncommon for supervision to be canceled to make room for a perceived client need or client appointments. On occasions such as these, supervision may be canceled if not rescheduled.

Supervisors may be responsible for the supervision of clinicians at multiple sites. Also, clinicians operating independently may struggle with finding local supervisors who have expertise in specific types of service provision or due to their geographically remote area of practice, there may be no supervisors nearby. These are all examples of situations when face-to-face supervision may not be possible or easily accessible to clinicians.

Play therapy supervision often includes play- and art-based activities both for therapist self-awareness and reflection, and also as part of case conceptualization. "When we reflect we can review our beliefs and attitudes, discover what assumptions we are making and explore our mind maps . . . becoming reflective is then a crucial element in being open to unlearning old beliefs, actions and strategies, and then becoming open to new learning. Once our new neural networks become well developed we become reflexive" (Shohet, 2011, p. 92).

So this is the challenge when supervision is needed or wanted—how can it be arranged if time and/or space interferes with the face-to-face opportunity? The answer for some supervisors and supervisees is the use of technology in supervision. In the past, technology in supervision might mean a telephone or a microphone for bug in the ear training (Gallant, Thyer, Bailey, 1991) where a supervisor watched the client session from a one-way mirror and directed the supervisee in their therapeutic interactions. Hill, Stahl, and Roffman (2011) stated that "we have found that immediate feedback tends to be better than delayed feedback (e.g., stopping a role-playing exercise and having the trainee do it again with a little shaping is more helpful than delayed feedback" (p. 368).

Taped sessions were also utilized in the 1940s. "These recorded interviews have proven extremely valuable in the training of advanced students . . . they give a vivid and clear-cut picture of various client attitudes which is much more meaningful than anything the counsellor can obtain through abstract descriptions. Probably the most significant use of our recordings is in the process of supervision. It is the unanimous testimony of counsellors that they have gained a great deal and have been able to correct many mistakes . . . [allowing] the inexperienced and experienced counsellor alike a new understanding of the therapeutic process" (Rogers, 1942, pp. 429-431). Rogers concluded that the use of these relatively new mechanical devices provides for the first time a sound basis for the investigation of therapeutic processes, and for the teaching and improvement of therapeutic techniques. Therapy need no longer be a vague, therapeutic skill nor need no longer be an intuitive gift (as cited in Armstrong, Barletta, & Pelling, 2009, p. 341).

The Internet, computer software, and the decreased cost of long-distance fees, has provided accessibility opportunities for synchronous and asynchronous supervision. Asynchronous supervision can include both video sent via mail or uploaded to a web space such as a private Youtube channel. Some supervisors will view weekly session tapes such as Theraplay, which is a parent-child therapy that is based primarily on the work of Bowlby (1988). Activities focused in the domains of structure, challenge, nurture, and engagement (Munns as cited in Bowers, 2014) selected and facilitated first by the therapist, and then by the parent (with therapist support). When sessions are videotaped, a supervisor can provide written feedback on therapist and client interactions and provide feedback back to the therapist via email or post.

Other supervisors will review tapes and discuss the play therapy sessions via phone, Skype, or web conferencing (Fraser, 2016). Hill, Stahl, and Roffman (2007) stated that trainees learn to use skills more successfully from observing videotapes and transcribing and coding helping sessions at various points in time and reflecting on their experiences than from just instruction, modeling, practice, and feedback (as cited in Wolf, 2007, p. 368).

Group Supervision Applications

Group supervision can also occur via group conferencing with phone or web based applications. Such applications can provide the opportunity for group supervisees to practice taking on the teaching role. Power points, photos of sand trays, or client work can be shared in real time with screen-sharing tools. Additional time needs to be set aside for all group members to log in and to practice, using application tools as noted in the next section. Supervisor agreements or contracts need to include informed consent including confidentiality discussions and payment arrangements, as well as agreements around processes especially if there are conflicting beliefs between supervisor and supervisee around client intervention. Malpractice insurance information should be shared as well as clarity around what code of ethics each clinician adheres to. This is particularly important information to review if supervisee and supervisee hold different memberships in regulated colleges for their profession.

Skype data apparently goes through an external server so this will not meet HIPPA requirements. It is free and anywhere there is reliable Internet. Sessions can be recorded with additional software; it goes through an external server and therefore, sharing of files may not meet HIPPA requirements. It works best with sound-canceling head phones and it is important to inform supervisees of the limits of confidentiality.

Facetime (Apple Application): It is easily accessible if both the supervisor and the supervisee have Apple products; the clinician and the supervisor need to ensure that the location where they are using this product is secure (e.g., not in public spaces). There is no taping capability and not all individuals own Apple products.

Private Youtube channel: This can be locked after the supervisor views the sessions. Sessions are shared using a link; the supervisor and the supervisee need to ensure privacy and ensure that accurate consent is achieved from clients so that they are aware how and when and with whom their taped sessions are being shared. It is important to inform supervisees of the limits of confidentiality given their faces and voice are also being taped.

Online meeting programs such as Zoom.us, Adobe.com, and gotomeeting.com: Feedback can be provided immediately with the option of screen sharing, report sharing, and so forth; teaching video clips can be viewed by all meeting members who can engage in real time reflection and discussion when using the free program known as Rabbit; privacy will need to be researched for each program given that new programs are constantly being updated and marketed, such as Go to Meeting, Zoom, and Rabbit.

Videotaping sessions and saving on CDs or on memory sticks only seen by the supervisee and the supervisor and can be kept for future teaching resource material if prior consent has been obtained; there is a longer time gap between recording and the receipt of feedback by the supervisee.

Google Docs allows the supervisor and the supervisee to both add to a document confidentiality. Over twenty-five clinical research studies on technology, assisted supervision and training (TAST) have been conducted since 2000, in training sites around the world, including Australia, Canada, England, Norway, and the United States (e.g., Reese et al., 2009). "Psychotherapy supervision and training are rapidly moving online" (Grossl et al., 2014, p. 282). The potential benefits of TAST are clear, including greatly increased flexibility, reduced travel costs, and the opportunity to address the limited availability of clinical training in rural, remote, and underserved areas.

An important consideration as a supervisor is how comfortable will the supervisee be using technology. This needs to be discussed, evaluated, and then if utilizing a specific technology for the first time, it would be important to integrate training time into the supervisory process. With practice and training using technology, Reese et al. found that "the supervisory relationship also did not appear to be affected by the videoconferencing format" (Grossl et al., 2014, p. 356).

This research is valuable in that many supervisees first queries if technology-assisted supervision is less valuable than face-to-face supervision.

Comments from This Writer's Supervisees

Greater Increased Flexibility

- "I can meet with my supervisor after I have put my children to bed and be in my pajamas if I choose."
- "I take advantage of distance supervision by phone so it supports my work/life balance."
- "I have access to more supervisors who may have various supervisory styles and areas of expertise if we can structure supervision using technology resources."
- "I am hearing impaired and need to see the face of my supervisor in order to read her lips. She was initially not comfortable using Skype but it is fine now. I appreciate that she was open to doing this as I really wanted to get her insight on cases I work on."
- "I tracked down a student of Margaret Lowenfeld's who supervises students. She lives in London and was open to supervising me by Skype. I couldn't afford the $200 an hour supervision fee, but if I could have, I would have had supervision from one of Lowenfeld's students by Skype."
- "I can connect with a supervisor who is in a different time zone and I can do it from home."
- "Supervision time shared with one other supervisee counts as individual supervision hours toward certification in my country, so I am able to not only have a supervision experience that is less costly, but my supervisor can initiate a conference call on her cell phone. The other supervisee and my supervisor are in different time zones, but we make it all work."
- "I had supervision and a training booked using zoom (an online meeting room) and then had a chance to go away with my partner for a week. I didn't want to cancel my supervision nor the training, and my partner had to go to some business meetings anyway, so I was able to connect with my supervisor even though I [am] halfway across the world. In many ways it was so very cool. I got the supervision I needed and then went and hung around the pool."

Reduced Travel Costs

- "I am in private practice and time and travel impacts the number of sessions I can have with clients. If I can have a supervision session in my place of work, with a supervisor who is in their place of work, then the supervisory process for me is less costly."

- "My supervisor has expertise in Sand tray therapy and I can't drive two hours to meet with her, but we can do sand tray supervision using a web-based program that is free for both of us. We just don't use actual client names or identifying information. I send photos of sand trays in advance and we can discuss these in real time."
- "I keep photos of sand trays in powerpoint (pp) presentations so I can share the pp with my supervisor and we talk about the sanitary by referring to the slide number of the presentation."
- "I sometimes don't have access to a car, so attending supervision using public transportation takes more time."
- "I live in an area that gets lots of snow in the winter. Distance supervision using technology ensures that I continue to have regular supervision and am not putting myself at risk driving in horrible weather."

Opportunity to Address Limited Availability of Clinical Training in Remote and Underserved Areas

- "I don't have reliable Internet in my community, and it is very slow; however, phone supervision has been really beneficial for my learning. I would rather see my supervisor's face so I could also tap into the nonverbal communication, but phone supervision is the answer to the challenges that I have."
- "I live in a small rural community and my supervisor lives in a city almost 1.5 hours from me. If she wasn't open to using technology, I fear I would not have a good support system for my caseload."
- "There are no Play therapy supervisors within eight hours of where I live/practice. If I didn't have supervision, I would be practicing without much-needed support."
- "The only supervisor near by is one at my place of work and I want to get supervision from more than one supervisor. I think it is helpful to gain different perspectives working with different populations."
- "My supervisor at work is not very supportive of Play therapy because he doesn't have any training in Play therapy. The board hired me for this expertise and I need to gain outside support because I won't get it from my work supervisor."
- "I am involved in group supervision and benefit from learning from the experience of group members I might not necessarily know without our distance supervision group, yet we all share the same interest in dyadic developmental psychotherapy, which is another therapy that addresses parent-child attachment. We also all have training in Theraplay as does the supervisor. It is wonderful to have a clinician

who has the experience in both models. Without this support, I would feel very isolated because I am the only clinician in my geographical area that has this expertise."

- "I am being supported to become a supervisor so that local therapists will have a local supervisor—until then we are forced to drive long distances or not have the expertise of a supervisor who has expertise in a specific intervention."

The only disadvantage of obtaining supervision from a supervisor outside of your area of practice or geographical area, is that the supervisor may not be well versed in the cultural implications of your work. For this reason, it may be also beneficial to investigate if there is also a local supervisor who you can connect with professionally. The Canadian Association for Play Therapy (www.cacpt.com) has a policy for therapists that has been certified by obtaining supervision outside of the country. Currently, that association expects clinicians to obtain a minimum of ten hours of supervision with a local supervision to ensure that cultural aspects of practice are both investigated and honored.

Safety and Security

In Canada, web-based consultation has already been implemented for remote medical consultation or with twenty-four hours a day medical consultation of a Telehealth nurse for patient medical concerns, both small and large. Whatever the technology that is utilized to provide support, training, and clinical consultation to supervisees, it is important that all parties have a commitment to making the process secure. For example, it is up to the supervisor to advise the supervisee to ensure that passwords are secure and strong but not used for multiple accounts. Like all online accounts, passwords should be changed regularly (Rousmaniere, Abbass, & Frederickson (2014). Identifying information should not be shared verbally or in writing, and all of the participants need to sign confidentiality agreements.

Even after we are mandated to gain supervision hours in order to be credentialed, it is important for all care providers and supervisors to plan to engage in supervision or in supervision on their supervision. Technology-assisted supervision tools can ensure that everyone working in the helping profession can join with a mentor or with a supervisor in order to practice safely with efficacy. A commitment to supervision not only ensures quality service for those clients we work with, but also self-care for the clinician. If utilizing a specific technology for the first time, it would be important to integrate training time into the supervisory process. "Competent supervisors must be attentive to the relational dynamics that shape the formation, course, and outcomes of supervision" (Johnson, Skinner, & Kaslow, 2014. p. 1074). Our experience is that supervision can be a very important part of taking care of oneself, staying open to learning and an indispensable part of the helper's well-being, ongoing self-development, self-arenas, and commitment to professional development (Hawkin, 2012).

So now you have to decide what tools you will be open to utilizing both as a supervisee and as a supervisor. If you were not previously open to the use of distance supervision, this chapter may have provided you with some examples that cause you to reflect on the benefits of technology tools. Whatever tools you utilize, you can be sure that both in client work and in supervision, they will change and adapt as technology changes and adapts. The reflective questions at the end of this chapter may help you and your supervisor or supervisee determine what tools will assist your supervisory relationship.

Reflective Questions

1. What are you hoping to gain from this supervisory relationship?
2. Why are you seeking supervision from this supervisor?
3. Is there someone close by who can provide you with the same support/mentorship/wisdom?
4. What stage of your profession are you in (new to the field, have some experience, or expert)?
5. What type of supervision are you or he or she comfortable utilizing: individual, group, phone, face-to-face, or online meeting room)?
6. What experience do you each (supervisor and supervise) have using various forms of supervision?
7. Are play-based interventions needed and been previously utilized?
8. If so—will the form of technology-proposed support play-based supervision?
9. Is there some adaptation of technology that can be found to support play-based supervision?
10. What resources do you both have available so you can try a different form of supervision?
11. Do you have an inexpensive long-distance plan and/or Internet plan?
12. Do you have a strong Internet connection?
13. Do you have privacy at home if you will be using technology outside of the workplace and outside of work hours?
14. Does your lap top or desktop computer have a camera and microphone?

15. Do you have a sound cancelling set of headphones?
16. Are you aware of the rules/regulations /policies of your regulatory body, insurance company, and/or the agency that you work for?
17. Do you have signed consent to share non- identifying client information with your supervisor?
18. Have you discussed a process with your supervisor/supervisee to problem solve any technology issues that arise that are getting in the way of the supervisory process?
19. How will you know that your supervisory process is effective?
20. What steps can you and your supervisor take if the technology tool is not effective?

REFERENCES

Armstrong, P., Barletta, J., & Pelling, N. (2009). *The practice of clinical supervision.* Bowen Hills, Qld: Australian Academic Press.

Bernard, J. M., & Goodyear, R. K. (2004). *Fundamentals of clinical supervision* (3rd ed). Boston: Pearson and Allyn and Bacon.

Blatner, A. (2000). *Foundations of psychodrama* (4th ed.). New York: Springer Publishing Compay.

Bowers, R. (2014). *Play therapy with families: A collaborative approach to healing.* Lanham: Jason Aronson, Inc.

Bowlby, J. (1988). *A secure base, parent-child attachment and healthy development.* New York: Basic Books.

Cleak, H., & Smith, D. (2012). Student satisfaction with models of field placement supervision. *Australian Social Work, 65*(2), 243–258.

Corey, G., & Corey, M. (1997). *Groups: process and practice.* Pacific Grove, CA: Brooks Cole.

Donald, E. J., Culbreth, J. R., & Carter, A. W. (2015). Play therapy supervision: a review of the literature. *International Journal of Play Therapy, 24*(2), 59–77. doi:10.1037/ a0039104

Drewes, A. A., & Mullen, J. A. (Eds.). (2008). *Supervision can be playful: Techniques for child and play therapist supervisors.* Lanham, MD: Rowman & Littlefield.

Fraser, T. (2014). *Supervision training course handouts.* Brampton. Canadian Association for Child and Play Therapy.

Fraser, T. (2016). *Supervision training course handouts.* Brampton. Canadian Association for Child and Play Therapy.

Grossl, A. B., Reese, R. J., Norsworthy, L. A., & Hopkins, N. B. (2014). Client feedback data in supervision: Effects on supervision and outcome. Training and *Education in Professional Psychology, 8,* 182–188.

Gallant, J. P., Thyer, B. A., & Bailey, J. S. (1991). Using bug-in-the-ear feedback in clinical supervision. Preliminary evaluations. *Research on Social Work Practice, 1*(2), 175–187.

Hawkin, S. (2012). *Supervision in the helping professions.* Berkshire, England. Open University Press.

Hill, C. E., Stahl, J., & Roffman, M. (2007). Training novice psychotherapists: Helping skills and beyond. *Psychotherapy: Theory, Research, Practice, Training, 44,* 364–370.

Johnson, W. B., Skinner, C. J., & Kaslow, N. J. (2014). Relational mentoring in clinical supervision: The transformational supervisor. *Journal of Clinical Psychology, 70*(11), 1073–1081.

Kadushin, A., & Harkness, D. (2014). *Supervision in social work.* New York: Columbia University Press.

Landreth, G. L. (2002). *Play therapy: The art of the relationship* (2nd ed.). New York: Brunner-Routledge.

Milne, D. (2009). *Evidence-based clinical supervision: Principles and practice.* Chichester, UK: BPS Blackwell.

Pool, J. (2010). Perspectives on supervision in human services: Gazing through critical and feminist lenses. *University of North Carolina: Greensboro, 14*(1), 60–70.

Rogers, C. R. (1942). The use of electronically recorded interviews in improving psychotherapeutic techniques. *American Journal of Orthopsychiatry, 12,* 429–434.

Rousmaniere, T., Abbass, A., & Frederickson, J. (2014). New developments in technology-assisted supervision and training: A practical overview. *Journal of Clinical Psychology, 70*(11), 1082–1093. doi:10.1002/jclp.2212

Ryde, J. (2011). Supervising psychotherapists who work with asylum seekers and refuges: A space to reflect where feelings are unbearable. In R. Shohet (Ed.)., *Supervision as transformation* (pp. 124–143). London: Jessica Kingsley Publishers.

Swank, J., & Lambie. G. (2016). Development of research competence scale. *Measurement and Evaluation in Counseling and Development 49*(2), 91-108.

Wolf, A. W. (2007). Internet and video technology in psychotherapy supervision and training. *Psychotherapy, 48*(2), 179–181. doi:10.1037/a0023532

Biography

Theresa Fraser is a child and youth care practitioner, play therapist supervisor, and registered psychotherapist in Canada. She has created supervisory training programs for CYCs, CPTs, and other helping professionals. Fraser has written many books, book chapters, peer reviewed articles, and magazine articles on topics related to trauma, play therapy, foster care, and supervision. She is a professor at Sheridan College in Ontario and can be reached at theresafraser@rogers.com

AUTHOR INDEX

Z

SUBJECT INDEX

CHARLES C THOMAS • PUBLISHER, LTD.

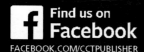